THE SPECTRUM OF PSYCHIATRIC RESEARCH

THE SPECTRUM OF PSYCHIATRIC RESEARCH

EDITED BY MICHAEL SHEPHERD

Professor of Epidemiological Psychiatry, Institute of Psychiatry, University of London

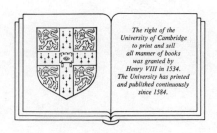

The right of the University of Cambridge to print and sell all manner of books was granted by Henry VIII in 1534. The University has printed and published continuously since 1584.

CAMBRIDGE UNIVERSITY PRESS

Cambridge

London New York New Rochelle

Melbourne Sydney

Published by the Press Syndicate of the University of Cambridge
The Pitt Building, Trumpington Street, Cambridge CB2 1RP
32 East 57th Street, New York, NY 10022, USA
10 Stamford Road, Oakleigh, Melbourne 3166, Australia

First published 1984

Printed in Great Britain at the
University Press, Cambridge

Library of Congress catalogue card number: 84–12662

British Library Cataloguing in Publication Data

The Spectrum of psychiatric research.
1. Psychiatry
I. Shepherd, Michael, *1923–*
616.89 RC454

ISBN 0 521 26585 1

UP

Contents

Preface vii
Editorials published in volumes 1–14 ix

NEUROSCIENCES

Cerebral mechanisms of mood and behaviour 3
D. G. Grahame-Smith
Endogenous opioid peptides and the control of pain 9
H. W. Kosterlitz
Pursuing the actions of psychotropic drugs: receptor sites and endogenous cerebral programmes 13
H. McIlwain
Cortical noradrenaline, attention and arousal 17
T. W. Robbins
Monoamines and the control of sexual behaviour 26
B. J. Everitt
Kuru 32
E. Beck and P. Daniel
The brain in Huntington's chorea 35
E. D. Bird
Plaques, tangles and Alzheimer's Disease 39
B. E. Tomlinson
The neuropathology of schizophrenia 50
J. R. Stevens

GENETICS

High risk for schizophrenia: genetic considerations 59
J. Shields
Immunogenetics and schizophrenia 63
D. F. Roberts and H. G. Kinnell
X-linked mental retardation 70
G. Turner
Chromosome loss and senescence 73
J. M. Martin

PSYCHOPHARMACOLOGY

Animal models for evaluating psychotropic drugs 79
R. Kumar
Pharmacogenetics and mental disease 86
G. S. Omenn and A. G. Motulsky
Pharmacokinetics and psychotropic drugs 91
S. H. Curry
Drug assays in neuropsychiatry 95
P. T. Lascelles
The benzodiazepines: recent trends 102
I. L. Martin

PSYCHOLOGY

Psychological theories and behaviour therapy 109
H. J. Eysenck
Anxiety and the brain: not by neurochemistry alone 112
J. A. Gray
Artificial intelligence 117
D. J. Hand
Cerebral laterality and psychopathology: fact and fiction 122
J. H. Gruzelier
Interhemispheric integration in man 131
M. Wyke
Psychological aspects of employment and unemployment 137
P. Warr
Neuropsychological studies of callosal agenesis 142
D. Milner

EPIDEMIOLOGY

Trends in the epidemiology of alcoholism 149
A. K. J. Cartwright and S. J. Shaw
Epilepsy: some epidemiological aspects 153
R. Neugebauer and M. Susser
Methodological issues in psychiatric case-identification 162
J. K. Wing
The epidemiology of life stress 168
M. Susser
Psychogeriatrics and the neo-epidemiologists 176
M. Shepherd
Clinical trials in psychiatry 180
A. L. Johnson

GENERAL PSYCHOPATHOLOGY AND CLINICAL ISSUES

The epistemology of normality 191
E. A. Murphy
Psyche and history 198
G. Rosen
Culture and schizophrenia 201
A. Jablensky and N. Sartorius
Hallucinations 213
P. D. Slade
The present status of anorexia nervosa 220
G. F. M. Russell
Research into the dementias 225
W. A. Lishman
The scientific status of electro-convulsive therapy 229
T. J. Crow
Type A behaviour and ischaemic heart disease 237
M. Marmot

Preface

Commissioned editorials have been a feature of *Psychological Medicine* since its inception in 1970, serving to supplement the reports of original research which constitute the core of the journal. They provide regular, authoritative reviews of the many branches of scientific inquiry that are related to psychiatry. The foundations of the series were laid in the early issues when a number of representative workers from the neurobiological, psychosocial and clinical sciences were invited to provide an overview of their disciplines in a psychiatric context. Since then more than 100 contributors have elaborated on these basic themes.

As a group the articles constitute an impressive testimony to the growing impact of scientific research on psychological medicine. And they go some way towards confronting the challenge presented by a distinguished professor of medicine in a controversial editorial entitled, *Research in Psychiatry: A View from General Medicine*: 'When recent Nobel Prizes in medicine have been awarded for, on the one hand, a combination of physiology, biochemistry and endocrinology of the brain (Schally & Guillemain), and on the other, for animal behavioural studies (Lorenz & Tinbergen), it is at present difficult to imagine a similar achievement in the field of psychiatry with the lead being taken by anyone with a psychiatric training' (Peart, 1977). Whether or not they have Nobelian aspirations contemporary psychiatrists must keep abreast of the relevant advances in science if they are to be more than what Peart calls 'purveyors of mumbo-jumbo at the worst and of brilliant dialectics at the best'. Unfortunately too much of this material has been and is being published in journals outside the purview of most psychiatrists whose reading habits, like those of most clinicians, tend to be restricted.

By monitoring such work the journal provides a unique service to its readers. Indeed, so popular has the series become that there has been a stream of requests for separate publication of a batch of editorials. This selection covers only a third of the editorials published so far: the full list is given overleaf. In this form they constitute a guide to ongoing psychiatric research which is not readily available elsewhere. It is hoped that they will prove to be of value to the clinician, the research worker and the general reader.

December 1983

Michael Shepherd
Institute of Psychiatry
University of London

Peart, W. S. (1977). Research in psychiatry: a view from general medicine. *Psychol. Med.*, **9**, 205–206.

Editorials published in Volumes 1–14

Volume 1 (1970–71)
Biochemical Research in Psychiatry
R. Rodnight
Evaluation of Psychotherapy:
R. H. Cawley
How many psychiatric beds?
J. K. Wing
Psychiatric genetics:
L. S. Penrose
Psychophysiology and Psychiatry
P. H. Venables

Volume 2 (1972)
Social anthropology and psychiatry:
J. B. Loudon
Pharmacology and psychiatry
E. Marley
Psyche and history
G. Rosen
Neuropathology and psychiatry
J. A. N. Corsellis

Volume 3 (1973)
Contributions of sociology to psychiatry
D. Mechanic
Psychology in relation to psychiatry
O. L. Zangwill
Psychological studies in subnormality
Neil O'Connor
Neurology and psychiatry
C. D. Marsden
Psychiatry and the neurosciences
J. R. Smythies
Epidemiological psychiatry
B. Cooper
Decline of industrial psychiatry
H. B. Murphy

Volume 4 (1974)
Criminology, deviant behaviour and mental disorder
D. J. West
Pharmacogenetics and mental disorder
G. S. Omenn & A. G. Motulsky
Alcoholism as a disease:
D. L. Davies
Neuroendocrinology and mental illness
B. T. Donovan
Endocrinology and psychiatry:
J. L. Gibbons
The brain, ageing, and dementia:
A. D. Dayan
Animal models for evaluating psychotropic drugs:
R. Kumar

Volume 5 (1975)
Sleep research and mental illness
I. Oswald
Circadian rhythms and mental illness
G. A. Sampson & F. A. Jenner
Culture & schizophrenia
A. Jablensky
'Exotic' treatments and Western treatment
J. Leff
Psychological theories and behaviour therapy
H. J. Eysenck
Time to evaluate long-term neuroleptics
D. Watt
Ethology and development
S. A. Barnett

Volume 6 (1976)
Nutrition, growth and development
J. Tizard
Hallucinations
P. D. Slade
Classification of depressive illness
G. A. Foulds & A. Bedford
Dyslexia
W. Yule
Anti-convulsant drugs and mental symptoms
M. R. Trimble & E. H. Reynolds
Kuru
E. Beck & P. Daniel
The role of rating scales in psychiatry
M. Hamilton

Volume 7 (1977)
On some risks in risk research
N. Garmezy
High risk for schizophrenia:
James Sheilds
'De-institutionalization' and the community
Henry R. Rollin

Neo-Pavlovianism and clinical psychiatry
W. Horsley Gantt
The present status of anorexia nervosa
G. F. M. Russell
Transcultural psychiatry should begin at home
H. B. M. Murphy
Hormones and sexual behaviour
John Bancroft
Calcium metabolism and mental disorder
J. L. Crammer
Better community residential services for the mentally handicapped
Norma V. Raynes

Volume 8 (1978)
Trends in the epidemiology of alcoholism
A. K. J. Cartwright & S. J. Shaw
The future of alcoholism
Jim Orford
Pharmacokinetics and psychotropic drugs
Stephen H. Curry
Information systems in psychiatry
M. R. Eastwood, H. M. R. Meier & C. M. Woogh
Research into the dementias
W. A. Lishman
The brain in Huntington's chorea
Edward D. Bird
Life event stress and psychiatric illness
Gavin Andrews & Christopher Tennant
Non-verbal communication and mental disorder
Michael Argyle

Volume 9 (1979)
Endogenous opioid peptides and the control of pain
H. W. Kosterlitz
The doctors, their patients and their care
T. A. Madden
The current status of childhood autism
Lorna Wing
Research in psychiatry
W. S. Peart
Epilepsy: some epidemiological aspects
Richard Neugebauer & Mervyn Susser
Behavioural changes in temporal lobe epilepsy
Norman Geschwind
The scientific status of electro-convulsive therapy
T. J. Crow
The epistemology of normality
Edmund A. Murphy
Residential care of the elderly in Britain today
Caroline Godlove & Anthony Mann
Anxiety and the brain: not by neurochemistry alone
J. A. Gray
Schizophrenia and physical disease
J. A. Baldwin

Volume 10 (1980)
Choline, acetylcholine and dementia
R. M. Marchbanks
Methodological issues in psychiatric case-identification
J. K. Wing
Whence and whither 'liaison' psychiatry?
Geoffrey G. Lloyd
New approaches to pain
M. R. Bond
Pursuing the actions of psychotropic drugs
Henry McIlwain
Language and schizophrenia
Til Wykes
Type A behaviour and ischaemic heart disease
Michael Marmot
The ethological approach to aggression
P. J. B. Slater

Volume 11 (1981)
The epidemiology of life stress
Mervyn Susser
The clinical significance of dysprosody
Macdonald Critchley
Cerebral laterality and psychopathology
John H. Gruzelier
Epidemiology and depression
M. R. Eastwood & P. M. Kramer
Immunogenetics and schizophrenia
D. F. Roberts & H. G. Kinnell
Artificial intelligence
D. J. Hand
Monoamine oxidase inhibitor efficacy in depression and the 'cheese effect'
M. Sandler
Drug assays in neuropsychiatry
P. T. Lascelles
Where have all the catatonics gone
B. Mahendra
Dementia, depression and the CT scan
Robin Jacoby
GABA and acute psychoses
Brian Meldrum
Psychological aspects of employment and unemployment
Peter Warr

Volume 12 (1982)
Motor disorders in schizophrenia
C. D. Marsden
Interhemispheric integration in man
Maria Wyke
Chromosome loss and senescence
Judith M. Martin
Genotype-environment interaction in antisocial behaviour
Remi J. Cadoret
DSM-III and the future orientation of American psychiatry
Murray A. Morphy
Plaques, tangles and Alzheimer's disease
B. E. Tomlinson
The neuropsychiatric implications of low exposure to lead
Herbert L. Needleman
Transmitter amines in depression
G. Curzon
X-linked mental retardation
Gillian Turner
The benzodiazepines: recent trends
I. L. Martin
The neuropathology of schizophrenia
Janice R. Stevens
Use of the anticonvulsant carbamazepine in primary and secondary affective illness
R. M. Post
The irritable bowel syndrome: soma and psyche
M. J. Ford, Jenny Eastwood & M. A. Eastwood

Volume 13 (1983)
Clinical trials in psychiatry
Anthony L. Johnson
Jacques Lacan and French psychiatry
S. Lebovici
Why neuroepidemiology?
Rudy Capildeo, S. Haberman, Bernard Benjamin & F. Clifford Rose
The aetiology of anorexia nervosa
L. K. George Hsu
Follow-up studies of anorexia nervosa: a review of research findings
H.-C. Steinhausen & K. Glanville
The clinical pharmacology of appetite – its relevance to psychiatry
Trevor Silverstone
Models of depression in primates
Stephen J. Suomi
Relapse in schizophrenia: a review of the concept and its definitions
Ian R. H. Falloon, Grant N. Marshall, Jeffrey L. Boyd, Javad Razani & Cathy Wood-Siverio
The idiot savant: flawed genius or clever Hans?
B. Hermelin & N. O'Connor
Life events and psychological morbidity
Christopher Tennant
Folic acid, S-adenosylmethionine and affective disorder
E. H. Reynolds & G. Stramentinoli

Volume 14 (1984)
Psychogeriatrics and the neo-epidemiologists
Michael Shepherd
The problem of mild dementia
A. S. Henderson & Felicia A. Huppert
Cortical noradrenaline, attention and arousal
T. W. Robbins
Psychotherapy in the market-place
Greg Wilkinson
The lessons of platelet monoamine oxidase
R. H. Belmaker
Biological markers and psychosis
P. McGuffin
The fractionation of human memory
Alan Baddeley
Working memory
G. J. Hitch
Diseases of Civilisation
H. B. Murphy
Psychopharmacology Tomorrow: 1984 or The Little Prince?
C. Giurgea
DNA and Huntington's Chorea
D. C. Watt & J. Edwards
Rapid Eye Movement (REM) Sleep
J. C. Gillin
The history of Huntington's Chorea
M. Critchley
Affective Psychopathology in Huntington's Disease
K. Koehler & H. Sass
Scrapie and Alzheimer's Disease
M. Bruce

NEUROSCIENCES

Psychological Medicine, 1976, **6**, 523–528

Cerebral mechanisms of mood and behaviour[1]

There is also another class of philosophers who, having bestowed much diligent and careful labour on a few experiments, have thence made bold to educe and construct systems, resting all other facts in a strange fashion to conformity therewith.

Francis Bacon, *Novum Organon*, 1620

Despite Bacon's admonition I shall try to construct a vague framework for the consideration of the cerebral mechanisms of mood and behaviour. This will be done from the viewpoint of one mainly concerned with the mechanism of action of drugs which affect the mind, the neuropharmacology of neurotransmitter substances in the brain and their possible involvement in normal and abnormal mental function.

Drugs are exogenous molecules which interact with endogenous molecules and set in train a sequence of events by which a biological process is manipulated. When this molecular interaction is put to therapeutic ends a disordered physiological process is either returned to normal or altered in such a way that the symptoms or manifestations of the disease are ameliorated.

Two points follow from this which are relevant to the biology of normal and abnormal mental function which although self-evident are nonetheless worth stating:

(1) Whatever the rationale for the use of a drug in mental illness, if the drug can be shown by clinical trial to produce benefit, then at some level a potentially definable biological process is involved.

(2) This being so, an understanding of the actions of the drug, whether from studies in man, animals, intact organs, cells, particles or at the molecular level, might give some insight into the pathological processes involved in the mental illness.

There are several corollaries to this. When drugs worsen or change the quality of mental illness similar insight into the underlying processes may be gained by the study of drug action. If certain drugs produce in 'normal' people states of mind, altered behaviour or mental symptoms which mimic certain aspects of spontaneous mental illness, the study of the action of such drugs might lead to the understanding of the biology of the mental illness or symptoms which are mimicked.

It is surely this kind of reasoning which has caused so much attention to be focused upon the role of the brain monoamines, noradrenaline, dopamine and 5-hydroxytryptamine in the neurobiological mechanisms underlying schizophrenia (Grahame-Smith, 1973; Snyder *et al.* 1974), manic-depressive disease (Schildkraut, 1969; Shopsin *et al.* 1974; Van Praag, 1974), and the mental syndromes produced by reserpine and psychotomimetic drugs. Reference to Table 1 shows some general current hypotheses concerning the pharmacological actions of some drugs used in the treatment of mental illness or which produce mental syndromes, together with some over-simplified, but quite widely held beliefs linking their pharmacological actions to the aetiology of mental illness. The table does an injustice to the arguments and open-mindedness of the workers propounding the hypotheses but it is these shorthand conclusions which get taken up into the general body of knowledge and which from time to time need open examination.

There is a big snag in this whole approach which might be explained by an artificial analogy. Suppose we were as ignorant of the pathophysiology of heart failure as we are of brain function in mental illness. Suppose too that by serendipity a powerful diuretic was discovered and used empirically with benefit in this uncharted syndrome of 'heart failure'. Intensive investigation of the mode of action of this drug would reveal that its action was on the kidney and the conclusion might be

[1] Address for correspondence: Dr D. G. Grahame-Smith, MRC Unit and University Department of Clinical Pharmacology, Oxford.

TABLE 1

(*a*) Some current shorthand hypotheses concerning the role of monoamine function in the causation of mental illness based upon the mode of action of psychotropic drugs

Drug	Illness	Possible mechanism of action	Shorthand 'aetiological' conclusions
Phenothiazines Butyrophenones Thioxanthenes	Schizophrenia Mania	Dopamine receptor blockade (see Snyder, 1974)	Overactivity of dopaminergic systems
Tricyclic antidepressants	Depression	Inhibition of presynaptic monoamine reuptake → increased monoaminergic function (see Iversen, 1973)	Decreased monoaminergic function
Monoamine oxidase inhibitors	Depression	Decreased metabolism of monoamines → increased monoaminergic function (see Iversen, 1973)	Decreased monoaminergic function
Lithium	'Prophylaxis' of manic depressive disease Mania	Increased functional activity of 5-HT (see Green & Grahame-Smith, 1975)	Disturbance in 5-HT function
ECT	Depression	Increased sensitivity to behavioural actions of 5-HT and dopamine (Green & Grahame-Smith, 1976)	Decreased 5-HT or dopamine function or 'sensitivity'

(*b*) Drugs 'mimicking' certain aspects of mental illness, their mode of action, and conclusions on aetiology

Drug	Clinical effects	Action	Conclusions
Reserpine	Depression	Depletion of brain monoamines (see Iversen, 1973)	Depression 'due to' decreased monoaminergic function
LSD	'Psychotic' symptoms	5-HT agonist/antagonist (see Grahame-Smith, 1973)	Aspects of schizophrenia due to 5-HT dysfunction
Amphetamine	Syndrome-like paranoid schizophrenia	Dopamine release (see Snyder *et al.* 1974)	Aspects of schizophrenia due to dopaminergic overactivity

drawn that this syndrome of 'heart failure' was due to a primary disturbance in renal tubular sodium excretion. We now know that heart failure produces a secondary disturbance in renal sodium excretion and indeed this might be considered a 'normal' response to the altered haemodynamic state produced by heart failure. But although a renal abnormality is involved excessive attention upon it would distract from the primary cause of heart failure.

Consider schizophrenia in this light. Study of the neuropharmacological actions of phenothiazines and other neuroleptics has shown a very impressive correlation between the ability of these compounds to block the actions of dopamine in the brain and their antipsychotic potency. The similarity between amphetamine psychosis and paranoid schizophrenia coupled with the known actions of amphetamine to release brain dopamine also fits in this picture. This has led to the proposition of a 'dopamine hypothesis' for the causation of schizophrenia (see Snyder *et al.* 1974). I am not exactly sure what is meant by a 'dopamine hypothesis' except that it implies that, somehow or other, a disturbance of dopaminergic neuronal function is involved. That may be so, but it would be naïve at this stage to consider it a primary disturbance. The neuroleptics could be equally well acting at a secondary level (Grahame-Smith, 1973). Curare would prevent the physical violence ensuing from a schizophrenic paranoid delusion but it would be foolish to invoke therefore a 'peripheral cholinergic hypothesis' as a cause of paranoid schizophrenia. I can find nothing in the indirect evidence culled from drug studies implicating dopaminergic mechanisms in schizophrenia which convinces me that an abnormality in dopaminergic function is a primary aetiological factor in schizophrenia. In fact just as the kidney in heart failure is reacting in a normal physiological manner to the change in the haemodynamic state produced by heart failure it might be that the dopaminergic systems in the brain are over-functioning as a 'normal' response to some other more fundamental disturbance influencing them. The neuroleptics then would 'dampen down' this over-activity without affecting the primary disturbance. This reasoning is rather destructive, particularly as I have no idea what the primary disturbance might be, except to speculate upon two possibilities.

(1) A disturbance of sub-cortical systems lying at an even more 'primitive' level than the monoaminergic systems but requiring monoaminergic systems for its linkage to cortical functions.

(2) A subtle, neurohumoral mechanism acting within the brain, altering in a diffuse way the function of monoaminergic systems or the reactivity of neuronal systems to their action.

These are not entirely idle speculations for there are now neurobiological precedences upon which they may be based. In regard to the first it has been shown that in rats the abnormal syndrome of a distinctive form of hyperactivity produced by increasing brain 5-HT levels or by central 5-HT agonists depends for its expression upon brain dopaminergic function. If one interferes with dopaminergic function pharmacologically either by decreasing brain dopamine levels or by pharmacologically blocking the action of brain dopamine then the pharmacological stimulation of brain 5-HT receptors no longer brings about abnormal hyperactive behaviour (see Green & Grahame-Smith, 1975). Thus the precedence is set for dopaminergic function in some way playing a linking or permissive role in the expression of behavioural syndromes produced by the abnormal function of non-dopaminergic pathways.

The second speculation is more hazy but is based upon the effects which small polypeptides, such as thyrotrophin releasing hormone (TRH) (Green & Grahame-Smith, 1974), melanocyte stimulating hormone release inhibitory factor (MIF) (Plotnikoff *et al.* 1972), and inhibitors of brain protein synthesis, such as cycloheximide, have on the behaviour of rats and mice. These effects involve changes in the hyperactivity syndromes produced by raising brain 5-HT levels or by the administration of 5-HT agonists, the hyperactivity syndrome produced by raising brain dopamine levels with L-Dopa and a monoamine oxidase inhibitor, and also upon pentylenetetrazol produced convulsions and pentobarbital induced sleeping time. TRH potentiates the hyperactivity syndromes without having much effect on monoamine synthesis and turnover, potentiates pentylenetetrazol induced convulsions and shortens pentobarbital induced sleeping time. Cycloheximide on the other hand does the opposite (Green *et al.* 1975). The actions of TRH on these behavioural syndromes is not mediated by its action on the pituitary to release TSH, since its behavioural actions occur in hypophysectomized rats. These phenomena suggest that polypeptides like TRH and MIF may in some way modulate the activity of monoaminergic systems or the responses of other neuronal systems to their action. Cycloheximide may be acting by either preventing the synthesis of these putative neuro-modulating polypeptides or by preventing either the release of monoamines or the mediation of their action. However unclear the picture may be at the moment, there is sufficient evidence to consider systems internal to the brain, perhaps mediated by polypeptides, which modulate neuronal activity in monoaminergic systems or systems influenced by them. If indeed this turns out to be the case then an abnormality in such a neurohumoral control mechanism could result in over-activity or under-activity of neuronal systems such as those subserved by the monoamines. The cyclic nature of manic-depressive disease, the latency of action of tricyclic antidepressants, the waxing and waning nature of several psychiatric syndromes, the usual requirement of a *course* of ECT, are phenomena, the time course of which might be explained by gradual biochemical and pharmacological changes requiring more primary changes in protein/polypeptide synthesis.

It is possible to apply the same types of argument to the actions of tricyclic antidepressants, monoamine oxidase inhibitors and the known effect of reserpine to produce monoamine depletion in the brain and then to the 'serotonin' or 'noradrenaline' hypotheses of manic-depressive disease.

Here again the monoaminergic theories of aetiology are based upon rather shaky evidence. The evidence from the action of drugs could be equally applied to a monoaminergic function at a secondary level mediating some other more primary disturbance. Such abnormalities in CSF monoamine metabolites in depression as have been demonstrated (particularly the low levels of 5-HIAA and its poor rise on the administration of probenecid (see Van Praag, 1974)) need not necessarily imply a primary abnormality in monoaminergic function. Other criticisms of a biochemical nature can be levelled at the significance of monoamine metabolites in the CSF, particularly in regard to CSF 5-HIAA (Green & Grahame-Smith, 1975).

Having arrived at the monoamine systems and there being entirely convincing evidence that the drugs considered do have important effects on these systems which in the absence of alternative explanations might well explain their therapeutic activity, it is well to ask the general question 'What do these monoaminergic systems do?' As a general statement one cannot do better than Moore (1971):

> Highly integrated neural functions, such as those involving thought processes, which are generally considered to take place in cortical structures may be modified by primitive, chronically active sub-cortical neuronal systems (e.g. limbic and reticular activating systems). Accordingly a dysfunction of these delicately balanced primitive systems may result in derangement of mental processes and behaviour.

Because we know so little of the functional neuroanatomy of human thought processes, mood and behaviour, it is necessary to play the game of association between the effects of drugs in man, the known actions of drugs, the functional neuroanatomy of animal behaviour, and the effects of drugs with known actions on animal behaviour and to try by this game, by intuitive reasoning and with a fair share of serendipity, to come out with some sensible answers.

Crucial to all these considerations is of course the mode of action of the relevant drugs. This can be a very complex matter and we ourselves have been made aware of this complexity through our study of the effect of lithium, phenytoin, reserpine, phenothiazines, tricyclic antidepressants, dopamine depletion, inhibitors of brain protein synthesis and electroconvulsive shock on the hyperactivity syndrome in rats produced by raising brain 5-HT levels by the administration of tryptophan and a monoamine oxidase inhibitor or by the administration of 5-HT agonists such as 5-methoxy N,N-dimethyltryptamine or 5-methoxytryptamine (see Green & Grahame-Smith, 1976). Drugs may affect one or more of the following functions of 5-HT and its behavioural effect: the synthesis, compartmentation, release, re-uptake and immediate post-synaptic action, or the function of other neuronal pathways mediating or permitting the immediate post-synaptic action of 5-HT to be expressed as a behavioural response.

It is also gradually becoming apparent that the chronic effects of drugs are quite different and involve unsuspected pharmacological actions on monoamine metabolism and function. Two examples will illustrate this. Acute chlorpromazine administration undoubtedly blocks the action of dopamine in the brain and will inhibit the hyperactivity syndromes produced by increasing brain 5-HT or dopamine function in the brain. Chronic chlorpromazine treatment however leads to a situation in which, when chlorpromazine is stopped, the hyperactivity produced by increasing brain 5-HT or dopamine function is enhanced, suggesting that perhaps 5-HT or dopamine receptor supersenstitivity has been induced by chronic pharmacological inhibition, though there is little direct evidence yet that this is so. A second example involves the effects of electroconvulsive shock in rats. One electroconvulsive shock does not alter the hyperactivity response produced by increasing brain 5-HT or dopamine function. However, a daily electroconvulsive shock for 10 days or one electroconvulsive shock twice weekly for 4 weeks greatly enhances the hyperactivity response produced by increasing brain 5-HT and dopamine function. We have no idea yet of the mechanism by which these changes are brought about. One cannot help feeling though, that in view of all the other evidence implicating changes in monoamine function in the actions of drugs which alter mood and behaviour, that this action of electroconvulsive shock on monoamine function has some meaning in regard to the therapeutic effect of ECT in depression. The long-term changes produced by

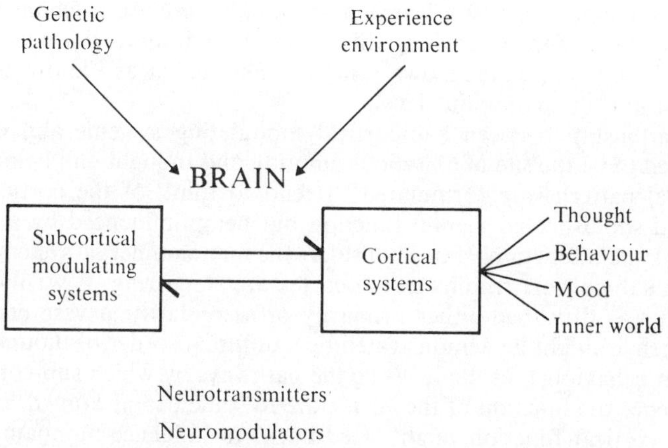

FIG. 1. Personal fantasy framework for the cerebral mechanisms of mood and behaviour.

drugs and other procedures are not unique in biochemical terms to the brain. The pituitary trophic hormones produce chronic changes in the target endocrine glands, often expressed as an increased secretory sensitivity to the action of the trophic hormone. Biochemical 'memory' is a common phenomenon.

How can all this be integrated into a general framework on which to consider the cerebral mechanisms of mood and behaviour. My personal viewpoint is summarized in Fig. 1 which is a grossly simplified working scheme.

I believe that general principles are now sufficiently well founded to allow certain statements to be made which bridge the gap which has so long existed between those whose views relied entirely upon psychological factors such as the effect of learning, experience and environment as being the sole factor involved in the production of mental states, to the exclusion of brain biology, and those who have relied solely upon brain biology as an explanation for all mental function.

One function of the brain is to record and process incoming information and experience. Undoubtedly there are neurobiological mechanisms underlying this recording, processing and retention and its effects upon pre-existing brain function. Exactly what these neurobiological mechanisms are we do not yet know but some little progress has been made in regard to the involvement of synthesis of new protein in simple memory (Cooper *et al.* 1970). The ability to record, process and retain incoming information obviously depends upon brain structure and function. Pathology, whether it be genetic or acquired, must affect these functions to some extent just as normal structure and normal function must be two of the determinants of the effect which experience has upon the existing brain function. This recording of experience in biochemical and pharmacological terms can be borne out by the effect stress has on monoamine synthesis and metabolism in animal brains and by the effect of drugs altering receptor sensitivity. The involvement of structure and function of the brain in its normal functions of recording experience, thinking, feeling and behaviour is of paramount importance in considering the neurobiology of psychiatric disease. To try and view psychiatric disease in isolation from the patient's environment, problems and past experience is as much biological nonsense as trying to understand angina without understanding that the heart is a muscular pump that works harder on exercise. Just as angina can be relieved by decreasing the amount of work that the heart has to do or by an adaptative change in collateral circulation, so one may presume that functional brain changes can be brought about to relieve anxiety and depression through environmental manipulation and psychotherapy. The 'psychological' and 'biological' factors in depression are brought together very well in a paper by Akiskal & McKinney (1973).

I see nothing inherently impossible in regard to the change in mind purported to be brought about by psychoanalysis. Readaptation and relearning presumably are the mechanisms of these forms of non-physical therapy. One of the interesting things about the brain is that through 'the inner world of the mind' it is able to manipulate its own function. This, as far as I know, does not occur in any other organ, at least not on a conscious level.

What of the relationship between sub-cortical modulating systems and cortical systems, the latter being presumed to be the site of conscious emotion and thought and being the site from which complex behavioural patterns are formulated? I tend to think of the cortical systems acting to subserve refined and sophisticated mental function but being influenced by a background of sub-cortical modulating system function. If one considers the monoaminergic systems, their ramifications from their nuclei in sub-cortical regions to the cortex are staggering. It would not be surprising if when their function was disturbed either primarily or secondarily, a very general abnormality in cortical function, such as might be demonstrated by a diffuse disorder of thought, a change of mood or general change in behaviour, resulted. While the pathways by which sub-cortical monoaminergic systems might influence the function of the cortex are to some extent known, much less seems to be known about how cortical function might 'feed-back' to influence monoaminergic function, but undoubtedly such mechanisms will be found to exist.

I would dearly love to be able to see into the future of psychiatry. How are psychiatrists going to cope with the increasing knowledge knitting together the interrelationships between experience, biological brain function and subsequent mental function and the introduction of psychotropic drugs of greater selectivity requiring a good deal of background knowledge for their proper use? It will be very interesting to see the subject evolve on this background.

D. G. GRAHAME-SMITH

REFERENCES

Akiskal, H. S. & McKinney, W. T. (1973). Depressive disorders: toward a unified hypothesis. *Science* **182**, 20–29.

Cooper, J. R., Bloom, F. E. & Roth, R. H. (1970). *The Biochemical Basis of Neuropharmacology*, Chapter 9. Oxford University Press: London.

Grahame-Smith, D. G. (1973). Pharmacological aspects of schizophrenia. *Biochemical Society Special Publications* **1**, 197–207.

Green, A. R. & Grahame-Smith, D. G. (1974). TRH potentiates behavioural changes following increased brain 5-hydroxytryptamine accumulation in rats. *Nature* **251**, 524–526.

Green, A. R. & Grahame-Smith, D. G. (1975). 5-hydroxytryptamine and other indoles in the central nervous system. In *Handbook of Psychopharmacology*, vol. 3 (ed. S. D. Iversen, L. L. Iversen & S. H. Snyder), pp. 169–245. Plenum Press: New York.

Green, A. R. & Grahame-Smith, D. G. (1976). The effect of drugs on the processes regulating the functional activity of brain 5-hydroxytryptamine. *Nature* **260**, 487–491.

Green, A. R., Heal, D. J. & Grahame-Smith, D. G. (1975). Lack of change in the sensitivity of rat caudate nucleus adenyl cyclase to dopamine when TRH and cycloheximide produce opposite effects on behavioural responses to certain centrally active drugs. In *Chemical Tools in Catecholamine Research*, vol. 2 (ed. O. Almgren, A. Carlsson & J. Engel), pp. 265–274. North Holland/American Elsevier.

Iversen, L. L. (1973). Monoamines in the mammalian central nervous system and the action of antidepressant drugs. *Biochemical Society Special Publications* **1**, 81–96.

Moore, K. E. (1971). In *Introduction to Psychopharmacology* (ed. R. H. Rech & K. E. Moore), p. 117. Raven Press: New York.

Plotnikoff, N. P., Prange, A. J., Breese, G. R., Anderson, M. S. & Wilson, I. C. (1972). TRH: Enhancement of DOPA activity by a hypothalamic hormone. *Science* **178**, 417–418.

Schildkraut, J. J. (1969). Rationale of some approaches used in the biochemical studies of the affective disorders: The pharmacological bridge. In *Psychochemical Research in Man* (ed. A. J. Mandell & M. P. Mandell). Academic Press: New York.

Shopsin, B., Wilk, S., Sathananthan, G., Gershon, S. & Davis, K. (1974). Catecholamines and affective disorders raised. A critical assessment. *Journal of Nervous and Mental Disease* **158**, 369–383.

Snyder, S. H., Banerjee, S. P., Yamamura, H. I. & Greenburg, D. (1974). Drugs, neurotransmitters and schizophrenia. *Science* **184**, 1243–1253.

Van Praag, H. M. (1974). Towards a biochemical typology of depression? *Pharmakopsychiatria* **7**, 281–292.

Psychological Medicine, 1979, **9**, 1–4

Endogenous opioid peptides and the control of pain[1]

In recent years it has become evident that peptides of relatively small molecular weight play an important role not only in the regulation of endocrine function but also in the control of certain pathways in the central nervous system. The discovery of peptides which mimic the actions of morphine is of particular interest since it may give an insight into the physiological modulation of responses to painful experiences. Two such pentapeptides, methionine-enkephalin (tyrosine-glycine-glycine-phenylalanine-methionine) and leucine-enkephalin (tyrosine-glycine-glycine-phenyl-alanine-leucine) were identified in extracts of pig brains (Hughes *et al.* 1975) and of other species. It is of interest that the sequence of methionine-enkephalin is present in the pituitary peptide β-lipotropin as amino acid residues 61–65.

Present evidence indicates that there are 2 independent peptidergic systems: one is characterized by the presence of the short-chain peptides, methionine-enkephalin and leucine-enkephalin, and is widespread throughout the central and peripheral nervous systems (Elde *et al.* 1976; Hughes *et al.* 1977; Simantov *et al.* 1977), whereas the other system contains the long-chain peptide, β-endorphin (β-lipotropin$_{61-91}$) and is centred around the hypothalamus–pituitary axis with extensions into the thalamus, midbrain, medulla and pons (Rossier *et al.* 1977*b*).

The investigation of the analgesic, or rather antinociceptive, properties of the opioid peptides is made difficult by the high sensitivity of the pentapeptides, the enkephalins, to the very rapid degrading actions of aminopeptidases and carboxypeptidases, whereas the long-chain peptides are resistant to these enzymes and have their activity more slowly reduced by an endopeptidase cleaving the molecule between amino acid residues 77 and 78. This property of the enkephalins makes the use of the ordinary antinociceptive tests unreliable, even if the peptides are administered directly into the cerebral ventricles. On the other hand, β-endorphin is a very strong and long-lasting antinociceptive agent (Feldberg & Smyth, 1977), even after intravenous administration to mice but not to rats (Tseng *et al.* 1976; Rossier *et al.* 1977*a*). In this context it is of interest that the affinity of β-endorphin to the receptor represented by [^{3}H]leucine-enkephalin or [^{3}H]methionine-enkephalin binding in brain homogenate is similar to that of methionine-enkephalin and leucine-enkephalin, whereas its affinity to the receptor represented by [^{3}H]naloxone or [^{3}H]naltrexone binding is considerably greater than that of methionine-enkephalin and particularly of leucine-enkephalin. In contrast to the opioid peptides, morphine has a much lower affinity to the binding site of [^{3}H]leucine-enkephalin than to that of [^{3}H]naloxone or [^{3}H]naltrexone (Lord *et al.* 1977).

The evidence that methionine-enkephalin and possibly leucine-enkephalin play an important role in the control of the modulation of the transmission of noxious and painful stimuli is based on electro-physiological experiments, on the relationship between substance P and enkephalin in the central nervous system and the antagonism by naloxone of the analgesic effects of electrical stimulation of the pericentral grey in intractable pain and of those of electro-acupuncture.

It has been shown (Duggan *et al.* 1977) that methionine-enkephalin and its amide have different effects on the responses of neurones of spinal laminae IV and V of spinal cats to noxious and innocuous skin stimuli. When administered in the substantia gelatinosa, the enkephalins predominantly reduce the responses to noxious stimuli with little effect on the responses to non-nociceptive stimuli. These observations are in good agreement with the immunohistochemical findings that methionine-enkephalin and substance P have a similar distribution in areas related to pain and analgesia (Hökfelt *et al.* 1977). Such areas are the periaqueductal grey, the marginal layer of the spinal trigeminal nucleus and the substantia gelatinosa of the dorsal horn of the spinal cord

[1] Address for correspondence: Professor H. W. Kosterlitz, University of Aberdeen, Unit for Research on Addictive Drugs, Marischal College, Aberdeen AB9 1AS, Scotland.

and, to a lesser extent, the medullary raphe nuclei. From lesion experiments it would appear that the enkephalinergic neurones in the dorsal horn are interneurones or propriospinal neurones with nerve terminals in laminae I and II, areas which are also very rich in substance P containing nerve terminals arising from primary afferent neurones. On the basis of these observations and the fact that D-Ala²-methionine-enkephalin amide inhibits the K^+-induced release of substance P from slices of spinal trigeminal nerve nuclei, the hypothesis has been put forward that presynaptic enkephalinergic neurones reduce the release of substance P from small diameter primary afferent fibres and thus modulate the transmission of nociceptive stimuli (Jessell & Iversen, 1977).

If the opioid peptides present in the central nervous system play a physiological role, it would follow that the opiate antagonists, naloxone and naltrexone, should increase pain perception in man and in animals. Perhaps surprisingly, the results of such investigations have not been consistent. Some authors have reported negative findings (El-Sobky *et al.* 1976; Goldstein *et al.* 1976), whereas others obtained increases in nociceptive responses (Jacob *et al.* 1974; Frederickson *et al.* 1976). Analysis of the reasons for these discrepancies should give an important insight into the nature and physiological significance of the postulated pain modulation by the enkephalinergic neurones.

More information on the effects of naloxone has been obtained from its interaction with the antinociception induced by electrical stimulation of different areas of the brain. For instance, the antinociceptive effect of stimulation of the periaqueductal grey of the brain stem of rats is blocked by naloxone (Akil *et al.* 1972), although this finding has not been unequivocally confirmed by other authors (Pert & Walter, 1976; Yaksh *et al.* 1976). Further, it has been shown that the analgesia produced by electrical stimulation of the periventricular and periaqueductal grey in patients with intractable pain is reversed by naloxone (Hosobuchi *et al.* 1977). Important findings were that an intensity of stimulation sufficient to induce pain relief does not seem to alter the acute pain threshold and that indiscriminate repetitive stimulation leads to tolerance to the analgesic effect of electrical stimulation and of narcotic analgesics. In cases of successful electrical stimulation, there is often an increase in the amount of opioid peptides in the cerebrospinal fluid (Terenius, 1978; J. Miles, J. Hughes & H. W. Kosterlitz, unpublished observations). Finally, it has been reported that the analgesic effects of acupuncture on the pain caused by electrical stimulation of teeth in man are abolished by naloxone (Mayer *et al.* 1977). On the other hand, naloxone has no effect on analgesia induced by hypnosis (Goldstein & Hilgard, 1975; Mayer *et al.* 1977).

The role of β-endorphin in physiological modulation of pain is still as uncertain as that of the enkephalins. As already mentioned, this peptide has powerful antinociceptive effects and it has been shown that in conditions of stress it is released from the pituitary into the blood stream together with corticotrophin (Guillemin *et al.* 1977). Under such conditions, the content of β-endorphin decreases in the hypothalamus but does not change in other areas of the brain. From a consideration of the levels of β-endorphin in the plasma, it is unlikely that the β-endorphin released into the blood stream is correlated with the mechanisms underlying pain suppression (Rossier *et al.* 1977*a*).

As far as therapeutic usefulness is concerned, the long-chain peptides have the disadvantage of the expense of their synthesis. Since the naturally occurring pentapeptides, methionine- and leucine-enkephalin, cannot be used because of their short biological survival, a very large number of analogues have been synthesized in numerous pharmaceutical laboratories. Such analogues may be potent antinociceptive agents after administration into the cerebral ventricles (e.g. D-Ala²-Met-enkephalin amide, Pert *et al.* 1976; NCH_3-Tyr-Gly-Gly-Phe-Met amide, Feldberg & Smyth, 1977; Tyr-D-Ala-Gly-Phe-D-Leu, Baxter *et al.* 1977). Other analogues are active after intravenous and subcutaneous injection (e.g. Tyr-D-Met-Gly-Phe-Pro amide, Székely *et al.* 1977), but only one or two compounds have an antinociceptive effect after oral administration (e.g. Tyr-D-Ala-Gly-NCH_3Phe-Met(*O*)-ol or FK 33–284, Sandoz; Roemer *et al.* 1977). In this context it is of importance that there are in the central nervous system several opiate receptors with different pharmacological characteristics; for instance, the δ-receptors have a higher affinity for the enkephalins than for morphine, whereas the μ-receptors have a higher affinity for morphine than for the enkephalins (Lord *et al.* 1977). It should be noted that most of the published analogues have a lower affinity for the δ-receptors than the natural enkephalins and a higher affinity for the μ-receptors; one of the few exceptions is Tyr-D-Ala-Gly-Phe-D-Leu (Lord *et al.* 1977; unpublished observations). This change in relative affinity may be of particular importance with regard to the non-analgesic actions of these compounds, such as their effects on respiration, mood, gastrointestinal motility and endocrine functions. At present, it is not possible to allocate different physiological roles to the different types of receptors.

As far as is known at present, all natural and synthetic opioid peptides are liable to produce tolerance and dependence. There is no evidence, however, that under physiological conditions animals or man are tolerant to, and dependent on, their own endogenous opioid peptides. The mechanisms which appear to prevent occurrence of such dependence are the sequestration of the opioid peptides in subcellular structures and the rapid destruction, particularly of the short-chain enkephalins, after their release from the nerve endings. These circumstances would limit the duration of exposure of the receptors to their ligands, thus avoiding the development of tolerance and dependence (Kosterlitz & Hughes, 1977).

H. W. KOSTERLITZ

REFERENCES

Akil, H., Mayer, D. J. & Liebeskind, J. C. (1972). Comparison chez le rat entre l'analgésie induite par stimulation de la substance grise peri-aqueducale et l'analgésie morphinique. *Comptes rendus hebdomadaires des séances de l'Académie des Sciences, Paris* **274**, 3603–3605.

Baxter, M. G., Goff, D., Miller, A. A. & Saunders, I. A. (1977). Effect of a potent synthetic opioid pentapeptide in some antinociceptive and behavioural tests in mice and rats. *British Journal of Pharmacology* **59**, 455–456P.

Duggan, A. W., Hall, J. G. & Headley, P. M. (1977). Enkephalins and dorsal horn neurones of the cat: effects on responses to noxious and innocuous skin stimuli. *British Journal of Pharmacology* **61**, 399–408.

Elde, R., Hökfelt, T., Johansson, O. & Terenius, L. (1976). Immunohistochemical studies using antibodies to leucine-enkephalin: initial observations on the nervous system of the rat. *Neuroscience* **1**, 349–351.

El-Sobky, A., Dostrovsky, J. O. & Wall, P. D. (1976). Lack of effect of naloxone on pain perception in humans. *Nature* **263**, 783–784.

Feldberg, W. & Smyth, D. G. (1977). C-fragment of lipotropin – an endogenous potent analgesic peptide. *British Journal of Pharmacology* **60**, 445–453.

Frederickson, R. C. A., Nickander, R., Smithwick, E. L., Shuman, R. & Norris, F. H. (1976). Pharmacological activity of met-enkephalin and analogues *in vitro* and *in vivo*. In *Opiates and Endogenous Opioid Peptides* (ed. H. W. Kosterlitz), pp. 239–246. North-Holland: Amsterdam.

Goldstein, A. & Hilgard, E. R. (1975). Failure of the opiate antagonist naloxone to modify hypnotic analgesia. *Proceedings of the National Academy of Sciences, Washington* **72**, 2041–2043.

Goldstein, A., Pryor, G. T., Otis, L. S. & Larsen, F. (1976). On the role of endogenous opioid peptides: failure of naloxone to influence shock escape threshold in the rat. *Life Sciences* **18**, 599–604.

Guillemin, R., Vargo, T., Rossier, J., Minick, S., Ling, N., Rivier, C., Vale, W. & Bloom, F. (1977). β-Endorphin and adrenocorticotropin are secreted concomitantly by the pituitary gland. *Science* **197**, 1367–1369.

Hökfelt, T., Ljungdahl, A., Terenius, L., Elde, R. & Nilsson, G. (1977). Immunohistochemical analysis of peptide pathways possibly related to pain and analgesia: enkephalin and substance P. *Proceedings of the National Academy of Sciences, Washington* **74**, 3081–3085.

Hosobuchi, Y., Adams, J. E. & Linchitz, R. (1977). Pain relief by electrical stimulation of the central gray matter in humans and its reversal by naloxone. *Science* **197**, 183–186.

Hughes, J., Smith, T. W., Kosterlitz, H. W., Fothergill, L. A., Morgan, B. A. & Morris, H. R. (1975). Identification of two related pentapeptides from the brain with potent opiate agonist activity. *Nature* **258**, 577–579.

Hughes, J., Kosterlitz, H. W. & Smith, T. W. (1977). The distribution of methionine-enkephalin and leucine-enkephalin in the brain and peripheral tissues. *British Journal of Pharmacology* **61**, 639–647.

Jacob, J. J., Tremblay, E. C. & Colombel, M.-C. (1974). Facilitation de réactions nociceptives par la naloxone chez la souris et chez le rat. *Psychopharmacologia* **37**, 217–223.

Jessell, T. M. & Iversen, L. L. (1977). Opiate analgesics inhibit substance P release from rat trigeminal nucleus. *Nature* **268**, 550–551.

Kosterlitz, H. W. & Hughes, J. (1977). Peptides with morphine-like action in the brain. *British Journal of Psychiatry* **130**, 298–304.

Lord, J. A. H., Waterfield, A. A., Hughes, J. & Kosterlitz, H. W. (1977). Endogenous opioid peptides: multiple agonists and receptors. *Nature* **267**, 495–499.

Mayer, D. J., Price, D. D. & Raffii, A. (1977). Antagonism of acupuncture analgesia in man by the narcotic antagonist naloxone. *Brain Research* **121**, 368–372.

Pert, A. & Walter, M. (1976). Comparison between naloxone reversal of morphine and electrical stimulation induced analgesia in the rat mesencephalon. *Life Sciences* **19**, 1023–1032.

Pert, C. B., Pert, A., Chang, J.-K. & Fong, B. T. W. (1976). [D-Ala^2]-Met-enkephalinamide: a potent, long-lasting synthetic pentapeptide analgesic. *Science* **194**, 330–332.

Roemer, D., Buescher, H. H., Hill, R. C., Pless, J., Bauer, W., Cardinaux, F., Closse, A., Hauser, D. & Huguenin, R. (1977). A synthetic enkephalin with prolonged parenteral and oral analgesic activity. *Nature* **268**, 547–549.

Rossier, J., French, E. D., Rivier, C., Ling, N., Guillemin, R. & Bloom, F. E. (1977*a*). Foot-shock induced stress increases β-endorphin levels in blood but not brain. *Nature* **270**, 618–620.

Rossier, J., Vargo, T. M., Minick, S., Ling, N., Bloom, F. E. & Guillemin, R. (1977*b*). Regional dissociation of β-endorphin and enkephalin contents in rat brain and pituitary. *Proceedings of the National Academy of Sciences, Washington* **74**, 5162–5165.

Simantov, R., Kuhar, M. J., Uhl, G. R. & Snyder, S. H. (1977). Opioid peptide enkephalins: immunohistochemical mapping in the rat central nervous system. *Proceedings of the National Academy of Sciences, Washington* **74**, 2167–2171.

Székely, J. I., Rónai, A. Z., Dunai-Kovács, Z., Miglécz, E., Bertzétri, I., Bajusz, S. & Gráf, J. (1977). (D-Met[2], Pro[5])-Enkephalinamide: a potent morphine-like analgesic. *European Journal of Pharmacology* **43**, 293–294.

Terenius, L. (1978). Significance of endorphins in endogenous antinociception. In *Advances in Biochemical Psychopharmacology*, vol. 18 (ed. E. Costa and M. Trabucchi), pp. 31–44. Raven Press: New York.

Tseng, L. F., Loh, H. H. & Li, C. H. (1976). β-Endorphin as a potent analgesic by intravenous injection. *Nature* **263**, 239–241.

Yaksh, T. L., Yeung, J. C. & Rudy, T. A. (1976). An inability to antagonize with naloxone the elevated nociceptive thresholds resulting from electrical stimulation of the mesencephalic central gray. *Life Sciences* **18**, 1193–1198.

Psychological Medicine, 1980, **10**, 399–402

Pursuing the actions of psychotropic drugs: receptor sites and endogenous cerebral programmes[1]

In discussing the logic of screening newly synthesized compounds as drugs, Creese (1978) writes: 'for example, the exact relationship between the mechanism by which a drug relieves a schizophrenic of auditory hallucinations and stops a rat from jumping up on a pole to avoid an electric shock (a common screen for antischizophrenic agents) is hard to discern'. It is, however, an important matter to pursue, for chemotherapeutic experience has shown (McIlwain, 1957) that success in finding drugs of value has followed the effective biological analysis of a system, rather than coming from less specifically oriented syntheses. Creese's (1978) account takes the hunt to extracellular receptor-binding sites as a means of providing biochemical points of action for psychotropic drugs in electrophysiological, pharmacological and behavioural studies. Correlations are shown between inhibition of stereotyped movements in the rat, and of neuroleptic binding to membrane preparations from the striatum; and between the binding and clinically effective doses of the drugs. These findings deepen the impression of a real connection between schizophrenic symptoms and the quoted aspects of animal behaviour, without indicating how this comes about.

EXTRACELLULAR NEUROTRANSMITTER-RECEPTORS

Further clues have, however, been given by the nature of the compounds with which neuroleptics interact at their receptors for, in several cases, these endogenous ligands are the catecholamines dopamine and noradrenaline. We thus arrive at a group of ideas on psychoses which implicate biogenic amines and receive support, for example, from the schizophrenia-like effects induced by amphetamines. As is noted by Matthysse (1975), these ideas have led to a number of catecholamine theories of the aetiology of schizophrenia whereby the illness might result from release of too much dopamine at central synapses; or the dopamine-receptors there might be hypersensitive; or systems which dopamine operates, or which are modulated by dopamine, might be defective. Following some discrepant data the latter ideas have been developed further to multi-transmitter and receptor theories, whereby a balance between catecholamine and acetylcholine or metabolites (Davis, 1975), or between catecholamines and endorphins (Volavka *et al.* 1979), was the factor disturbed in the illness: that is, the abnormality lay in one or more extracellular neurotransmitter-receptors, in ER, or in ER_1 plus $ER_2 \ldots ER_n$.

Additional hypotheses are still, however, needed to understand the particular symptom-pattern in schizophrenia, or the particular animal behaviour with which it is compared in the quotation (Creese, 1978) which begins this account. Thus, it must be supposed that the excess dopamine or the hypersensitive receptors occur at regions causing auditory hallucinations in man or at those facilitating or prompting pole-jumping in shocked rats: which is akin to rewriting the initial problem. This problem should, however, be broadened, for other sensory abnormalities which occur in schizophrenia are relieved by neuroleptics: for instance, abnormalities of sensory thresholds (Ungerstedt & Ljungberg, 1974); and other aspects of animal behaviour are affected by the drugs: for example, avoidance reactions in shuttle-box experiments (Andén, 1974). It is the relationship between endogenous components of animal behaviour and of perception which is hard to discern.

[1] Address for correspondence: Professor Henry McIlwain, Department of Biochemistry, Institute of Psychiatry, De Crespigny Park, Denmark Hill, London SE5 8AF.

EXTRACELLULAR RECEPTOR LOCATION

Experiments which localize neurotransmitter-receptors give some further enlightenment here. Animals in which localized damage was caused to dopamine neurons by stereotaxic injections of 6-hydroxydopamine showed no immediate motor disability, but lacked orienting reactions to visual, tactile and odour stimuli (Ungerstedt & Ljungberg, 1974). Deficits were shown also in more complex tasks, including maze-running for reward, and these deficits were restored by administering either the dopamine-precursor dihydroxyphenylalanine, or apomorphine which stimulated the relevant receptors.

These experiments attractively display how essential are the neurotransmitters and neurotransmitter-receptors to animal behaviour: as indispensable links between input stimuli and a complex behavioural output. The initial quotation (Creese, 1978), however, asks more: it seeks to discern mechanisms between two groups of observations concerning chemical substances and behaviour, and 'although behavioural biologists have long sought to decipher the chemical coding of behaviour the search for these codons has been elusive' (Reis, 1974). To judge by the experiments just discussed, the codons are not simply chemicals, but chemicals in particular cytological locations in cells carrying particular receptors and, understandably, much other metabolic machinery.

RECEPTOR-CONTROLLED PRODUCTS

Current investigation of neurotransmitter-receptors has led to extensive development of techniques for their measurement (Yamamura *et al.* 1978; O'Brien, 1979) and, indeed, to a feeling that here was a 'non-catalytic biochemistry' of cellular response. It is therefore to be emphasized that modification of enzyme catalysis is a major target of receptor control and that this applies *par excellence* to catecholamine receptors. Major products controlled by catecholamine receptors are cyclic nucleotides which very much have a life of their own in the brain (McIlwain, 1972; Newman & McIlwain, 1977). In particular, the nucleotides cyclic AMP and cyclic GMP when generated postsynaptically catalyse further changes which alter neuronal membrane potentials and increase or decrease cell-firing tendency.

Preconceptions about how the cyclic nucleotides acted caused some authors to write as though action of the nucleotides was extremely brief, and localized to immediately adjacent molecules at the cell-membrane point which received the neurotransmitter; but observations throughout have emphasized the limitations of such presuppositions. Concentrations of the nucleotides in the brain are altered by excitation and by neurotransmitters, and the nucleotides may persist in altered concentrations for some minutes after the perturbing stimuli have terminated (Newman & McIlwain, 1978). As one role of the cyclic nucleotides is as neurotransmitter-mediators, these observations are relevant to the modulation of cell-firing observed after cerebral stimulation, or after application of neurotransmitters: that is, the modification of cell-firing or firing tendency can be expected to persist for periods of up to some minutes after momentary transmitter-release. This is entirely parallel to the role of the same nucleotides in other cells or organs, when the responses which they mediate, e.g. glycogenolysis or lipid mobilization, may also last some minutes. Compared with most other mammalian organs, the brain is unusually rich in cyclic nucleotides and active in their metabolism, so that it may be judged that the nucleotides subserve functions which are highly developed in the brain.

Clues to the nature of such functioning have come by considering the role of the cyclic nucleotides in other cells and organs. Here they are 'second-messengers' which continue intracellularly the signal-transmission initiated at a cell-exterior by 'first-messengers' which are extracellularly acting humoral agents: for example, an agent acting at fat cells or muscle is also a catecholamine – adrenaline. Catecholamine-receptors here represent one set of transducers between humoral signal and cellular responses. But these responses do not necessarily occur at the points at which the cyclic nucleotides are generated; much occurs at lipid vesicles and glycogen granules, intracellular entities separated by (in cellular dimensions) appreciable distances from the extracellularly membrane-sited catecholamine receptors. The realm of the first-messenger humoral agents – hormone or neurotransmitter – is in these instances extracellular; that of the nucleotide second-messengers and their second-messenger receptors are intracellular. The nucleotide function especially developed in the brain may thus concern second-messenger transmission among different regions of its unusually elongated nerve cells.

INTRACELLULAR SECOND-MESSENGER RECEPTORS AND MOVEMENTS

Second-messengers also act at receptor-sites, distinct from those of first-messengers but again susceptible to chemical characterization and cellular localization. On seeking cyclic-nucleotide combining entities in various fractions of cerebral tissues, it was found that intracellular receptors occurred at neuronal membrane sites, including postsynaptic sites, and also cytoplasmically (Walter *et al.* 1978; McIlwain, 1978, 1980; Newman *et al.* 1980). The best-established points of cyclic nucleotide generation are at the postsynaptic region of synaptic junctional complexes. Translocation of nucleotide is thus involved within a given junction and between junctions; and also between junctions and cytoplasmic regions and other organelles accessible from the cytoplasm.

Intracellular movements in the brain are highly organized: some 10 % of the soluble protein of the brain is tubulin, much of which *in situ* is organized as longitudinal tubules in the axons and dendrites of constituent cells and which has there a function in the intracellular transport of substances and particles. Cyclic nucleotides and their precursors, and neurotransmitters and their precursors, in some cases vesiculated, are among the entities transported (see Newman & McIlwain, 1978). Note, however, that the cytoplasmic movement of neurotransmitters, or of first-messengers generally, is of very different status from the cytoplasmic movement of the cyclic nucleotides as second-messengers. Neurotransmitters have been observed moving towards nerve-terminals where later they may be released and only after their release may act. Nucleotides have been observed moving along axons and dendrites and are then already in the cytoplasmic regions which are their sphere of action. Thus, when the nucleotides undergo cytoplasmic transport, they are enabled to act successively at a number of intracellular receptor sites, $IR_1 \ldots IR_n$, along their route of movement and during their life-time of some minutes.

The long dendritic branches of large cerebral neurons are especially significant regions in considering the movements of cyclic nucleotides (McIlwain, 1976, 1979). They carry many hundreds of terminals; a given neuron often makes multiple synapses with a given dendritic branch. Second-messenger nucleotide generated postsynaptically at axosomatic or at dendritic junctions may proceed along the dendrite and activate such of the successive postsynaptic or other regions as are sensitive to it: that is, those which carry the appropriate second-messenger receptors. Details of the activation, and consideration of other components of cyclic nucleotide systems which also undergo cytoplasmic movements, have been given elsewhere (McIlwain, 1977, 1978).

INTRACELLULAR RECEPTORS AND ENDOGENOUS CEREBRAL PROGRAMMES

An outcome of the movement of cyclic nucleotides intracellularly along dendritic receptor-arrays is thus a temporal modulation of cell-firing or firing tendency, which corresponds to the spatial pattern of nucleotide-sensitive regions, $IR_1 \ldots IR_n$, along the dendrite. Supporting evidence has been quoted (McIlwain, 1977) from observation of prolonged effects on cell-firing rates in eight separately studied cerebral systems, including instances of concomitant changes in cyclic nucleotide content and firing rate following the stimulation of noradrenergic innervation. The action of dopamine on cerebellar Purkinje cells and on caudate nucleus cells was to alter their pattern of firing (Bloom, 1975, 1978), actions also given by cyclic nucleotides. Responses to dopamine, but not to cyclic AMP, were antagonized by several antipsychotic phenothiazines, including chlorpromazine and fluphenazine. These drugs thus act as components ER in the sequence (1):

$$\text{Dopamine–}ER_1 \ldots ER_n\text{–Intracellular messenger–}IR_1 \ldots IR_n. \qquad (1)$$

Sequence (1) involves several other reactants, detailed elsewhere (McIlwain, 1977); its components $IR_1 \ldots IR_n$ are considered to condition the normal firing pattern of the neuron concerned and to be formed or positioned during development while the organism involved is receiving sensory input, environmental and proprioceptive. That noradrenergic innervation of the cerebral cortex which has been found necessary to programmed performance in rats (Anlezark *et al.* 1973) can be interpreted in terms of its providing intracellular messenger which 'reads' the component $IR_1 ... IR_n$. Such components, comprising series of nucleotide-sensitive receptors in the many available dendritic branches, offer mechanisms both for endogenous motor programmes and also for constructing the internal model of environmental events that is believed to be necessary to perception and memory.

The mechanisms sought by Creese (1978) in the initial quotation of this account involve the material bases for programmed series of endogenous cerebral activities, as manifested by signs and symptoms of hallucinations in man and by behavioural responses in animals. Activation of components $IR_1 ... IR_n$ of sequence (1), which conceptually links these phenomena, has been noted above to have consequences detectable electrophysiologically, and the emitted cerebral events of Weinberg *et al.* (1974) may also represent such an output. In certain schizophrenics hallucinatory activity was reported to be correlated with a particular pattern seen electrically in the septum (Bloom, 1978). Study of intracellular and extracellular receptor-sites, of receptor-controlled products and of their translocation can now offer vantage-points for discernment of behavioural mechanisms and of potential therapeutic approaches. Receptors, so prominent in the theoretical writing of Paul Ehrlich around 1900, did not feature much in his selection or synthesis of drugs (see McIlwain, 1957); as indicated above, however, chemotherapists now have the advantage of extensively developed techniques for measurement of receptor sites, and increasing attention could well be given to applying such measurements to the later stages of sequence (1).

HENRY MCILWAIN

REFERENCES

Andén, N. E. (1974). Antipsychotic drugs and catecholamine synapses. *Journal of Psychiatric Research* **11**, 97–104.

Anlezark, G. M., Crow, T. J. & Greenaway, A. P. (1973). Evidence that noradrenergic innervation of the cerebral cortex is necessary to learning. *Journal of Physiology* **231**, 119–120.

Bloom, F. E. (1975). The role of cyclic nucleotides in synaptic function. *Review of Physiology, Biochemistry and Pharmacology* **74**, 1–103.

Bloom, F. E. (1978). Modern concepts in electrophysiology for psychiatry. In *Biochemistry of Mental Disorders* (ed. E. Usdin and A. J. Mandell), pp. 31–52. Dekker: New York.

Creese, I. (1978). Receptor-binding as a primary drug screening device. In *Neurotransmitter Receptor Binding* (ed. H. I. Yamamura), pp. 141–170. Raven: New York.

Davis, J. M. (1975). Critique of single-amine theories. *Research in Nervous and Mental Disease* **54**, 333–346.

McIlwain, H. (1957). *Chemotherapy and the Central Nervous System*. Churchill: London.

McIlwain, H. (1972). Regulatory significance of the release and action of adenine derivates in cerebral systems. *Biochemistry Society Symposium* **36**, 69–85.

McIlwain, H. (1976). An extended messenger-role in the brain for cyclic AMP. *FEBS Letters* **64**, 271–273.

McIlwain, H. (1977). Extended roles in the brain for second-messenger systems. *Neuroscience* **2**, 357–372.

McIlwain, H. (1978). Synaptic mediators and the structuring of cerebral activity. *Progress in Neurobiology* **11**, 189–203.

McIlwain, H. (1979). Intracellular synaptic mediators and the endogenous simulation of neural input to the brain. In *Brain Mechanisms in Memory and Learning* (ed. M. A. B. Brazier), pp. 71–79. Raven: New York.

McIlwain, H. (1980). Brain: intracellular and extracellular purinergic receptor-systems. In *Purinergic Receptors* (ed. G. Burnstock). Chapman & Hall: London (in the press).

Matthysse, S. W. (1975). Epilogue. In *Catecholamines and Schizophrenia* (ed. S. W. Matthysse and S. S. Kety), pp. xv–xviii. Pergamon: Oxford.

Newman, M. & McIlwain, H. (1977). Adenosine as a constituent of the brain and of isolated cerebral tissues, and its relationship to the generation of adenosine 3′5′-cyclic monophosphate. *Biochemical Journal* **164**, 131–137.

Newman, M. & McIlwain, H. (1978). Cellular site and state of combination of adenosine 3′5′-cyclic monophosphate persisting after excitation of cerebral tissues. *Biochemical Journal* **170**, 73–79.

Newman, M. E., Patel, J. & McIlwain, H. (1980). Protein-bound cyclic AMP and histone kinase activities in cerebral cortical preparations. Submitted for publication.

O'Brien, R. D. (1979). *The Receptors: a Comprehensive Treatise. I. General Principles and Procedures*. Plenum: New York.

Reis, D. J. (1974). Consideration of some problems encountered in relating specific neurotransmitters to specific behaviours or disease. *Journal of Psychiatric Research* **11**, 145–148.

Ungerstedt, U. & Ljungberg, T. (1974). Central dopamine neurons and sensory processing. *Journal of Psychiatric Research* **11**, 149–150.

Volavka, J., Davis, L. G. & Ehrlich, Y. H. (1979). Endorphins, dopamine and schizophrenia. *Schizophrenia Bulletin* **5**, 227–239.

Walter, V., Kanof, P., Schulman, H. & Greengard, P. (1978). Adenosine 3′5′-monophosphate receptor proteins in mammalian brain. *Journal of Biological Chemistry* **253**, 6275–6280.

Weinberg, H., Grey Walter, W., Cooper, R. & Aldridge, V. J. (1974). Emitted cerebral events. *EEG and Clinical Neurophysiology* **36**, 449–456.

Yamamura, H. I., Enna, S. J. & Kuhar, M. J. (1978). *Neurotransmitter Receptor Binding*. Raven: New York.

Psychological Medicine, 1984, **14**, 13–21

Cortical noradrenaline, attention and arousal[1]

Since Marthe Vogt discovered the presence of noradrenaline (NA) in the central nervous system in the mid 1950s, this brain neurotransmitter has been implicated in a plethora of functions, ranging from the control of blood pressure to neuronal plasticity, memory and learning. Most interest has focused on the so-called dorsal noradrenergic ascending bundle (DNAB) which arises from cell bodies in the locus coeruleus of the dorsal pons. Utilizing novel histochemical techniques, Swedish research workers demonstrated that this nucleus not only had descending projections to the spinal cord and cerebellum, but also ascending projections to cortical areas such as the neocortex and hippocampus (Dahlström & Fuxe, 1964; Ungerstedt, 1971). It is the latter projections especially which have captured the imagination of neuroscientists and will be the main subject of this brief review. Part of the reason why this 'veteran' neurotransmitter substance is still engendering a good deal of interest, even in the vanguard of the neuropeptides, is that genuine advances are emerging in the understanding of its possible roles in brain function. Another reason is that many psychoactive drugs are known to modulate activity of this ascending NA system. For example, opiates such as morphine, and antidepressants such as desipramine, reduce the activity of coeruleal NA neurones, although through different receptor mechanisms (see Olpé *et al.* 1983). In addition, central NA mechanisms are thought to modulate the behavioural effects of peptides such as arginine vasopressin, which has been used to treat human memory disorders (Kovacs *et al.* 1979). Indeed, changes in DNAB activity have been directly implicated both in Alzheimer's disease and in Korsakoff's psychosis (see Crow, 1981).

One consequence of the likely clinical relevance of studying central NA mechanisms has been the continuing emergence of a number of sophisticated neuropharmacological tools for analysing further their nature and functions. Thus, there are now available NA neurotoxins such as 6-hydroxydopamine (6-OHDA) and DSP-4, as well as drugs which affect the pre-synaptic release and uptake of NA (e.g. amphetamine and imipramine) and a host of agonists and antagonists for adrenergic receptors of different types together with sensitive receptor assays. This sophistication has undoubtedly contributed in a major way to the advances to be described.

There is still a good deal we do not know about the basic neuroanatomical and neurophysiological features of nucleus locus coeruleus and the DNAB. For example, the nature of the afferents to locus coeruleus and the organization of the DNAB are still a matter of debate. Early findings suggested that there was little discrete organization of the various NA projections of locus coeruleus. For example, a single cell body could give rise to both ascending and descending axons. However, some recent evidence has suggested a degree of topographical organization of the projection so that certain spatially-grouped collections of cell bodies project predominantly to some forebrain areas, whereas other groups project elsewhere. Nevertheless, Morrison & Magistretti (1983) have contrasted the rather diffuse innervation of neocortex by the DNAB with that of other cortical afferents.

EARLY PROPOSALS FOR DNAB FUNCTION

The peculiar features of organization of the DNAB suggested to some workers that it had a rather general function. Clearly, messages relayed to at least a fair proportion of NA cell bodies would result in impulses simultaneously being transmitted to widespread portions of brain as far afield as the cerebellum and neocortex. In functional terms this supported an early proposal by Jouvet

[1] Address for correspondence: Dr Trevor W. Robbins, Department of Experimental Psychology, University of Cambridge, Downing Street, Cambridge CB2 3EB.

(1974), among others, that the DNAB was implicated in arousal: that is to say, a non-specific tonic state of neural activity which modulates not only the sleep/waking cycle, but also the efficiency of performance in the waking state. Arousal itself depended not only upon endogenous determinants but also upon the non-specific, intensive aspects of stimulus input including novelty, as opposed to its informational or 'cue' properties. Electrophysiological recordings from single units show activity in locus coeruleus cells to be highest during waking, at intermediate levels in slow-wave sleep, and at its lowest levels during REM sleep, an ordering which correlates with the behavioural degrees of arousal associated with these three states. However, there is also a good deal of evidence showing that the DNAB may not play an essential role in sleep regulation, and there is little doubt that a unidimensional concept of arousal is now in any case of little explanatory value. For example, Eysenck (1982), in a review of the evidence from experimental psychology, suggests that increasing arousal is linearly related to efficiency of certain aspects of performance except at very high levels which disrupt performance through anxiety, thereby generating the ubiquitous inverted U-shaped function relating arousal level to performance.

Other theorists had turned their attention to more specific functions of DNAB. It was known that rats would self-administer apparently rewarding trains of intracranial stimulation to those portions of brain rich in catecholamine-containing neurones, including of course the DNAB. Stein (1968) proposed that NA was the reward neurotransmitter, whereas Crow (1968) and Kety (1970) seized on the possibility that cortical NA provided the necessary reinforcing impact for learning to occur. Although early results involving electrolytic destruction of locus coeruleus supported this interpretation, later lesions produced by 6-OHDA resulting in more selective and profound loss of cortical NA failed to alter acquisition in the rat, at least of simple associations such as learning to press a lever for food on a continuously reinforced basis, or of learned taste aversion (Mason & Iversen, 1979).

DNAB AND NEURAL PLASTICITY

Notwithstanding the apparent lack of involvement in learning *per se*, some remarkable effects of central NA mechanisms have been shown on synaptic plasticity in response to altered environmental input, particularly in development. For example, Kasamatsu and colleagues (for a review, see Kasamatsu, 1983) have employed the well-known model of binocularity in cat visual cortical cells to investigate the possible role of the neocortical NA innervation in the changes in ocular dominance produced by monocular deprivation during the post-natal critical period for the development of binocular cells. Noradrenergic depletion produced by 6-OHDA injected either intraventricularly, or by a sophisticated method of local perfusion of cortical zones, reduced the plasticity of visual cortical cells following monocular deprivation: that is to say, ocular dominance of these cells failed to develop fully. In contrast, the ocular dominance could be restored by infusion of exogenous NA in a dose-related manner. Moreover, Kasamatsu found that the recovery of binocular vision (i.e. the reversion from ocular dominance) which followed only brief periods of monocular deprivation could be retarded by NA depletion and accelerated by infusions of NA itself. Thus, the expected change in binocularity was opposite to that in the earlier studies and so represented a general change in plasticity rather than a particular effect on ocularity. Infusion of the β-adrenergic receptor blocker propanolol, but not α-adrenergic blockers, could mimic the effects of 6-OHDA, suggesting that this change in plasticity was mediated by β receptors. Furthermore, the involvement of β rather than α receptors makes it likely that the effects on plasticity are not mediated via some effects of the DNAB on the regulation of cerebral blood flow.

Using a completely different, more behavioural model, Sutherland *et al.* (1982) have obtained analogous results. They found that damage to the medial cortex in rats resulted in impaired acquisition of a spatial task, but only if the lesions were made when the rat was adult. If instead the brain damage was inflicted early in development, then the animals were able to recover from its effects and exhibit normal spatial learning. This behavioural recovery, however, was prevented by the intraventricular administration of 6-OHDA to the neonatal rats. Therefore, this set of findings again suggests that NA affects cortical plasticity, especially in the developmental stage.

Although these findings give the impression that cortical NA has special functions in the development of neural connections early in life, this may be misleading. After all, animals are equipped with the DNAB for the whole of their lives; indeed, it is of interest that depletion of cortical NA appears to be implicated as a correlate of pre-senile dementia. Moreover, there are examples of apparent changes in plasticity, in electrophysiological terms, within hippocampus produced by DNAB destruction in adult rats (e.g. Bliss *et al.* 1981). In addition, Kasamatsu and colleagues themselves elegantly showed that plasticity in adult rats could be altered by central manipulations of cortical NA. Even more recently Keverne & de la Riva (1982) have shown that a 'short term olfactory memory' manifested in endocrine terms as the 'Bruce effect' in adult mice can be abolished by 6-OHDA depletion of NA from the olfactory bulb. In the Bruce effect the blockade of pregnancy occurs only by an odour from a strange male mouse while in the NA-depleted females the response also occurs by the odour of the stud male. Thus, the noradrenergic mechanism apparently sets into motion a relatively short-term olfactory memory which protects the female from the pregnancy block which would otherwise be induced by her stud male.

Most of these studies do not specify the nature of the conditions or stimuli producing activity in NA-containing cells. It seems most unlikely that NA is simply a modulatory neurohumour unresponsive itself to environmental conditions. Presumably, its effects on plasticity are normally mediated by induced activity in central NA neurones. How specific are the conditions producing such activity? For example, in the case of the olfactory memory described above, it is possible that cervical stimulation may be the trigger which increases NA turnover and thus facilitates 'memory'-formation in the olfactory bulb (E. B. Keverne, personal communication). However, evidence described below suggests that the central NA mechanisms may be influenced by far more general classes of stimuli. In that case, the specificity of the effect of 6-OHDA lesions of olfactory bulb (and visual cortex in the case of Kasamatsu's experiments) may depend on the specificity of the neurones within the cortical areas to which the ascending NA neurones project.

In summary, these experiments have provided a confirmation of the Crow and Kety propositions that cortical NA modulates the long-term effects of experience on cortical function, although not to the extent of demonstrating definitive alterations in learning processes resulting from the changing impact of reinforcement conveyed by the ascending DNAB neurones.

DNAB, ANXIETY AND STRESS

An alternative, but no less specific, theory of dorsal bundle function was that activity within it was produced by stress, including, for example, anxiety produced by signals of punishment or non-reward. Gray (e.g. 1982) has argued that one of the means by which the minor tranquillizers (e.g. benzodiazepines) alleviate anxiety is by reducing activity in the DNAB. A related but thorny issue is the likely involvement of the DNAB in the phenomena related to depression. One well-known animal model of depression – learned helplessness – has long been associated with NA depletion, particularly in the coeruleal NA system (see Weiss *et al.* 1982). This depletion might be seen to result from a failure to replete the central NA system following the large increases in turnover produced by stressors such as unpredictable, inescapable electric shocks.

Previously, this NA depletion has been linked with the behavioural hypoactivity accompanying learned helplessness, although some workers have claimed that this hypoactivity is ancillary to a primary cognitive impairment in that model (see Gray, 1982, ch. 12 for a review). However, given the likely involvement of cortical NA in syndromes such as Alzheimer's disease and Korsakoff's psychosis, it seems quite possible that cortical NA depletion would also lead to cognitive impairment, especially in view of the types of deficit produced by DNAB lesions in animals. These deficits, which are described below, do not include behavioural hypoactivity, and infusions of low doses of NA into dense projections of the DNAB, such as the dentate gyrus of the hippocampus, do not produce the opposite effect of behavioural hyperactivity (Flicker & Geyer, 1982). Therefore, the intriguing link between the motor retardation of the learned helplessness model and the locus coeruleus may not involve its cortical projection. Although the locus coeruleus NA system may well respond in a unitary fashion to stress, the different effects of the latter on learning and memory and on motor performance, for example, may result from the diverse influence of the coeruleal NA system on a variety of terminal regions, subcortical as well as cortical, which are specialized for those different functions. Activity in the DNAB may then enable the organization of a coordinated response to stress over a range of different behavioural and physiological functions.

ELECTROPHYSIOLOGICAL APPROACHES TO DNAB FUNCTION

Although it is the case that stressors such as electric shock can elevate NA turnover in the DNAB, a similar change in turnover can be elicited by other stimuli, not obviously aversive or stressful, such as rewarding intracranial stimulation (for a review, see Robbins & Everitt, 1982). This fact, together with observations that cells in locus coeruleus respond electrophysiologically to polymodal, non-noxious inputs (Aston-Jones & Bloom, 1981), again raises the possibility that the DNAB mediates general arousal as a function of stimulus intensity, novelty and learned salience, but not of detailed information about stimulus characteristics. In support of this Watabe *et al.* (1982) have shown how visual input from a variety of sources converges onto locus coeruleal cells and how such cells may respond to novel light flashes, but not to specific stimuli such as spots or slits. Earlier, the arousal possibility was mentioned, but was thought not to explain satisfactorily the complex role of the DNAB in sleep nor to recognize the inadequacy of monolithic constructs of arousal. To these doubts can be added the evidence that DNAB lesions produce only transient effects on cortical arousal as measured by the EEG (see Robbins & Everitt, 1982). However, cortical EEG under baseline conditions is a fairly crude measure of the synaptic operations in neocortex and it may be more useful to consider the participation of NA in the evoked single cell responses to specific sensory inputs.

Bloom (1979) has argued that one of the functions of the DNAB is to extend in temporal terms the impact of environmental events, thus presumably converting phasic events into longer term tonic influences. He discusses an 'enabling' or 'biasing' mode of operation of the DNAB which enhances the response of the target cell to its other afferent responses without altering it directly. These ideas are based on the pioneering observations of Segal & Bloom (e.g. 1976) who demonstrated that the electrical stimulation of locus coeruleus or microiontophoresis of NA onto pyramidal cells of the hippocampus enhanced the inhibitory effect of an auditory tone on hippocampal firing or, alternatively, enhanced the excitatory effect of the same stimulus when predictive of food.

Foote *et al.* (1975) have also shown that microiontophoresis of NA onto cells in the auditory cortex of the squirrel monkey changed the pattern of firing to species-specific vocalizations. Noradrenaline generally inhibited evoked firing, but did so to a greater extent for the background firing rate. This and other observations have led to the ideas that exogenously applied NA increases the signal to noise ratio (S/N) of the evoked responses. Analogous effects have been found in somatosensory cortex (Waterhouse & Woodward, 1980) and Kasamatsu & Heggelund (1982), studying single cell responses in cat visual cortex to visual stimulation during iontophoresis of NA, also recently found that the increased S/N notion could satisfactorily summarize findings of diverse excitatory, as well as inhibitory, responses to NA. Thus this effect of cortical NA extends over at least three sensory modalities and seems to enhance the effects of stimuli that are specific for the cortical region studied.

THE DNAB AND SELECTIVE ATTENTION: RECENT FINDINGS

Extrapolating these electrophysiological findings to behavioural function is a perilous step which may not yet be completely justified. On balance, it would seem sensible to place the effects in a functional context at some level. One obvious possibility is that the change in S/N ratio reflects alterations in sensory processing. However, just as little evidence has been found of motor impairment following DNAB lesions, there has also been little suggestion so far of sensory impairment. Recent work by Everitt *et al.* (1983) and by Carli *et al.* (1983), using visual and auditory discrimination of temporal frequency and spatial localization of brief, dim visual stimuli, has revealed no impairments in performance of rats with DNAB lesions. Mason & Iversen (1979), arguing initially from indirect evidence, suggested alternatively that DNAB-lesioned animals have instead an attentional inability to screen out irrelevant stimuli. This is an ingenious proposal, but it does depend crucially upon how an irrelevant stimulus is defined. The most straightforward definition is a familiar stimulus that is only randomly correlated with reward. However, one might also possibly include stimuli (of the same or different sensory modality) which are redundant in predicting reward and novel, distracting stimuli of potential relevance which are extraneous to a particular task.

In brief, there have been several tests of this hypothesis, with rather conflicting results. One of the most important papers supporting the attentional hypothesis is that of Mason & Lin (1980). In this article, a number of paradigms, well-known to learning theorists, are used to assess the extent to which rats have learned not to attend to stimuli that have in the past been unpredictive of reward. When such stimuli are subsequently made relevant, this will be advantageous to a rat unable to ignore these formerly irrelevant stimuli and hence will lead to a faster acquisition of response to them. Thus, under certain conditions, *better* acquisition should be predicted in rats with DNAB lesions. Although this facilitation of acquisition has been seen in a few experiments, it has in general proved difficult to obtain. For example, some of our own work has used a discrimination task in which there are two modalities, visual and auditory, and the rat was rewarded with food for discriminating fast or slow frequency flashes (or bleeps) in one modality, while ignoring the fast or slow stimuli in the other. Then, the previously irrelevant dimension was made relevant and *vice versa*, so that the DNAB-lesioned rat should have a clear advantage in shifting attention. However, we found that, unfortunately, the DNAB-lesioned rats were slower to learn the basic task which would invalidate any interpretation of faster reversal on their part because of their different training experiences (Robbins *et al.* 1982) (in fact, they were not in any case faster to reverse). This result would still support an attentional hypothesis if there was no difference in learning between the DNAB and sham-operated animals in the simple discrimination with only one modality present, but we have also found an acquisition impairment under those conditions (Everitt *et al.* 1983). Most of the DNAB rats did eventually learn, but of course this is entirely consistent with a modulatory rather than an essential role of the DNAB on stimulus processing of the type discussed by Bloom (1979). Control experiments ruled out the possibility of sensory or motivational impairment. For example, if the rats were trained to criterion before surgery, then there was no significant behavioural decrement by the cortical NA depletion: the deficit was in acquisition, not performance. We were surprised to find such apparently clear-cut deficits in acquisition, given the previous evidence. However, the temporal discrimination task was a difficult one, taking many sessions to learn, and the task may have been sufficiently sensitive to show an impairment following the marked capacity for recovery of function that is known to follow damage to the DNAB. It is also possible that the deficit was more apparent because of some special feature of the task, such as reliance on discrimination of temporal frequency, which may be a particularly 'cortical' type of function. However, we have now noted several other recent reports of acquisition failure after DNAB lesions (see Robbins *et al.* 1982).

These recent findings force us to reconsider the 'attentional hypothesis' because, although it is entirely possible that the deficits result from an attentional failure (that is, the discriminative stimuli fail to gain access to central associative mechanisms), it is also possible that the deficits result from a direct impairment of associative processes, as mooted by Crow and Kety. In order to test further the attentional hypothesis, extra pressure must be placed on selective attentional mechanisms in a situation in which the rat cortically depleted of NA and the sham controls are initially at the same level of performance. One way of achieving this is to present the discriminative stimuli with a shorter interval between them than is usual and, indeed, this does impair the performance of the DNAB-lesioned rat more than its control counterpart (Everitt *et al.* 1983; Carli *et al.* 1983). The other main means of disturbing performance is to introduce distracting stimuli. Interpolation of distractors simultaneously with the relevant discriminanda leads surprisingly to little disruption of performance, even in DNAB-lesioned rats. However, we have recently found, employing a task requiring the localization of brief visual target stimuli randomly at one of five locations, that playing loud (85 dB) bursts of white noise just prior to the onset of the target visual stimuli can significantly impair the accuracy of detection of the visual target in the DNAB-lesioned but not the sham control rats (Carli *et al.* 1983). The interpolated white noise has other effects on performance: it increases the likelihood of premature, inappropriate responses (i.e. it makes the rats adopt a riskier criterion for responding), and it significantly hastens long reaction times in response to the light. Thus, it would appear that the white noise in some way arouses or activates motor performance. However, both of these effects are equivalent in the sham controls and DNAB-lesioned rats and it is only in the accuracy of detection that the latter perform worse. This suggests a quite specific behavioural impairment, and we shall speculate on this below.

The extreme measures we took to demonstrate a significant differential effect of distraction on the DNAB-lesioned rats make the type of attentional deficit shown by these animals seem less likely to be one of ignoring stimuli only randomly correlated with reward. On the whole, the DNAB-lesioned rat seems able to do this perfectly well. Of course, it is possible, as with the deficits in acquisition we observed, that the relatively small (though significant) effects result because of neurochemical recovery processes occurring within the DNAB. This requires further investigation. In addition, it would be worthwhile to attempt to activate or depress the coeruleo-cortical NA pathway by more acute manipulations (e.g. Flicker & Geyer, 1982) to gain a more complete picture of the role of the DNAB in these attentional situations.

THE DNAB, ATTENTION AND AROUSAL

In accounting for these behavioural results we have made use of comparisons between the human experimental literature on attentional changes resulting from the manipulation of different environmental conditions. For example, the 5-choice visual localization test described above is obviously similar to Leonard's 5-choice serial reaction task, which is frequently used to assess the effect of environmental conditions and change in arousal produced, for example, by white noise and various drugs in human subjects (see Eysenck, 1982).

In our version of the continuous performance test it is notable that the stimulant *d*-amphetamine produces similar effects to those of white noise in normal rats: that is, over a wide dose range it has no effects on accuracy but increases premature responding and hastens reactions. It is now generally thought that the majority of the behavioural effects of *d*-amphetamine are mediated by central dopaminergic rather than noradrenergic mechanisms (which may, however, have a modulatory role). Complementing this fact, we have shown that dopamine (DA) depletion from the nucleus accumbens produces a slower response but no change in accuracy (Robbins *et al.* 1982). Therefore, it seems likely that the central NA and DA systems have rather different roles in controlling performance on this task. When arousing distractors, such as white noise, induce impulsive responding and threaten to disrupt discriminative performance, activity in the DNAB may maintain accuracy. However, from these preliminary results, the central mesolimbic DA system seems to be implicated in activating responding, making it both more likely and faster in execution, but not necessarily also guiding its accuracy. A distinction may then be made between mediation of the effects of *arousal* by cortical NA, and *activation* of behaviour by central DA mechanisms. This distinction, which runs counter to old unitary notions of arousal, may be analogous to Broadbent's concept of 'upper' and 'lower' arousal mechanisms (Broadbent, 1971) in which the upper mechanism monitors performance under conditions of supra-optimal activation of the lower mechanism (produced, for example, by white noise) and helps to prevent the disruptive effects of arousal on discrimination. The DNAB may then normally contribute to the functioning of this upper mechanism by enhancing inhibitory effects and preventing the organism from becoming overdistractible (see Fig. 1). This would appear to be broadly consistent with the electrophysiological studies of the DNAB reviewed above and with the findings that stressful stimuli increase NA turnover. An obvious prediction of the model is that the DNAB does not in itself mediate stress,

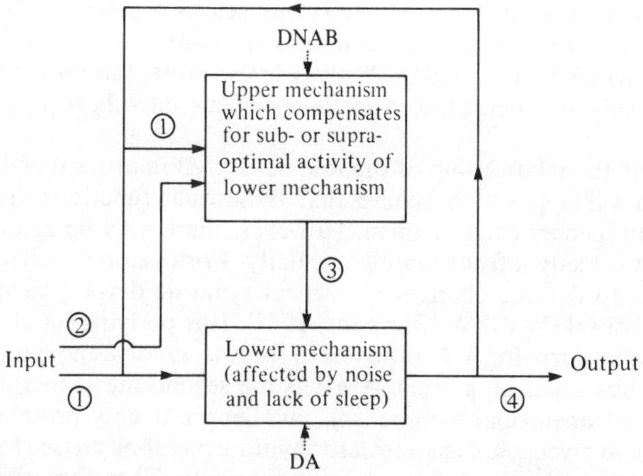

FIG. 1. Schematized diagram of the proposed 'upper' and 'lower' arousal mechanisms. Examples of the types of conditions influencing the lower mechanism are given on the figure. Stimulus input is hypothesized to have two main aspects: non-specific and arousing, produced by intense, or salient stimuli; and specific, involving informational properties such as spatio-temporal patterning. Both aspects are available to the upper mechanism, but only the arousing aspects to the lower mechanism. The latter controls primarily speed and probability of responding rather than response selection itself. The DNAB mediates arousal to the upper mechanism whereas the central DA systems may contribute to the activation of performance by the lower mechanism. For further description, see text. ①, non-specific arousal, drive (intensive aspects); ②, informational (discriminative aspects); ③, response selection or choice; ④, speed and likelihood of response.

but rather becomes active during stressful situations inducing high arousal, to preserve attentional selectivity. I would expect, in general, that impairments resulting from DNAB damage would most readily be seen under conditions of over-arousal of the lower mechanism, since the compensatory ability of the upper mechanism is lost. I would expect the lower mechanism to be aroused by salient arousing stimuli, including perhaps autonomic feedback, and to be mediated in part by activity in the central dopaminergic system. In contrast, the upper mechanism may also help to compensate for performance decrement produced by sub-optimal levels of arousal arising, for example, from lack of sleep. We can then perhaps explain why DNAB lesions in conjunction with adrenalectomy have such a devastating effect on avoidance performance in the rat (e.g. Ögren & Fuxe, 1974) because, not only are the basic arousal processes of the animal deranged by adrenalectomy, but the upper mechanism which normally compensates for such deficiencies is also impaired.

There are many results which this speculative model probably cannot easily explain without extra assumptions. For example, in order to explain the selective effect of DNAB lesions on acquisition rather than performance, described above, it is necessary to assume that acquisition conditions involve higher levels of arousal than the conditions obtaining during the more automatic processes involved in performance. We would obviously have to predict, in parallel with this, elevated NA turnover in the DNAB during acquisition compared with performance.

Although I have emphasized the 'protective' effects of the DNAB on attention at elevated levels of arousal, it is also possible, given the possible exaggeration of effects of salient stimuli described by Segal & Bloom (1976), that *beneficial* effects of arousal upon learning and memory are also mediated through the upper mechanism, as arousal apparently can improve long-term (though not short-term) memory in man (see Eysenck, 1982). We have no space here to review the effects of NA manipulations upon the consolidation of long-term memory traces, but there is some evidence that a reduction in central NA activity plays a central role in the effects of various amnesic agents such as electroconvulsive shock (Gold & Sternberg, 1978). It is also possible that the apparently positive effects on memory of neuropeptides such as arginine vasopressin are also mediated by activity in the DNAB corresponding to enhanced levels of arousal, as Sahgal & Wright (1983) have recently argued.

I have tried to indicate how this account of DNAB function incorporates various hypotheses about DNAB function involving learning, arousal, stress and selective attention. The fact that it has not proved possible to provide conclusive evidence in favour of any one of these hypotheses may reflect their inter-relatedness, which I have tried to clarify. Furthermore, this more integrated account may explain how the relatively few neurones in locus coeruleus have been implicated in all of these functions.

A remaining puzzle is the relationship of the role of DNAB in arousal and in synaptic plasticity. Kasamatsu (1983) himself appears to believe that these dual functions are not directly related, although the DNAB influences each of them. However, there may be grounds for believing that changes in arousal can directly affect synaptic plasticity. For example, rearing animals in enriched environments can lead to definite changes in cortical synaptic development which some authors attribute to elevated arousal (Walsh & Cummins, 1975). It is perhaps significant that the effects of NA on plasticity and on improving S/N ratios both seem to involve the β receptor, which is linked to adenylate cyclase, thus generating cyclic AMP as the second messenger. Cyclic AMP is known to be connected with intraneuronal metabolism, involving not only protein kinases that mediate phosphorylation, but also glycogenolysis and carbohydrate metabolism (see Morrison & Magistretti, 1983), both of which may be implicated in neuronal plasticity. Therefore, the possibility arises that the metabolic and neuronal effects of cortical NA are quite closely related. This possibility would doubtless please Duffy, one of the earlier proponents of arousal as an important neural process, who believed that arousal or activation could be defined in terms of metabolic activity in the tissues: 'The level of activation of the organism may be defined as the extent of the release of potential energy, stored in the tissues of the organism, as this is shown in activity or response' (Duffy, 1962, p. 17). This bold statement may still have some relevance today, although we have come some way from the behavioural notion of arousal as Duffy intended, and we must not be distracted from specifying in much more detail the processes underlying this transduction.

T. W. ROBBINS

I thank Dr B. J. Sahakian and Dr E. B. Keverne for critically reading the manuscript and my collaborators, especially Dr B. J. Everitt, Dr M. Carli, Dr P. J. Fray and J. Evenden, for discussion. The author's recent experimental work upon which this editorial is based was supported by MRC grant G979/1150/N.

REFERENCES

Aston-Jones, G. & Bloom, F. E. (1981). Norepinephrine-containing locus coeruleus neurones in behaving rats exhibit pronounced responses to non-noxious environmental stimuli. *Journal of Neuroscience* **1**, 887–900.

Bliss, J. V. P., Goddard, G. V., Robertson, H. A. & Sutherland, R. J. (1981). Noradrenaline depletion reduces long term potentiation in the rat hippocampus. In *Cellular Analogues of Conditioning and Neural Plasticity* (ed. O. Feher and F. Joo), pp. 175–185. Advances in Physiological Science Vol. 36. Pergamon Press: Oxford.

Bloom, F. (1979). Is there a neurotransmitter code in the brain? In *Neurotransmitters* (ed. P. Simon), pp. 205–213. Advances in Pharmacology and Therapeutics Vol. 2. Pergamon Press: Oxford and New York.

Broadbent, D E. (1971). *Decision and Stress.* Academic Press: New York.

Carli, M., Robbins, T. W., Evenden, J. & Everitt, B. J. (1983). Effects of lesions to ascending noradrenergic neurons on performance of a 5-choice serial reaction task in rats: implications for theories of dorsal noradrenergic bundle function based on selective attention and arousal. *Behavioural Brain Research* **9**, 361–380.

Crow, T. J. (1968). Cortical synapses and reinforcement. *Nature* **219**, 736–737.

Crow, T. J. (1981). Biochemical aspects of memory. In *Metabolic Disorders of the Nervous System* (ed. F. Clifford Rose), pp. 369–375. Pitman: London.

Dahlström, A. & Fuxe, K. (1964). Evidence for the existence of monoamine-containing neurons in the central nervous system. I. Demonstration of monoamines in the cell bodies of brain stem neurones. *Acta Physiologica Scandinavica* **62**, Suppl. 232, 1–55.

Duffy, E. (1962). *Activation and Behaviour.* Wiley: London.

Everitt, B. J., Robbins, T. W., Gaskin, M. & Fray, P. J. (1983). The effects of lesions to ascending noradrenergic neurones on discrimination learning and performance in the rat. *Neuroscience* **10**, 397–410.

Eysenck, M. W. (1982). *Attention and Arousal.* Springer-Verlag: Berlin.

Flicker, C. & Geyer, M. A. (1982). Behavior during hippocampal microinfusions, I. Norepinephrine and diversive exploration. *Brain Research Reviews* **4**, 79–103.

Foote, S. L., Friedman, R. & Oliver, A. P. (1975). Effects of putative neurotransmitters on neuronal activity in monkey cerebral cortex. *Brain Research* **86**, 229–242.

Gold, P. E. & Sternberg, D. B. (1978). Retrograde amnesia produced by several treatments; evidence for a common neurobiological mechanism. *Science* **201**, 367–369.

Gray, J. A. (1982). *The Neuropsychology of Anxiety.* Oxford University Press: Oxford.

Jouvet, M. (1974). Monoaminergic regulation of the sleep–waking cycle in the cat. In *The Neurosciences, Third Study Program* (ed. F. O. Schmidt and F. G. Worden), pp. 499–508. MIT Press Cambridge, Mass.

Kasamatsu, T. (1983). Neuronal plasticity maintained by the central norepinephrine system in the cat visual cortex. In *Progress in*

Psychobiology and Physiological Psychology, Vol. 10 (ed. J. M. Sprague and A. N. Epstein), pp. 1–112. Academic Press: New York.

Kasamatsu, T. & Heggelund, P. (1982). Single cell responses in cat visual cortex to visual stimulation during iontophoresis of noradrenaline. *Experimental Brain Research* **45**, 317–324.

Kety, S. S. (1970). The biogenic amines and the central nervous system: their possible roles in arousal, emotion and learning. In *The Neurosciences, Second Study Program* (ed. F. O. Schmidt), pp. 324–336. Rockefeller University Press: New York.

Keverne, E. B. & de la Riva, C. (1982). Pheromones in mice: reciprocal action between the nose and brain. *Nature* **296**, 148–150.

Kovacs, G. L., Bohus, B. & Versteeg, D. H. G. (1979). The effects of vasopressin on memory processes: the role of noradrenergic neurotransmission. *Neuroscience* **4**, 1529–1537.

Mason, S. T. & Iversen, S. D. (1979). Theories of dorsal bundle extinction effect. *Brain Research Reviews* **1**, 107–137.

Mason, S. T. & Lin, D. (1980). Dorsal noradrenergic bundle and selective attention. *Journal of Comparative and Physiological Psychology* **94**, 819–832.

Morrison, J. H. & Magistretti, P. J. (1983). Monoamines and peptides in cerebral cortex. *Trends in Neuroscience* **6**, 146–151.

Ögren, S. & Fuxe, K. (1974). Learning, noradrenaline and the pituitary-adrenal axis. *Medical Biology* **52**, 399–405.

Olpé, H.-R., Jones, R. S. G. & Steinmann, M. W. (1983). The locus coeruleus actions of psychoactive drugs. *Experientia* **39**, 242–249.

Robbins, T. W. & Everitt, B. J. (1982). Functional studies of the central catecholamines. *International Review of Neurobiology* **23**, 303–365.

Robbins, T. W., Everitt, B. J., Fray, P. J., Gaskin, M., Carli, M. & de la Riva, C. (1982). The roles of the central catecholamines in attention and learning. In *Behavioral Models and the Analysis of Drug Action* (ed. M. Y. Spiegelstein and A. Levy), pp. 109–134. Elsevier: Amsterdam.

Sahgal, A. & Wright, C. (1983). A comparison of the effects of vasopressin and oxytocin with amphetamine and chlordiazepoxide on passive avoidance behaviour in rats. *Psychopharmacology* **80**, 88–92.

Segal, M. & Bloom, F. E. (1976). The action of norepinephrine in the rat hippocampus. IV: The effect of locus coeruleus stimulation on evoked hippocampal activity. *Brain Research* **107**, 513–525.

Stein, L. (1968). Chemistry of reward and punishment. In *Psychopharmacology: a Review of Progress 1957–1967* (ed. D. H. Efron), pp. 105–123. US Government Printing Office: Washington, D.C.

Sutherland, R. J., Kolb, B., Whishaw, I. Q. & Becker, J. B. (1982). Cortical noradrenaline depletion eliminates sparing of spatial learning after neonatal frontal cortex damage in the rat. *Neuroscience Letters* **32**, 125–130.

Ungerstedt, U. (1971). Stereotaxic mapping of the monoamine pathways in rat brain. *Acta Physiologica Scandinavica* **367** (Suppl.), 1–49.

Walsh, R. N. & Cummins, R. A. (1975). Mechanisms mediating the production of environmentally-produced brain changes. *Psychological Bulletin* **82**, 986–1000.

Watabe, K., Nakai, K. & Kasamatsu, T. (1982). Visual afferents to norepinephrine-containing neurones in cat locus coeruleus. *Experimental Brain Research* **48**, 66–80.

Waterhouse, B. D. & Woodward, D. J. (1980). Interaction of norepinephrine with cerebro-cortical activity evoked by stimulation of somatosensory afferent pathways. *Experimental Neurology* **67**, 11–34.

Weiss, J. M., Bailey, W. H., Goodman, P. A., Hoffman, L. J., Ambrose, M. J., Salmon, S. & Charry, J. M. (1982). A model for neurochemical study of depression. In *Behavioral Models and the Analysis of Drug Action* (ed. M. Y. Spiegelstein and A. Levy), pp. 195–233. Elsevier: Amsterdam.

Psychological Medicine, 1983, **13**, 715–720

Monoamines and the control of sexual behaviour[1]

The availability of large numbers of drugs in the 1960s and 1970s resulted in an explosion of psychopharmacological studies of motivated behaviour, including sexual behaviour. The effects of some drugs, particularly those affecting serotonin and dopamine, on patterns of sexual activity in males and females of a number of non-human species were impressive and encouraged the belief, held by many, that these cerebral monoamines were of special importance in regulating the expression of sexual motivation. Before summarizing the major consequences of manipulating monoaminergic activity in the brain, it is important to point out that such experimental investigations were undertaken within a conceptual framework which acknowledged that sexual behaviour is hormone-dependent. Thus, it was well known that gonadal steroids critically determine whether or not a male or female displays sexual activity in the presence of an appropriate stimulus. That the hypothalamus is a major target for these behavioural effects of sex steroids was similarly widely accepted, but the precise mechanism of action remained largely a mystery. It was the latter problem which the consequences of aminergic manipulations appeared to address although, as we shall see, the narrow interpretation of the results of many of these psychopharmacological experiments was, in retrospect, misleading.

It was Meyerson, in a series of innovative experiments, who first showed that inhibiting serotonin (5-HT) synthesis enhanced the display of 'heat' in female rats (Meyerson, 1964). Indeed, the effect was so great that progesterone, the hormone which together with oestradiol controls oestrous behaviour in this species, could be replaced by drugs causing 5-HT depletion. Conversely, elevating 5-HT levels prevented the display of oestrus normally induced by the ovarian hormones. These results have been confirmed subsequently in a number of species and have been extended to include the male – for example, castrated male rats treated with doses of testosterone too low to restore their sexual behaviour can be rendered sexually active by injection of 5-HT-depleting drugs or receptor antagonists (Malmnäs, 1973). The interpretation of these data, still held by many, was that hormones induce changes in sexual behaviour by depressing 5-HT transmission – indeed, Meyerson spoke of 5-HT neurones as a 'heat inhibition system' and continues to present experimental evidence directly linking progesterone and 5-HT in female rats. There is no doubt that decreasing 5-HT concentrations in the brain can have profound effects on sexual behaviour and not only in rodents.

Thus, treatment of female rhesus monkeys made unreceptive by hormone withdrawal with para-chlorophenylalanine (PCPA), an inhibitor of tryptophan hydroxylase and hence 5-HT synthesis, greatly increases their receptivity, an effect prevented by restoring 5-HT levels by treatment with 5-hydroxytryptophan (Gradwell *et al.* 1975). Indeed, there have also been reports that PCPA or another 5-HT-depleting compound, para-chloromethamphetamine, increases 'libido' in men, although the behavioural analysis and rationale for such drastic treatments leave much to be desired (see Everitt, 1976).

Manipulating dopamine (DA) transmission profoundly alters the expression of sexual behaviour. The availability of an array of relatively specific DA receptor agonists and antagonists has allowed an exploration of dopaminergic functions to proceed more rapidly than is the case for 5-HT. In the male DA receptor blockade virtually abolishes sexual behaviour: ejaculation, intromission and mounting patterns are decreased by doses of drugs which do not markedly interfere with locomotor activity and which are much lower than those inducing catalepsy (Malmnäs, 1973: Baum & Starr,

[1]Address for correspondence: Dr Barry J. Everitt, Department of Anatomy, University of Cambridge, Downing Street, Cambridge CB2 3DY.

1980). Conversely, DA agonists (e.g. apomorphine, amphetamine) enhance sexual activity (Paglietti *et al.* 1978). Thus, ejaculation occurs after fewer intromitted mounts, post-ejaculatory refractory periods are said to decrease, and mounting activity is in general greatly increased. It has even been reported that so-called 'sexually sluggish' rats, who rarely if ever copulate, can be made sexually potent by treatment with these drugs. There have been some attempts to relate improved sexual performance in men to enhanced DA activity. For example, in the late 1960s and early 1970s it was claimed that patients with Parkinson's disease receiving *l*-dopa showed a marked recrudescence of their sexual interest and capacity. More careful analysis, however, revealed that this effect was only a reflection of the reversal of akinesia and their generally improved motor performance and not a specific action of *l*-dopa on sexual behaviour alone (see Everitt, 1976). This, as we shall see, was an important and often missed conclusion.

In the female, the situation is slightly complicated by the fact that, in most species, sexual behaviour comprises active and inactive (immobile) patterns which serve to incite the male's interest and then allow intromission, respectively. These patterns have been termed proceptive (an expression of the female's readiness to mate – her 'motivation') and receptive (the ease with which she assumes the receptive posture, lordosis, and hence allows the male to intromit). Drugs which enhance DA activity enhance proceptive patterns – as they do, by analogy, in the male – but diminish receptive patterns probably because the attendant motor activation is inconsistent with immobility (Everitt *et al.* 1974, 1975; Caggiula *et al.* 1979). Conversely, DA receptor blockade markedly attenuates proceptivity but enhances the display of lordosis. Indeed, female rats, for example, will remain immobile in the lordosis posture for 30–60 s instead of the normal 1 s necessary for an intromitted mount to occur (Everitt *et al.* 1974, 1975; Caggiula *et al.* 1979).

These, then, are major effects of DA manipulations on sexual behaviour. Initially it was largely ignored that the same drug treatments also markedly affected the expression of all other forms of goal-directed behaviour (e.g. eating, drinking, aggression, etc.). Hence, rather specific hypotheses concerning dopamine systems and sexual behaviour were proposed (as they were for other forms of behaviour) and it was some time before more broadly based views of dopaminergic function in the control of behaviour were aired. I return to this below.

In contrast to the success of psychopharmacological experiments on DA and 5-HT, those involving noradrenergic (NA) manipulations have been difficult to interpret. This may be largely because many of the drugs have severe effects on the periphery via the autonomic nervous system – for example, alpha-Na receptor acting drugs – which make any possible central actions difficult to define. The advent of neurotoxins with which to lesion central NA neurones has been of major importance, therefore, in revealing their behavioural functions (see below).

The problem facing psychopharmacologists armed with so much data on the effects of drugs on sexual behaviour was interpretation. Specifically, it is necessary to define the relationship between monoaminergic neurones in the brain (which, presumably, are affected by aminergic drugs) and the hypothalamic hormone-dependent mechanisms known to regulate sexual behaviour. Much was, and still is, made of the fact that the hypothalamus receives a rich monoaminergic innervation. Furthermore, castration and subsequent treatment with sex steroids (oestradiol, testosterone, progesterone) results in substantial changes in the levels and turnover of DA, NA and 5-HT. These correlations between steroid hormones and hypothalamic amines form in large measure the basis of assertions that the two are causally linked in the context of sexual behaviour. Indeed, it has recently been shown that sex steroids can induce alterations in the binding of NA, 5-HT and DA in the hypothalamus and elsewhere (see Everitt *et al.* 1983). Thus, these hormones may alter the expression of sexual behaviour by a direct action on amine receptors thereby indirectly modulating NA, DA and 5-HT transmission.

This remains an area of intense research effort, and it is a particularly interesting one since it may explain how widespread and diffusely projecting systems of neurones, which NA, DA and 5-HT neurones undoubtedly are, may have their actions channelled specifically at some points in time. In this case, only those axons terminating in areas which are addressed by steroid hormones would have the consequences of transmitter release modified and only at those times when steroid hormone secretion is optimal. Axons terminating elsewhere (and these may even arise from the same neurones, since the axons of monoamine neurones branch widely) would, presumably, be unaffected by this process. However, a problem for this view is that few reports have convincingly demonstrated that aminergic drugs exert their behavioural actions within hormone-sensitive areas of the brain. Indeed, if we focus our attention on the preoptic area (in males) and the ventromedial nucleus (in females) there are few data to suggest that aminergic manipulations here affect sexual behaviour. Conversely, aminergic manipulations elsewhere do, particularly with regard to the DA system.

It is the advent of neurochemical neurotoxins and accurate information on the distribution of monoamine neurones which has allowed a more refined investigation of their behavioural importance. The neurotoxins include: 6-hydroxydopamine (6-OHDA) which may be used to destroy either NA or DA neurones or both, depending on where it is placed; 5,6- and 5,7-dihydroxytryptamine which may be used more or less specifically to destroy 5-HT neurones; and, more recently, excitotoxic amino acids such as ibotenic acid or aspartate which have the unique property of destroying neuronal cell bodies when injected intracerebrally but leaving axons passing through the area unaffected. These compounds have made it possible to make neurochemically specified lesions in the brain, a distinct improvement over the 'burn and run' of electrolytic and related lesion techniques. But neurochemical neurotoxins are not without their drawbacks – for example, it has proved difficult to make specific lesions in terminal areas receiving a mixed innervation, while local plasticity changes following such lesions make interpretation of behavioural effects problematical, particularly in the long term. However, selective lesions to ascending (and descending) axons may be achieved in the brainstem to yield neurochemically specific denervation of relatively restricted structures, and these have resulted in valuable behavioural data.

Before considering some of these data it is pertinent to mention briefly the organization of monoaminergic neurones in the brain (see Hökfelt *et al.* 1983; Steinbusch, 1981; Lindvall & Björklund, 1978). Dopaminergic neurones lie largely in the midbrain within the substantia nigra and adjacent ventral tegmental area. The forebrain areas receiving the densest innervation from these cells are the neostriatum, including the nucleus accumbens, septal nuclei, amygdala and frontal cortex. The hypothalamus has intrinsic DA neurones lying periventricularly, particularly in the arcuate nucleus, while the preoptic area receives a DA input from cells in the zona incerta. Noradrenergic (and adrenergic) neurones lie in the ventro-lateral reticular formation of the medulla and, within the dorsal vagal complex, they innervate largely sub-cortical structures, especially the hypothalamus, and also septal nuclei and amygdala. Noradrenergic cells in the pontine locus coeruleus also innervate similar sub-cortical structures but, in addition, they uniquely provide the hippocampus and neocortex with NA terminals. Both groups of NA neurones branch widely, such that relatively few cells innervate virtually the entire neuraxis. This characteristic is shared with 5-HT neurones which lie in the raphé nuclei of medulla, pons and midbrain. Only cells in the latter (dorsal and median raphé) contribute substantially to ascending systems which provide the hypothalamus (particularly suprachiasmatic nuclei), thalamus (particularly lateral geniculate nuclei), striatum, septum, hippocampus and neocortex with a 5-HT innervation. The question to be answered here, then, is how such widespread ascending reticular formation-like projections are involved with the expression of sexual behaviour. It seems unlikely at present that sub-divisions of these systems are specifically involved with sexual behaviour *per se*. They are more likely to subserve much more general or fundamental functions since this would explain why single monoaminergic manipulations affect the expression of so many forms of behaviour, as well as endocrine and physiological processes. The real challenge, then, is to define the nature of these amine-dependent processes and how they interface, if they do, with the hormone-dependent events which are specifically related to the expression of sexual behaviour.

Ungerstedt's demonstration that many features of the lateral hypothalamic syndrome of adipsia, aphagia and akinesia could be produced by 6-OHDA lesions of the nigrostriatal DA pathway has been of seminal importance in revealing the behavioural functions of DA (Ungerstedt, 1971). Both types of lesion also impair, not surprisingly in retrospect, sexual behaviour – particularly in the male. Here we see then, quite clearly, what was often not taken into account in psychopharmacological experiments: the depression of central DA levels/transmission, especially in the striatum, markedly impairs the expression of virtually all forms of goal-directed behaviour and not just sexual behaviour (see Robbins & Everitt, 1982). With respect to the latter, it is important to note that the striatum is not a hormone-sensitive structure and, thus, we must come to terms with the fact that dopaminergic manipulations can affect the expression of sexual behaviour without *directly* affecting its hormonal determinants. Much has been written about the nature of DA-dependent functions of the striatum and these have been variously described as such fundamental processes as 'sensory–motor integration' and 'activation'. Space precludes a detailed discussion of these views (but see Robbins & Everitt, 1982), but if we accept, as it is reasonable to do, that DA-depleted animals cannot respond to environmental cues (whether due to sensory, motor or activational impairments) then the problem of DA function in the control of sexual behaviour is easier to define. Thus, the expression of sexual behaviour depends critically on exposure of the hypothalamus to sex steroids. It also depends, as do all other forms of motivated behaviour, on the integrity of the DA system and, hereby, upon the integrity of striatal processes. Is there a relationship between the two? For example, are the sensory–motor functions of the striatum biased towards sexual patterns when the hypothalamus is exposed optimally to sex hormones and the animal is in the presence of appropriate environmental cues (e.g. an individual of the opposite sex)? Little is known about where such interactions between these two systems might occur, although the abundant preoptic and hypothalamic projections to the limbic midbrain area, where many DA neurones lie, would appear to be a natural focus. Some data do suggest that hypothalamic and DA mechanisms interact: thus, the marked decline in sexual performance following preoptic area lesions in male rats can be reversed by systemic treatment with the DA agonist lisuride (Hansen *et al.* 1982). Exact interpretation of this result requires more experimentation, but it is consistent with the possibility that recruitment of the DA system might be impaired after hypothalamic lesion, so preventing the sex hormone-related bias in response priorities, and that this was essentially circumvented by direct activation of the DA system by the DA agonist. The possibility of interactions between hypothalamic and striatal DA-dependent mechanisms should undoubtedly be explored experimentally. However, it should not detract from the possibility of more direct DA-steroid hormone interactions occurring intrahypothalamically. Changes in DA receptor sensitivity attendant upon oestradiol or testosterone treatment in both steroid and non-steroid target areas of the brain emphasize that both interactions might occur and that the story is not a simple one.

Noradrenergic neurones in the brainstem appear from electrophysiological studies to be concerned with sensory events. Those within the dorsal vagal (solitary) complex seem especially to receive visceral afferent inputs and those in the ventro-lateral medulla may receive somatosensory information from fibres running in the anterolateral columns. These groups, rather than locus coeruleus neurones, are mentioned here because of their dominant projections to the hypothalamus and limbic forebrain. Furthermore, a number of these NA neurones appear to be targets for sex steroids, notably oestradiol (Heritage *et al.* 1977). Selective lesions of the lateral tegmental NA neurones by 6-OHDA in female rats results in a dissociation of proceptivity and receptivity which reveals their possible importance in sensory processing (Hansen *et al.* 1981). Thus, proceptive responses (which probably reflect the female's sexual 'motivation') are unimpaired by the lesion. By contrast, receptive responses (lordosis) which depend exclusively on tactile stimulation of the perineum and vagina by the male during a mount are much reduced. Hence, it would appear that these NA neurones are important in enabling behavioural responses to tactile cues associated with coitus. Indeed, the same lesions disrupt the induction of pseudopregnancy following cervical stimulation in this species, so emphasizing how different types of response, though both dependent on the same types of sensory information, are equally impaired by damage to a single system (Hansen *et al.* 1981). This principle is an extremely important one since it helps to explain how a diffusely projecting system of neurones can affect different behavioural and other processes rather selectively, provided that they have in common dependence, for example, on a particular category of sensory stimulus. Thus, 6-OHDA lesions to NA terminals in the main and accessory olfactory bulbs profoundly affect the selective processing of olfactory cues following coitus in the mouse (which determines the olfactory block to pregnancy – the 'Bruce effect') and following parturition/cervical stimulation in the sheep (which determines subsequent mother–infant bonding) (Keverne & de la Riva, 1982; Keverne *et al.* 1982). The brainstem noradrenergic systems, then, can modify the expression of at least sexual and maternal behaviour as well as endocrine responses to coital events by mediating, in some way yet to be defined, the consequences of somatic and/or visceral sensory stimulation. It will be intriguing to discern whether noradrenergic influences on feeding, aggression and other forms of behaviour can also be viewed in a similar context.

If we come full circle to discuss, finally, 5-HT mechanisms in the control of sexual behaviour we see that this system of neurones remains an enigma. The advent of 5-HT neurotoxins has not, to any great extent, revealed more clearly the functions of 5-HT-containing neural systems. There is no doubt, however, that animals bearing 5-HT denervations of the hypothalamus and limbic forebrain generally display increased levels of sexual behaviour (and also aggressive and ingestive behaviour) (Everitt, 1978). Much interest has focused on the dense 5-HT innervation of the suprachiasmatic nuclei since they are very much involved in the genesis of circadian rhythms. Recently, a circadian rhythm in oestradiol sensitivity and hence sexual activity has been demonstrated in the female rat, with peak levels occurring at night (Hansen *et al.* 1978). Lesions of the suprachiasmatic nuclei abolish this rhythm and result in high levels of sexual receptivity both during the day and night – a situation also seen after systemic 5-HT-depleting treatments (e.g. with PCPA) (Hansen *et al.* 1978). It may be, then, that one way in which 5-HT neurones may affect the display of sexual behaviour is by contributing to the regulation of circadian rhythms in steroid sensitivity. However, this has not been demonstrated directly, and it is entirely possible that these neurones are more involved with regulating the responsiveness of several areas of the brain to sensory inputs arriving through more direct channels – as has been suggested, for example, for the responsiveness of lateral geniculate neurones to visual inputs.

To summarize a field of research where so little is definite is impossible. It is probably more pertinent to re-emphasize that the widespread systems of monoamine neurones are of fundamental importance in regulating the selection (NA and perhaps 5-HT) and expression (DA) of goal-directed behaviour. Defining the neural processes they subserve is a task that has only just begun, although real advances have been made with respect to the functions of dopaminergic and noradrenergic neurones. When considering sexual behaviour itself, it is clear that the dominant question to be answered is how the unique, hormone-dependent mechanisms are related to the processes subserved by the monoamine systems and here, indeed, is a fertile area of research. It has recently been suggested that hypothalamic gonadotrophin releasing hormone (GnRH) containing neurones may represent a steroid hormone-sensitive link between the two, since their cell bodies lie in a region (the preoptic area) highly responsive to sex steroids and their axons project to the midbrain, where aminergic and/or descending neural systems may be influenced (Kawano & Daikoku, 1981). Certainly, intracerebral infusion of GnRH seems quite specifically to activate sexual behaviour, at least in female rats (Sakuma & Pfaff, 1983). This trilogy of amine, peptide and steroid has long been the focus of functional studies of the control of anterior pituitary function and may, it seems, have its counterparts in the brain (see Everitt *et al.* 1983).

BARRY J. EVERITT

The research reviewed here was supported by a Medical Research Council Programme Grant (PG733722). I thank Elisabet Björklund for her help in preparing the manuscript.

REFERENCES

Baum, M. J. & Starr, M. S. (1980). Inhibition of sexual behaviour by dopamine antagonists or serotonin agonist drugs in castrated male rats given estradiol of dihydrotestosterone. *Pharmacology, Biochemistry and Behaviour* 13, 57–67.

Caggiula, A. R., Antelman, S. R., Chiodo, L. A. & Lineberry, C. G. (1979). Brain dopamine and sexual behaviour. Psychopharmacological and electrophysiological evidence for an antagonism between active and passive components. In *Catecholoamines: Basic and Clinical Frontiers*, Vol. 2 (ed. E. Usdin, I. Kopin, and J. Barchas), pp. 1766–1767. Plenum Press: New York.

Everitt, B. J. (1976). Cerebral monoamines and sexual behaviour. In *Textbook of Sexology* (ed. H. Musaph and J. Morey), pp. 429–448. Elsevier North-Holland: Amsterdam.

Everitt, B. J. (1978). A neuroanatomical approach to the study of monoamines and sexual behaviour. In *Biological Determinants of*

Sexual Behaviour (ed. J. B. Hutchison), pp. 555–574. Wiley: Chichester.

Everitt, B. J., Fuxe, K. & Hökfelt, T. (1974). Inhibitory role of dopamine and 5-hydroxytryptamine in the sexual behaviour of female rats. *European Journal of Pharmacology* **29**, 187–191.

Everitt, B. J., Fuxe, K., Hökfelt, T. & Jonsson, G. (1975). Role of monoamines in the control by hormones of sexual receptivity in the female rat. *Journal of Comparative and Physiological Psychology* **89**, 556–572.

Everitt, B. J., Herbert, J. & Keverne, E. B. (1983). Neuroendocrine anatomy of the limbic system. In *Progress in Anatomy* (ed. V. Navaratnam). Cambridge University Press: Cambridge (in the press).

Gradwell, P. B., Everitt, B. J. & Herbert, J. (1975). 5-hydroxytryptamine in the central nervous system and sexual receptivity of female rhesus monkeys. *Brain Research* **88**, 281–293.

Hansen, S., Södersten, P., Eneroth, P., Srebro, B. & Hole, K. (1978). A sexually dimorphic rhythm in oestradiol-activated lordosis behaviour in the rat. *Journal of Endocrinology* **83**, 267–274.

Hansen, S., Stanfield, E. J. & Everitt, B. J. (1981). The effects of lateral tegmental noradrenergic neurons on components of sexual behaviour and pseudopregnancy in female rats. *Neuroscience* **6**, 1105–1117.

Hansen, S., Köhler, C., Goldstein, M. & Steinbusch, H. V. M. (1982). Effects of ibotenic acid-induced neuronal degeneration in the medial preoptic area and the lateral hypothalamic area on sexual behaviour in the male rat. *Brain Research* **239**, 213–232.

Heritage, A. S., Grant, L. D. & Stumpf, W. D. (1977). ^{3}H-estradiol in catecholamine neurons of the rat brain stem; combined localisation by autoradiography and formaldehyde-induced fluorescence. *Journal of Comparative Neurology* **176**, 607–630.

Hökfelt, T., Johansson, O., Fuxe, K. & Goldstein, M. (1983). Catecholamine neurons-distribution and cellular localization as revealed by immunohistochemistry. In *Catecholamines*, Vol. 2 (ed. V. Trendelenburg and N. Weiner). Springer-Verlag: Berlin (in the press).

Kawano, H. & Daikoku, S. (1981). Immunohistochemical demonstration of LHRH neurons and their pathways in the rat hypothalamus. *Neuroscience* **32**, 179–186.

Keverne, E. B. & de la Riva, C. (1982). Pheromones in mice: reciprocal interaction between the nose and brain. *Nature* (*London*) **296**, 142–150.

Keverne, E. B., Poindron, P., Levy, F. & Lindsay, D. R. (1983). Vaginal stimulation: an important determination of maternal bonding in sheep. *Science* (*New York*) **219**, 81–83.

Lindvall, O. & Björklund, A. (1978). Organization of catecholamine neurons in the rat central nervous system. In *Handbook of Psychopharmacology*, Vol. 9 (ed. L. L. Iversen, S. D. Iversen and S. H. Snyder), pp. 139–231. Plenum Press: New York.

Malmnäs, C. O. (1973). Monoaminergic influence on testosterone-activated copulatory behaviour in the castrated male rat. *Acta Physiologica Scandinavica* **395**, Suppl., 1–128.

Meyerson, B. J. (1964). Central nervous monoamines and hormone-induced estrous behaviour in the spayed rat. *Acta Physiologica Scandinavica* **241**, Suppl., 1–32.

Paglietti, E., Pellegrini-Quarantotti, B., Merev, G. & Gessa, G. L. (1978). Apomorphine and *l*-dopa lower ejaculation threshold in the male rat. *Physiology and Behaviour* **20**, 559–562.

Robbins, T. W. & Everitt, B. J. (1982). Functional studies of central catecholamines. *International Review of Neurobiology* **23**, 303–365.

Sakuma, Y. & Pfaff, D. W. (1983). Modulation of the lordosis reflex of female rats by LHRH, its antiserum and analogs in the mesencephalic central gray. *Neuroendocrinology* **36**, 218–224.

Steinbusch, H. (1981). Distribution of serotonin immunoreactivity in the central nervous system of the rat: cell bodies and terminals. *Neuroscience* **4**, 557–618.

Ungerstedt, U. (1971). Adipsia and aphagia after 6-hydroxydopamine induced degeneration of the nigro-striatal dopamine system in the rat brain. *Acta Physiologica Scandinavica* **367**, Suppl., 95–122.

Psychological Medicine, 1976, **6**, 343–345

Kuru

In 1957 Gajdusek & Zigas described the clinical features of a disease, kuru, hitherto unknown to Western medicine. Kuru was seen exclusively amongst the inhabitants of the Eastern Highlands of New Guinea. This neurological disease, with marked psychiatric features, was confined to members of the Fore people and their nearest neighbours, with whom they intermarry, and had at that time reached epidemic proportions, causing more than half of all recorded deaths in the region. It is believed that the first case appeared around the turn of the century.

'Kuru' is the Fore word for shivering or trembling as with cold or fear and a fine tremor is one of the diagnostic signs of the disease. Clinically kuru has an insidious onset, with ataxia and disturbance of balance. These disturbances are often first noted by a relative before the patient becomes aware of them. Many patients recall having headaches before the first signs of the disease appear. Ataxia becomes progressively more severe and is soon accompanied by a fine tremor involving the trunk, head and extremities. Within a few months the patient is no longer able to walk or stand without support. Speech slowly becomes unintelligible and in the later stages of the disease patients are quite unable to talk. There is a tendency to jerky eye movements but no true nystagmus. The patients show a blunting of their personality and an emotional lability. Gajdusek does not regard dementia as a prominent feature of kuru, though Hornabrook (1968) considers that it develops in the later stages of the disease. Dysphagia develops after a time and this contributes to the severe wasting seen in the last stages of the disease. The course taken by the illness is stereotyped, with little variation between different patients and there is no response to any form of treatment. Death usually occurs partly from starvation, partly from decubitus ulceration within 9–24 months after the onset of clinical signs, but cases of only 3–6 months duration have been recorded. Convulsions, paralysis and sensory impairment do not occur, although pyramidal signs may sometimes be present during the terminal stage. When the disease was first described, the majority of cases occurred amongst young women and children of both sexes, but in the course of the last 15 years the incidence in children has become lower, more cases are observed in adults and the number of cases seen is decreasing rapidly.

Abnormalities in the urine, blood and CSF have not been found, nor have antibodies to any of the known encephalitides been demonstrated. Histopathological studies by, amongst others, Klatzo *et al.* (1959), Fowler & Robertson (1959), Beck & Daniel (1965), Beck *et al.* (1969) showed that the condition was a subacute degeneration of the central nervous system. In the cerebral cortex many nerve cells are lost and others show degeneration, the grey matter is spongy and there is proliferation and hypertrophy of fibrous astrocytes and some microglial reaction. The limbic cortex, i.e. cingular, insular and parahippocampal cortex, is particularly severely affected while elsewhere areas of the cortex may appear essentially normal and show a well-preserved cytoarchitecture. Alzheimer's neurofibrillary tangles and senile plaques have not been observed. Large vacuoles are seen in many of the big neurons in the striatum and an increased amount of neurosecretory material is found in the tuber cinereum; the latter pointing to some nerve fibre degeneration in the hypothalamo-neurohypophysial tract. There is no inflammatory reaction and the cerebral white matter is not demyelinated. Sharply demyelinated plaques, such as are seen in disseminated sclerosis, have never been observed.

The severest changes, by far, are found in the cerebellum, which shows atrophy of its foliae, particularly noticeable in the phylogenetically old vermis and flocculo-nodular lobe. Microscopically there is a severe loss of granule cells, degeneration of Purkinje cells and a dense fibrillary gliosis; the molecular layer contains numbers of microglial cells in all stages of phagocytic activity. Another feature in most cases is the presence of amyloid plaques throughout the cerebellar cortex and the subcortical white matter. These plaques resemble the so-called 'burned-out' stage of the senile plaque (Terry & Wiśniewski, 1970; Wiśniewski & Terry, 1973) but lack the contingent of degenerating neurites which are typical of the 'classical or mature' senile plaque (Krücke *et al.*, 1973). The brainstem nuclei which have afferent cerebellar connexions such as the pontine nuclei, inferior olives and medial vestibular nuclei, show degenerative changes. The cortico-spinal tracts are degenerated in about half the cases. Like the clinical signs, the histopathological changes are stereotyped and the distribution of the lesions within the limbic cortex, striatum and hypothalamus as well as those within the cerebellum and its connexions is essentially the same in all cases.

The pathological changes that are found in the nervous system explain most of the signs seen in the disease and some of the symptoms. The severe degeneration of the cerebellum accounts for the ataxia and tremor, the degenerated vestibular nucleus for the disturbance of balance, while the degeneration of the cerebral cortex accounts for the speech defects, the emotional and personality changes and for the dementia, when this is present.

The pathogenesis of kuru remained an enigma until Hadlow in 1959 made a suggestion that was to have important results. He was impressed by the similarities in the histological changes in the brains of sheep with natural scrapie and those in the brains of patients with kuru. Since it had been found to be possible to transmit scrapie from affected sheep to normal sheep and to goats by inoculation Hadlow suggested that it might be worth while to attempt to transmit kuru to primates. In 1963, Gajdusek took up Hadlow's suggestion and inoculated chimpanzees with brain material from cases of kuru. After a prolonged incubation period the inoculated animals developed a kuru-like syndrome (Gajdusek *et al.*, 1966). Clinically the animal becomes withdrawn and lethargic and develops increasing signs of ataxia which lead to frequent falls and stumbles. Occasionally shivering-like tremors are seen. Terminally the animal is no longer able to sit up without support and has to be hand-fed; its facial expression becomes vacant and there is usually some visual impairment. To date the duration of the disease from the appearance of the first clinical signs to a moribund stage ranges between 1 and 15 months, the incubation time between 10 and 39 months. Since these early experiments kuru has been transmitted to chimpanzees from 11 different patients; it has also been transmitted serially through chimpanzees up to the fifth passage, with incubation times decreasing to an average of 12 months. Later, transmission to New World and rhesus monkeys was achieved.

The inoculum has been prepared from brain, from kidney, spleen or liver, it has been given intracerebrally or by a peripheral route, stored at -70 °C for 2 years, diluted as high as 10^{-7}, filtered through a 220 nm gradocol membrane and heated to 85 °C for 30 min; finally it has been prepared from long-maintained explant cultures of kuru brain tissue. All these varieties of inoculum have induced the experimental disease, which throughout has remained clinically and pathologically remarkably constant (Lampert *et al.*, 1972). Although much work has been done in trying to discover the nature of the transmissible agent no virus or virus-like structure has been identified with the electron microscope.

It seems possible that the disease was originally spread by inoculation, for at the time of its highest incidence there were ceremonies in which ritual cannibalism played a part and the tissues of those dead of kuru were handled by the living. Thus the opportunity of 'self-inoculation' through cuts and abrasions was great.

Attempts have been made to find out whether other degenerative diseases of the brain associated with mental abnormalities can be transmitted to animals by inoculation and material from cases of Alzheimer's and Pick's disease and from Creutzfeldt-Jakob disease have been used by Dr Gajdusek. So far, only Creutzfeldt-Jakob disease has been shown to be transmissible (Gibbs *et al.*, 1968), and it is interesting that the histopathology of this condition closely resembles that of experimental kuru (Beck *et al.*, 1969). It may be noticed that Klatzo *et al.* (1959) originally likened the histopathology of kuru to that of Creutzfeldt-Jakob disease.

Recent experiments suggest that Creutzfeldt-Jakob disease may be transmissible to mice and it is hoped that progress in elucidating the basic causes of these degenerative diseases of the brain, which are associated with such distressing mental changes, will advance more rapidly than it has done in the past, when the only animal available for experimental work was the rare and expensive primate.

ELISABETH BECK
PETER DANIEL

REFERENCES

Beck, E. & Daniel, P. M. (1965). Kuru and scrapie compared: are they examples of system degeneration? In *Slow, Latent and Temperate Virus Infections*, pp. 85–93. National Institute of Neurological Diseases and Blindness Monograph, no. 2 (U.S. Department of Health, Education and Welfare).

Beck, E., Daniel, P. M., Alpers, M., Gajdusek, D. C. & Gibbs, C. J. Jr. (1969). Neuropathological comparisons of experimental kuru in chimpanzees with human kuru. In *Pathogenesis and Etiology of Demyelinating Diseases*. Add. ad *International Archives of Allergy, and Applied Immunology* (*Basel*) **36**, 553–562.

Fowler, M. & Robertson, E. G. (1959). Observations on kuru: pathological features in five cases. *Australian Annals of Medicine* **8**, 16–26.

Gajdusek, D. C., Gibbs, C. J. Jr. & Alpers, M. (1966). Experimental transmission of a kuru-like syndrome to chimpanzees. *Nature, London* **209**, 794–796.

Gajdusek, D. C. & Zigas, V. (1957). Degenerative disease of the central nervous system in New Guinea: the endemic appearance of kuru in the native population. *New England Journal of Medicine* **257**, 974–978.

Gibbs, C. J. Jr., Gajdusek, D. C., Asher, D. M., Alpers, M. P., Beck, E., Daniel, P. M. & Matthews, W. B. (1968). Creutzfeldt-Jakob disease (spongiform encephalopathy): transmission to the chimpanzee. *Science* **161**, 388–389.

Hadlow, W. J. (1959). Scrapie and kuru. *Lancet* ii, 289.

Hornabrook, R. W. (1968). Kuru: a subacute cerebellar degeneration. The natural history and clinical features. *Brain* **91**, 53–74.

Klatzo, I., Gajdusek, D. C. & Zigas, V. (1959). Pathology of kuru. *Laboratory Investigation* (*New York*) **8**, 799–847.

Krucke, W., Beck, E. & Vitzthum, H. G. (1973). Creutzfeldt-Jakob disease: some unusual morphological features reminiscent of kuru. *Zeitschrift für Neurologie* **206**, 1–24.

Lampert, P. W., Gajdusek, D. C. & Gibbs, C. J. Jr. (1972). Subacute spongiform virus encephalopathies. Scrapie, kuru and Creutzfeldt-Jakob disease: a review. *American Journal of Pathology* **68**, 626–646.

Terry, R. D. & Wiśniewski, H. (1970). The ultrastructure of the neurofibrillary tangle and the senile plaque. In G. E. W. Wolstenholme & M. O'Connor (eds.), *Alzheimer's Disease and Related Conditions*, pp. 145–165. Churchill: London

Wiśniewski, H. M. & Terry, R. D. (1973). Re-examination of the pathogenesis of the senile plaque. In H. M. Zimmerman (ed.), *Progress in Neuropathology*, vol. II, pp. 1–26. New York and London: Grune & Stratton.

Psychological Medicine, 1978, **8**, 357–360

The brain in Huntington's chorea[1]

The primary genetic defect in Huntington's chorea has not yet been identified, but some new insight into the brain abnormalities that exist in this tragic disorder has come from recent findings of histopathological and neurochemical changes in post-mortem brain.

Although atrophy occurs throughout the whole brain in chorea, the greatest loss of cells occurs in the basal ganglia (Corsellis, 1976). The increased number of glial cells seen particularly in the caudate nucleus and putamen have been counted by Lange *et al.* (1976), who found the total glial cell number in each nucleus to be the same as in normal brain; however, the concentration of glial cells is increased due to the loss of neuronal cells. The basal ganglia at death weigh approximately 50% of normal, whereas the whole brain weight is usually reduced by about 20%. Loss of cortical cells occurs in layers 3, 5 and 6, and although the atrophy is not as marked as in the basal ganglia, this accounts for most of the whole brain weight loss.

Since an increased number of post-mortems have been carried out on patients dying with Huntington's chorea during the last few years, Professor Corsellis and his colleagues have found that about 7% of the cases diagnosed as having Huntington's chorea have some other neurological condition. The condition most often mis-diagnosed as Huntington's chorea is Alzheimer's disease. The confusion may occur because this disorder can also be dominantly inherited and may sometimes present with abnormal movements. However, the rapid progression of the dementia that dominates the clinical presentation in Alzheimer's disease ought to distinguish these 2 disorders. Three cases in the series diagnosed as Huntington's chorea had cerebellar changes consistent with the autosomal dominant form of cerebellar ataxia. It is important that every patient diagnosed as having Huntington's chorea have this confirmed eventually by autopsy, and the neuropathological report subsequently filed in the clinical notes, since these records will continually be examined by future physicians caring for the offspring.

Although the disorder is most frequently first diagnosed when choreiform movements begin between the ages of 37 and 47 years, an examination of the atypical clinical features and the brain when the disorder presents at the 2 age extremes may provide some insight into the biochemical genetics of this disorder.

The juvenile form of this disease is thought to reflect a genetic variant, since rigidity rather than chorea is usually present. Epileptic convulsions may also occur in children, and these manifestations may occur before either parent is suspected of having Huntington's chorea. The progression of the disease in children is rapid, with death usually occurring within 10 years from the onset of symptoms. Juvenile chorea tends to occur sporadically among families; however, it is clear that the juvenile cases will most often have inherited the disorder from their father (Merritt *et al.* 1969). It has been noted that the offspring of affected males have the onset of their disease and die almost a decade earlier than their father, whereas the offspring of affected females have their onset and death at the same age as their mother (Bird *et al.* 1974). It seems very likely that there must be an inherited sex-related factor modifying the disorder. The biochemical defect which is inherited as an autosomal dominant may have the same penetrance in all cases regardless of age but the amount of inherited modifying factor may vary and determine the rate of cell death in the brain. In children the onset is often 2 decades earlier than their affected parent and the cell death is obviously very rapid. Histopathological examination reveals extreme atrophy of the basal ganglia, with the caudate nucleus often reduced to a thin ribbon (Byers *et al.* 1973).

With the onset of choreiform movements in the sixth or seventh decade there is a very slow

[1] Address for correspondence: Dr Edward D. Bird, Addenbrookes Hospital, Department of Neurological Surgery and Neurology, Hills Road, Cambridge CB2 2QQ.

progression of the disease without the development of dementia that is associated with chorea under the age of 50 years. Elderly choreic patients often live for more than 20 years with their chorea and usually die from natural causes. The basal ganglia will not appear as atrophic as in the younger, more typical, cases. Cell death must be progressing at a very slow rate. The late onset of this mild form of Huntington's chorea without mental deterioration tends to maintain this pattern through several family generations, a useful and encouraging point to remember when counselling the offspring.

Psychotic features may precede the onset of choreiform movements by as much as a decade. These behaviour abnormalities are more common in families in which the onset of chorea is earlier than usual, with psychotic features often occurring in the late teens or early twenties. Patients may be admitted to a psychiatric hospital with the diagnosis of schizophrenia and 10 years later, when the choreiform movements appear or when another member of the family develops chorea, the diagnosis becomes clear.

Several chemical transmitters and related enzymes are fairly stable in post-mortem brain and a number of these have been measured in human brain. Brain cooling has been shown to start immediately after death and, provided the cadaver has been placed in a refrigerator, this rate of cooling progresses until the centre of the brain reaches 4 °C, usually about 24 hours after death (Spokes & Koch, 1978). Enzyme activities usually decline to some stable level during this first 24 hours. Control tissues are handled similarly and since it usually takes 24 hours to complete the administrative post-mortem details, cases will usually be autopsied after stability has been attained. The pre-mortem conditions of the patient are more difficult to control. Choreic patients are usually in a psychiatric hospital receiving neuroleptic drugs for some months or years before death. They often develop bronchopneumonia prior to death. Although most of the control brain tissues used for comparison in the past have been from non-neurological cases dying from natural causes, a recent large collection of brain tissues from patients dying in mental hospitals with the diagnosis of schizophrenia can serve as another group for comparison.

Perry *et al.* (1973) were the first to report that the concentration of gamma-aminobutyric acid (GABA), a neuroinhibitory transmitter, was decreased in the caudate nucleus and putamen of post-mortem brain from patients dying with chorea. Bird & Iversen (1974, 1976) found that the biosynthetic enzyme for GABA, glutamic acid decarboxylase (GAD), was decreased in the striatum and substantia nigra but not in the frontal cortex of the brain from choreics. The activity of tyrosine hydroxylase (T-OH), the biosynthetic enzyme for dopamine (DA), however, was normal in the striatum or even increased, particularly in the substantia nigra (Bird & Iversen, 1976).

We have focused considerable attention on the substantia nigra, an area which has had little histopathological examination in the past, since it is always normally pigmented. The substantia nigra is divided into 2 regions, the more dorsal region being the zona compacta which is normally darkly pigmented and contains the cell bodies of the dopamine neurones whose axons form a pathway to the striatum. Dendrites extend from the dopamine cell body throughout both regions of the substantia nigra. The less pigmented ventral region of the substantia nigra, the zona reticulata, receives axons from neuroinhibitory GABA cells in the striatum, and the terminals of these axons are in contact with the dendrites from the dopamine cells. The dopamine concentration in the zona compacta is normally twice that of the zona reticulata (Hornykiewicz, 1963) and concentration of GABA is two-fold higher in the reticulata zone than the compacta zone (Kanazawa & Toyokura, 1975). The substantia nigra in the brain from a patient with chorea is often more darkly pigmented than normal and the zona reticulata is much more atrophic than the zona compacta because of the loss of striatal afferents.

These pathological and neurochemical findings in Huntington's chorea correlate well with the clinical features in this disorder, since loss of neuroinhibition in the substantia nigra could result in excessive dopaminergic activity that is known to be associated with the abnormal movements. Pharmacologic agents used to reduce these movements are usually those which interfere with the post-synaptic receptor for dopamine, e.g. phenothiazines and butyrophenones, or agents which interfere with the storage of dopamine in dopaminergic terminals, e.g. tetrabenazine (Nitoman).

Whether the administration of GABA-like drugs would be therapeutic in chorea would depend on the integrity of the natural receptors for GABA. Enna *et al.* (1976), using radio-active labelled GABA as a ligand, have shown that the density of GABA receptors in the substantia nigra is increased two-fold. Other evidence suggests that the receptors for GABA are located on the dendrites of the dopamine cells, so Enna's study does correlate with the increased concentration of dopamine neurones in the substantia nigra in the brain from choreics.

The activity of choline acetyltransferase (ChAc), the biosynthetic enzyme for acetylcholine, is also decreased in the basal ganglia from some cases who die with chorea (Bird & Iversen, 1974). This decrease is related to the degree of basal ganglia atrophy and is especially marked in the juvenile cases. The cholinergic neurone probably serves as one of the sites for post-synaptic receptors for dopamine and, therefore, the loss of this cell type may explain why the juvenile cases, and indeed many of the adult cases, develop rigidity as the terminal event in their disease. This may also explain why L-DOPA administration to rigid choreics is not effective.

Other clinical indications of the imbalance between GABA and dopamine concentrations may be reflected through the hypothalamus where dopamine acts as a transmitter for cells that produce a number of releasing factors. Gonadotropic releasing factor (GnRF) is under catecholamine control and has been used clinically to treat infertility. GnRF is significantly increased in the hypothalamus of the post-mortem brains from female choreics (Bird *et al.* 1976), and this may explain the increased fertility of the choreic female when compared to her non-affected sibling (Reed & Palm, 1951). The increased libido that many choreic women have may also be due to an increased production of GnRF. Increased serum growth hormone concentration (Phillipson & Bird, 1976) and decreased serum prolactin (Hayden *et al.* 1977) have been reported in patients with chorea, findings consistent with excess dopaminergic activity. There will no doubt be other neuroendocrine alterations discovered in the future that will be secondary to the altered GABA/dopamine ratio in the brain.

Many of the various clinical manifestations of Huntington's chorea have been shown to be associated with specific histological and neurochemical findings in the brain. These clinical features are common to other neurologic and psychiatric disorders and, therefore, future collaboration between clinicians and basic scientists in the examination of post-mortem brain should help to elucidate the defects in a wide spectrum of diseases.

EDWARD D. BIRD

REFERENCES

Bird, E. D. & Iversen, L. L. (1974). Huntington's chorea: post-mortem measurement of glutamic-acid decarboxylase, choline acetyltransferase and dopamine in basal ganglia. *Brain* **97**, 457–472.

Bird, E. D. & Iversen, L. L. (1976). Neurochemical findings in Huntington's chorea. In *Essays in Neurochemistry and Neuropharmacology* (ed. M. B. H. Youdim, W. Lovenberg, D. F. Sharman and J. R. Lagnado), pp. 177–195. John Wiley & Sons: London.

Bird, E. D., Caro, A. J. & Pilling, J. B. (1974). A sex related factor in the inheritance of Huntington's chorea. *Annals of Human Genetics* (*London*) **37**, 255–260.

Bird, E. D., Chiappa, S. A. & Fink, G. (1976). Brain immuno-reactive gonadotropin-releasing hormone in Huntington's chorea and in non-choreic subjects. *Nature* **260**, 536–538.

Byers, R. K., Gilles, F. H. & Fung, C. (1973). Huntington's disease in children: neuropathologic study of four cases. *Neurology* (*Minneapolis*) **23**, 561–569.

Corsellis, J. A. N. (1976). Ageing and the dementias. In *Greenfield's Neuropathology* (ed.W. Blackwood and J. A. N. Corsellis), p. 822. Edward Arnold: London.

Enna, S. J., Bennett, J. J. Jr, Bylund, D. B., Snyder, S. H., Bird, E. D. & Iversen, L. L. (1976). Alterations of brain neurotransmitter receptor binding in Huntington's chorea. *Brain Research* **116**, 531–537.

Hayden, M. R., Paul, M., Vinik, A. I. & Beighton, P. (1977). Impaired prolactin release in Huntington's chorea: evidence for dopaminergic excess. *Lancet* ii, 423–426.

Hornykiewicz, O. (1963). Die topische Lokalisation und das Verhalten von Noradrenalin und Dopamin (3-Hydroxy-tyramin) in der Substantia nigra des normalen und Parkin-sonkranken Menschen. *Wiener klinischer Wochenschrift* **75**, 309–312.

Kanazawa, I. & Toyokura, Y. (1975). Topographical study of the distribution of gamma-aminobutyric acid (GABA) in the human substantia nigra: a case study. *Brain Research* **100**, 371–381.

Lange, H., Thorner, G., Hopf, A. & Schroder, K. F. (1976). Morphometric studies of the neuropathological changes in choreatic diseases. *Journal of the Neurological Sciences* **28**, 401–425.

Merritt, A. D., Conneally, P. M., Rahman, N. F. & Drew, A. L. (1969). Juvenile Huntington's chorea. In *Progress in Neuro-genetics*. Vol. 1 of the Proceedings of the Second International Congress of Neuro-genetics and Neuro-ophthalmology of the World Federation of Neurology (ed. A. Barbeau and J.-R. Brunette), pp. 645–650. Excerpta Medica: Amsterdam.

Perry, T. L., Hansen, S. & Kloster, M. (1973). Huntington's chorea, deficiency of gamma aminobutyric acid in brain. *New England Journal of Medicine* **288**, 337–342.

Phillipson, O. T. & Bird, E. D. (1976). Plasma growth hormone concentration in Huntington's chorea. *Clinical Science and Molecular Medicine* **50**, 551–554.

Reed, S. C. & Palm, J. D. (1951). Social fitness versus reproductive fitness. *Science* **113**, 294–296.

Spokes, E. G. & Koch, D. J. (1978). Post-mortem stability of dopamine, choline acetyltransferase and glutamic acid decarboxylase in the mouse brain under conditions simulating handling of human autopsy material. *Journal of Neurochemistry* (in the press).

Psychological Medicine, 1982, **12**, 449–459

Plaques, tangles and Alzheimer's disease[1]

For the purpose of this review, Alzheimer's disease and senile dementia of Alzheimer type will be considered as the same disease process, a view broadly accepted at this time.

For total satisfaction in morphological diagnosis, both plaques and tangles need to be present in large or considerable numbers in the neocortex. In most pre-senile cases both are present in vast numbers: in many cases below the age of 80 years a similar picture exists but, in extreme old age, demented subjects may have many plaques but a few or no demonstrable tangles occur (Tomlinson *et al.* 1970; Terry, personal communication) and, occasionally, in the pre-senium or senium relatively few or no plaques may be found in the presence of large numbers of tangles (Corsellis, 1976*a*). Both these appearances have been accepted as variants of Alzheimer's disease, but perhaps some reservations about such a decision are necessary.

Since the original reports of Kidd (1963, 1964), Terry (1963), Terry *et al.* (1964) and Krigman *et al.* (1965), the ultrastructure of plaques and tangles has been largely agreed. Plaques which are visible on light microscopy, and vary from 15 to 200 μm in diameter, are clusters of abnormal, enlarged nerve processes and terminals surrounding a central mass of amyloid fibrils, and associated with some astrocytic processes and microglia. The enlarged terminals (often termed neurites) are ballooned by lamellar lysosomes, abnormal mitochrondria and paired helical filaments (PHF) identical with those which form the neurofibrillary tangle. The smallest (earliest) plaque not visible on light microscopy is said to consist of three or four distended neurites with no evidence of amyloid fibrils, and the oldest is a mass of amyloid with few surrounding neurites remaining (Terry & Wisniewski, 1970).

Gonatas *et al.* (1967) and Gonatas & Gambetti (1970) considered the majority of neurites as pre-synaptic (or axonal) and emphasized the presence of changes which suggest regenerative activity. Terry & Wisniewski (1970) identified apparently normal synapses on the neurites and regarded the post-synaptic element as largely normal; Ishii (1976), however, identified both abnormal pre- and post-synaptic terminals as well as abnormal synapses.

Tangles consist of large clusters (Kidd, 1963; Wisniewski *et al.* 1976*a*) of PHF each 10–13 nm wide, which measure around 22 nm at their widest and are reduced to approximately 10 nm at intervals of 80 nm. In affected neurons bundles of PHF fill much of the cell soma, displacing and intermingling with otherwise apparently normal cytoplasmic elements. Although total agreement was reached on the interpretation of the fibrils as PHF rather than twisted tubules only after a number of years (Wisniewski *et al.* 1976*a*), reports were largely consistent that tangles were made up of such structures. Gibson *et al.* (1976), however, illustrated abnormally large numbers of straight tubules as well as the twisted variety. Mixtures of both straight and twisted filaments as well as tangles of both varieties have been reported by Yagashita *et al.* (1981); and Oyanagi (1979) also observed 15 nm straight filaments in some dendrites. Shibayama & Kitoh (1978) have also observed both straight and paired helical filaments in a case of atypical senile dementia. The mixture of straight and helically wound filaments clearly needs bearing in mind in chemical and immunological studies of these structures. Perhaps the only other well established abnormality in the neuron affected by tangle formation is a diminution in the size of the nucleolus (Dayan & Ball, 1973), though additionally, in the hippocampus only, tangles frequently occur along with granulovacuoles in the same cell, the latter being an additional neuronal alteration which occurs in higher concentration in Alzheimer's disease than in normal old subjects (Woodard, 1962, 1966; Tomlinson & Kitchener, 1972).

[1] Address for correspondence: Professor B. E. Tomlinson, Department of Pathology, Newcastle General Hospital, Newcastle upon Tyne NE4 6BE.

The ultrastructure of the tangles in Alzheimer's disease is not unique to that condition and normal old age. Identical tangles are found in large numbers in the cortex and deep grey matter in the Parkinsonism dementia complex of Guam (Malamud *et al.* 1961; Hirano *et al.* 1961; Hirano, 1974), in the anterior temporal cortex and substantia nigra in dementia pugilistica (Corsellis *et al.* 1973; Wisniewski *et al.* 1976*b*), in the substantia nigra and locus coeruleus of post-encephalitic Parkinsonism (Wisniewski *et al.* 1970*a*), in the cortex of occasional cases of subacute sclerosing pan-encephalitis (Manydbur *et al.* 1977; Paula-Barbosa *et al.* 1979), and extensively in the majority of cases of Down's syndrome surviving to middle life (Olson & Shaw, 1969; Burger & Vogel, 1973; Solitare & Lamarche, 1966; Jervis, 1948). In the latter subjects, senile plaques are also present in large numbers and the appearances are indistinguishable histologically from Alzheimer's disease. Clearly, therefore, PHF develop in a variety of unrelated conditions as divergent as repeated cerebral trauma and virus infection; it need hardly be emphasized that three of the disorders mentioned above are of proven or suspected viral origin, and that a genetic factor is suggested by their occurrence in Down's syndrome. In sporadic motor neuron disease and progressive supranuclear palsy, the tangles differ from the above conditions in consisting predominantly of bundles of straight fibres and not PHF.

Tangles and plaques, though far more frequent in the cortex than elsewhere, occur in the deeper brain structures. Plaques outside the cortex are probably most numerous in the mamillary bodies, but do occur in the basal ganglia, hypothalamus, upper brain stem and cerebellum, the latter rarely. Tangles may be seen in small numbers in any deep nuclear mass, in the substantia nigra and locus coeruleus, but rarely in Alzheimer's disease or normal old age in the lower stem, cerebellum or spinal cord.

The variations in findings in demented old subjects, plus the the well-known occurrence of neocortical plaques and hippocampal tangles in the majority of old people who are not demented, raise many questions about the relationship of plaques and tangles with each other, their formation and relationship with the dementing process and old age, and the relationship of old age and Alzheimer's disease.

Plaques and tangles are common in old age in intellectually well-preserved old subjects, but with major differences in the numbers of plaques and the numbers and distribution of tangles, compared with demented subjects (Tomlinson, 1972, 1977; Tomlinson *et al.* 1968, 1970; Matsuyama & Nakamura, 1978). A few plaques are found in the cortex in a small number of subjects from the fourth decade on; a steep rise in incidence occurs in the seventh and eighth decade, and by the ninth decade, 75–80% of normal subjects have some plaques (Tomlinson, 1972), though in most subjects they are small in number, and often concentrated in the deep cortical layers. Usually the greatest number are found in the amygdaloid complex and hippocampal gyrus, and a much smaller number in the deep nuclear masses and hypothalamus. Occasionally, in a non-demented old person, plaque numbers reach similar proportions and overlap the levels of plaques found in the demented group (Tomlinson & Henderson, 1976).

The situation concerning tangles is different. A few affected cells can be found in the hippocampal pyramidal layer in all patients above 50 years (Ball, 1976), the other most involved areas being the uncal cortex and the subiculum and, occasionally, the hippocampal gyrus. The number of cells affected in the hippocampus increases with age but does not reach the massive numbers found in Alzheimer's disease (Ball, 1976). Tangles in normal subjects are, however, absent or scarce in the neocortex (Tomlinson *et al.* 1968; Tomlinson, 1979; Matsuyama & Nakamura, 1978), being found in this situation in large numbers only in demented cases.

The relationship between plaques and tangles is unknown. In normal old age there can be no direct anatomical connection between the localized tangles in the hippocampus and the widely scattered plaques which are commonly found in the neocortex. In Alzheimer's disease, when tangles and plaques are intermingled in great numbers in the neocortex together, it is tempting to postulate that the axons of tangle-bearing neurons terminate in the abnormal bulbous sproutings which constitute the bulk of the plaque, but there is no direct evidence for this and it is even possible that the nerve terminals forming the plaque only arise in neurons unaffected by tangle formation. Furthermore, the occurrence of some older demented subjects with numerous neocortical plaques and very few neocortical tangles and, more rarely, with numerous tangles and few plaques suggests that these two phenomena, though frequently occurring together in Alzheimer's disease, are not closely related structurally and may arise independently. The occurrence of tangles in the absence of plaques in post-traumatic dementia, in the Parkinsonism–dementia syndrome, and in post-encephalitic Parkinsonism illustrates their independent occurrence in other conditions.

Though forming the chief morphological markers of Alzheimer's disease, the role played by plaques and tangles in the symptomatology of Alzheimer's disease is also unknown. The grossly abnormal neurites of plaques, intermingled or clustered around a mass of amyloid, would seem most unlikely to perform a normal function so far as conduction and transmission of nervous impulses are concerned, despite possessing apparently normal synapses. The presence of the latter sustains the hope that the synapses of the plaque might be susceptible to pharmacological influence and that, if the process of plaque formation can be reversed (and the amyloid reabsorbed), something approaching normal structure might result. Neurofibrillary tangles constitute abnormal fibrillary proteins, but whether they have an abnormal function in themselves, are physiologically inactive, or reduce function by interfering with the flow of material from cell soma to axons, dendrites and terminals, is not known. Nevertheless, several studies, starting with that of Corsellis (1962), have shown the association of dementia with the presence of large numbers of neocortical plaques and tangles by comparison with non-demented subjects, the conclusion being drawn (Roth *et al.* 1966; Blessed *et al.* 1968; Tomlinson *et al.* 1970; Constantinidis, 1978; Constantinidis *et al.* 1978) that it is the quantity and distribution of these structures, not their mere presence, which distinguishes Alzheimer's disease from non-demented patients. Blessed *et al.* (1968) showed a tendency for plaque formation to be greater in the more severely demented subjects and found (Tomlinson *et al.* 1970) that all patients with many neocortical tangles were demented. Tomlinson *et al.* (1970) also found greater quantities of tangles in the anterior temporal lobes in the majority of cases of Alzheimer's disease; Ball (1976) quantified the greater numbers of tangles by detailed, serial section analysis. Constantinidis (1978) found that numerous neocortical tangles were associated with aphasia, apraxia and agnosia in 91% of cases, whereas these instrumental disorders only occur in 32% of cases when neurofibrillary tangles are limited to the hippocampus and neighbouring temporal cortex, and in only 16% of cases if tangles are present only in small numbers in the hippocampus. When senile plaques are present alone only 12% of demented cases show instrumental signs. Blessed (personal communication), in a recent study of pathological and clinical data from the Newcastle study, found that parietal lobe symptomatology (aphasia–apraxia–agnosia) is closely related to the presence of numerous neocortical tangles in old demented subjects, but that demented old subjects with only large numbers of senile plaques were largely free of such symptomatology. In pre-senile Alzheimer's disease numerous neocortical tangles are invariable, and marked parietal lobe signs are usually a prominent feature of the disease. In the senile group with parietal lobe signs many neocortical plaques and tangles are usually present; with parietal lobe signs absent, neocortical tangles are usually few or absent. If these findings (and those of Constantinidis, 1978) are confirmed, there may be considerable merit in agreeing on a clinical and pathological nomenclature to distinguish these two sub-varieties of dementing syndromes in old age.

The growing evidence of abnormalities in various components of the cholinergic transmitter system in Alzheimer's disease (Davis & Maloney, 1976; Perry *et al.* 1977; Spillane *et al.* 1977; White *et al.* 1977) may also be partly related to or reflected by plaque formation. Thus a significant decline in cholineacetyl-transferase occurs with increasing plaque numbers in the neocortex of non-demented and demented old people (Perry *et al.* 1978); Perry & Perry (1980) also showed significant correlations between plaque numbers and decreasing acetylcholinesterase. The diminution of these enzymes is in contrast to the normal levels of the muscarinic acetylcholine receptor (Perry *et al.* 1977; Davies & Verth, 1978), the latter finding again fitting with the apparent ultrastructural integrity of the synapse, despite the presence of grossly abnormal pre-synaptic terminals.

Thus considerable indirect evidence exists that plaques and tangles of Alzheimer's disease may have relevance to some features of the actual dementing process. A considerable body of evidence (De Fendis, 1974; Karczmar, 1975) links the cerebral cholinergic system with many behavioural patterns (sleep, arousal, sensory, emotion and learning activities) which are frequently severely disturbed in Alzheimer's disease. So far, however, the evidence is no more than indirect, and therapeutic attempts to correct the cholinergic defect have been without significant or lasting benefit (Loew, 1980), though slight improvement has been claimed in some mild and moderate cases of presumed Alzheimer's disease treated with choline and lecithin (Christie *et al.* 1979; Etienne *et al.* 1979); it is clearly essential to explore all reasonable avenues of rectifying the levels of the proven decreased components of the cholinergic system by the use of rigorously controlled trials.

Whereas no evidence on the functional effects of plaques in experimental animals exists, evidence relating to disturbed behaviour and neuronal function in animals with neurofibrillary degeneration induced by the intracranial application of aluminium salts has accumulated (Crapper, 1976). The tangles so produced are not helically twisted paired filaments, but 10 nm straight filaments (Terry & Pena, 1965). Animals so treated have a 7–10 day asymptomatic period, although neurofibrillary degeneration is present by the fourth day and is extensive by the ninth (Crapper & Dalton, 1973*a*, *b*). Previously normal cats, however, showed some motor incoordination, impairment of short-term memory and deterioration of an acquired avoidance response within 7–10 days of the aluminium injection; motivational mechanisms, EEG and visual evoked potentials were not affected until a late stage of the neurological illness. Even in the late stages of the encephalopathy, when neurofibrillary tangles were present in almost all spinal cord motor neurons, axon conduction velocity is unaffected in the sciatic nerve, as is the electromyogram and muscle and peripheral nerve histology (Crapper, 1973). Motor neuron resting potential and antidromic spikes recorded on individual neurons showing neurofibrillary tangles did not differ from normal (Crapper, 1973). Furthermore, axonal transport in similarly affected rabbits is normal (Liwnicz *et al.* 1974). Single neuron sampling (Crapper & Tomko, 1975; Tomko & Crapper, 1974) within the visual cortex of aluminium treated animals showed a reduction in spontaneous discharge rate probably related to a failure of post-synaptic potentials, this failure probably being restricted to cells with neurofibrillary degeneration.

Is plaque or tangle formation related to the cortical neuron loss thought by many to be severe in Alzheimer's disease, and how good is the evidence for such neuron loss? In the pre-senile form, the brain is almost invariably severely atrophied, and its weight is often around or below 1000 g. Total cortical and white matter volume is also reduced (Corsellis, 1976*b*; Hubbard & Anderson, 1981), so that the absolute volume of neuron-bearing cortex is diminished. Since plaques in many instances occupy a considerable volume of the cortex, cortical atrophy would be more severe without them and the volume of neuron-bearing cortex still further reduced. Counts of neurons per unit area or volume of cortex from histological preparations have been few and have yielded varying results, though the majority of reports have favoured some degree of neuron loss (Colon, 1972; Shefer, 1973; Terry *et al.* 1980; Brun & Gustafson, 1976) with some areas slightly, but others heavily, affected. Neuron loss is undoubtedly severe in the anterior temporal lobes of many subjects but cell loss in many cortical areas, particularly in the senile cases (Tomlinson & Henderson, 1976; Terry *et al.* 1980), may have been over-estimated in the past. However, taking cortical volume loss into account and the neuron loss per unit volume found by most observers using quantitative sampling techniques, the average case of pre-senile Alzheimer's disease seems likely to have lost some 30–40% more neurons than has the normal subject by that age. Considering the almost uniform agreement from quantitative studies, that cortical neurons are lost throughout life in normal subjects (Brody, 1955, 1970; Tomlinson & Henderson, 1976; Colon, 1972; Shefer, 1973), the additional loss sustained in pre-senile Alzheimer's disease is likely to result in a brain which has lost in excess of 60% of its original cortical nerve cells. Cortical neuron loss in young and middle-aged adults cannot, however, be due to plaque and tangle formation, since both occur rarely during that period. Further, plaque formation cannot, initially at least, produce cell loss, since the abnormal neurites of the plaques clearly need functioning neurons to support them. Indeed, since the terminals are grossly enlarged (hypertrophied rather than atrophied), the parent neurons may be sustaining a higher metabolic demand than normal. Also, Terry *et al.* (1980) failed to find any correlation between plaque counts and neuron numbers in the cortex in SDAT. No good evidence therefore exists to associate plaque formation directly with neuron loss, unless the neurites of a plaque represent attempted regeneration or sprouting of axons as a response to diminishing numbers of nerve processes resulting from neuron and dendritic loss initiated by some other means. Such a hypothesis ignores the presence of amyloid within plaques, something which appears fundamental to our understanding of plaque genesis.

Unfortunately, we do not know the cells of origin of the neurites within a plaque or whether the clusters of neurites forming a plaque arise from many, few, or even a single neuron, though the latter seems unlikely. In the absence of such knowledge, there is no way in which the neurons whose terminals end in plaques can be studied, and we remain ignorant of the morphology, neurochemistry and physiological behaviour of the neurons involved in plaque formation.

There is, equally, no certain relationship between tangle formation and neuron loss or tangle formation and the dendritic abnormalities demonstrated in normal ageing and demented subjects (Scheibel *et al.* 1975; Scheibel, 1978). Dendritic and bouton loss in some cortical pyramidal cells is quantitatively greater in Alzheimer's disease than in age-matched controls (Mehraein *et al.* 1975), but it is not established that the neurons with tangles are also those with grossly abnormal dendritic trees. It is highly unlikely that the cells with grossly abnormal dendritic processes demonstrated in normal old age are the site of tangle formation, since within the neocortex in normal old age neurofibrillary tangles are scarce and often not demonstrable at all. Similarly, it is not known whether tangle formation contributes to neuronal death and loss, though it is certain that it has nothing to do with neuron loss in normal subjects in the cortex and a number of other sites (Brody, 1955, 1976; Colon, 1972; Tomlinson & Henderson, 1976; Corsellis, 1976*b*; Tomlinson & Irving, 1977; Henderson *et al.* 1980), including the locus coeruleus (Brody, 1976; Tomlinson *et al.* 1981).

The pathogenesis and life history of human plaques and tangles are also unknown. Electron microscopic evidence suggests that the earliest evidence of plaque formation is a small cluster of abnormal terminals which, as they continue to grow in number, become associated with increasing amounts of amyloid to form what has been described as the mature plaque (Terry & Wisniewski, 1970). Acceptance of this view has implications for the role of amyloid in plaque formation, since some observers in the past have seen amyloid deposition as the primary lesion which stimulates plaque formation (Schwartz, 1970). If the amyloid of plaques results from an antigen–antibody response in the cerebral tissues with subsequent damage to neighbouring axons, then we have a logical beginning from which the development of plaques can be studied (Terry & Wisniewski, 1970). The nature of the amyloid of plaques is not yet established. Ishii & Haga (1976) obtained positive reactions to immunoglobulins in amyloid fibrils in plaques. However, evidence that different mechanisms may be involved in the deposition of amyloid in cerebral vessels and plaques in demented subjects has been presented by Torack & Lynch (1981), who demonstrated immunoglobulins in the amyloid of three cases of congophilic angiopathy but considered an endogenous substrate more likely in the amyloid of plaques. Powers & Spicer (1977) and Powers & Skeen (1980) have indeed demonstrated similarities between plaque and apud amyloid. Johnson *et al.* (1981) have produced evidence that plaque and vessel amyloid may share a common antigen with neurofibrillary tangles. It cannot be assumed at this time that the amyloid content of plaques in normal and demented old subjects have the same chemical constituents or origins, or that all the plaque amyloid occurring in different cases in Alzheimer's disease is identical. It is not certain that plaque amyloid has the same origins or chemical constitution as vascular amyloid (Torack & Lynch, 1981) and the latter is common, though not constant, in Alzheimer's disease and normal old age (Wright *et al.* 1969; Morimatsu *et al.* 1975). Vascular amyloid is present in many subjects with Alzheimer's disease, but may be absent even when plaques are extremely numerous (Mandybur, 1975; Mountjoy *et al.* 1982), and there is certainly no constant relationship between the two. Thus plaque amyloid may be heterogeneous in origin and chemical constitution, as seems likely with the two types of amyloid already identified in the senile heart (Cornwell & Westermark, 1980). To establish whether or not this is so is of fundamental importance since, whatever the connection between plaque amyloid and the surrounding neurites, the close association cannot be coincidental. The possibly heterogeneous nature of amyloid in plaques and vessels has to be considered in any investigation into cerebral amyloid, as does the difficulty in extraction procedures, of establishing what proportion comes from vessel walls or from plaques. Certain forms of amyloid are known to be secreted with tumours, such as the medullary thyroid carcinoma (Glenner *et al.* 1973). The possibility therefore arises that plaque amyloid may result from neurosecretion or from the modification of neuropeptides. Our lack of knowledge of the morphological characteristics of neuropeptides means that we cannot exclude them as precursors of plaque amyloid or even as constituents of neurofibrillary tangles. Indeed, the neuropeptide, substance *P*, has been shown to form polyuric fibrillary aggregates with ultrastructural dimensions in the same range as has been reported for amyloid fibrils (Perry *et al.* 1981). The origin of the paired helical filaments of the human tangle is also uncertain, with evidence supporting a possible derivation from human neurotubules (Iqbal *et al.* 1974, 1975, 1978; Schlaepfer, 1978; Grundke-Iqbal *et al.* 1979) and neurofilaments (Gambetti *et al.* 1980, 1981) being reported. Perhaps through different mechanisms or under different circumstances, PHF may derive from either or both of these components of the normal neuron.

Once the plaque and the tangle have formed within the human brain, do they ever disappear? Here, again, we have no certain knowledge. An increase in the incidence of plaques within normal subjects throughout life and the involvement of increasing numbers of tangles in the anterior temporal lobes do not demonstrate their indestructability. The vast numbers of plaques and tangles in Alzheimer's disease establish that the majority of such people die without reabsorption or disintegration of many plaques and tangles. However, in the anterior temporal lobes and some other areas of the brain (Brun & Gustafson, 1976) there is suggestive evidence that the end result of massive tangle and plaque formation, and whatever other destructive processes occur in Alzheimer's disease, may lead to the final disintegration of cortical tissue. This occurs in only restricted cerebral sites and is not a striking feature in the majority of cases. One would have to conclude therefore that plaques and tangles probably have an extremely long life-cycle and that, once formed, they are probably present for many years, but they are not necessarily permanent or irremovable.

The view has frequently been advanced that Alzheimer's disease represents an exaggeration or acceleration of the normal ageing process. A threshold limit of plaque formation has been conceived below which the majority of old subjects are well-preserved intellectually and above which the majority show evidence of dementia. This might be true without supporting the view that Alzheimer's disease represents an acceleration of normal ageing. Such a proposition is not supported by some of the other morphological features of the disease and is far too restrictive of thought about the origin of Alzheimer's disease to be allowed as a dominant hypothesis. The study of neocortical tangle formation lends no support to the proposition since there is no continuum in appearances within the cortex of non-demented subjects and cases of Alzheimer's disease. In non-demented old subjects tangles are rare in the neocortex, whereas in Alzheimer's disease they are often present in vast numbers and are an inevitable marker of dementia. Some factor which is absent in normal old age therefore stimulates neocortical tangle formation. It is very unlikely that with increasing longevity we are all destined to develop Alzheimer's disease. In extreme old age sufficient neurons may be lost and dendritic abnormalities occur for dementia to develop on that basis alone, but present evidence is against the possibility that Alzheimer's disease would acount for an ever increasing proportion of cases. Erlich & Davis (1980) found a diminution in the incidence of dementia above the age of 90 years; they found no evidence for an inevitable accumulation of plaques and tangles with increasing age. Unfortunately, their histological observations were made on hippocampal sections only, an inadequate procedure in research and morphological diagnosis in Alzheimer's disease. Indeed, in the ninth and tenth decades dementia, although usually of the Alzheimer type morphologically, presents an increasing number of cases with plaque formation only (Terry, personal communication), and a small, but increasing, number which have no obvious morphological basis. Beyond the tenth decade dementia may result from other factors of which we have no knowledge. Some subjects may be genetically resistant to tangle and plaque formation and therefore to Alzheimer's disease, and it is possible that the susceptible population to this disorder is largely wiped out by the tenth decade.

So far no animal has been found which naturally, or under experimental conditions, develops both tangles and plaques. A few plaques, similar on light microscopy to the human variety, have been found in ageing dogs (Brunmuhl, 1956; Pauli & Luginbühl, 1971) and Wisniewski *et al.* (1970*b*) confirmed their ultrastructural similarity to the human (primitive) plaque, though they failed to find abnormal fibrils in the neurites. Wisniewski *et al.* (1973) found similar plaques in ageing rhesus monkeys, including PHF, though neurons showing tangles were not identified. Indeed, tangles consisting of PHF do not appear to have been identified in any animal as a spontaneously occurring phenomenon.

Experimentally induced tangles, mostly by methods unlikely to have direct relevance to the tangles of Alzheimer's disease, are only similar to the human variety on light microscopy, consisting of straight filaments. This applies to tangles induced by the intracerebral inoculation of aluminium phosphate (Klatzo *et al.* 1965; Terry & Pena, 1965), by cochicine (Wisniewski & Terry, 1967) and mitotic spindle inhibitors (Schochet *et al.* 1968; Wisniewski *et al.* 1968), the latter substances being tubulin binding agents, as are a number of other substances capable of producing tangles experimentally (Ghetti, 1980). Interest in aluminium as a possible aetiological agent was heightened by the report of raised brain aluminium levels in patients with Alzheimer's disease (Crapper *et al.* 1976) and by the experimental production of tangles by systemic aluminium (De Boni *et al.* 1976). McDermott *et al.* (1977), however, failed to confirm increased aluminium concentrations in Alzheimer brains; furthermore, patients with dialysis encephalopathy associated with much higher levels of brain aluminium (McDermott *et al.* 1978) show neither tangles nor plaques (Burkes *et al.* 1976), a fact confirmed in our laboratory. Contradictory evidence has also arisen from studies of tangle-bearing neurons in Alzheimer's disease. Using X-ray spectrometry, Peri & Brody (1980) found foci of aluminium within the nuclei of tangle-bearing neurons, whereas Duckett & Galle (1980) were unable to provide an indication of aluminium in the pathogenesis of tangles by electron-microprobe studies. Unlikely as any aetiological role would appear, the aluminium concentration in normal and Alzheimer brains needs further investigation.

Tangles in post-encephalitic Parkinsonism and in subacute sclerosing pan-encephalitis demonstrate their formation following virus infections in humans. One animal model in which neuritic plaques can be predictably produced is now available since Bruce & Fraser (1975) and Bruce *et al.* (1976) showed plaque formation in certain strains of mice infected with particular strains of scrapie agent. Some of these plaques are ultrastructurally similar to the human variety (Wisniewski *et al.* 1975), though lacking PHFs. The effects of the genetic constitution of mice on the inoculation period of scrapie (Dickinson *et al.* 1968, 1969) have been elucidated to the extent of the identification of two alleles responsible for the shortening or prolongation of the incubation period after injection with a particular scrapie agent, and identification of scrapie agent properties responsible for plaque formation now appears likely. The relevance of these observations to any disease of man is purely speculative, but the presence of transmissible agents with prolonged incubation period in man (Kuru and Creutzfeldt–Jakob disease) and with other similarities to scrapie (with abundant plaques in two-thirds of the cases of Kuru and 10% of cases of Creutzfeldt–Jakob disease) must stimulate investigation of the possibility that Alzheimer's disease, with its late onset (and therefore perhaps after long incubation), might be similarly determined by genetic and 'infective' agent factors. Major variations exist in the incubation period, clinical manifestations and pathological changes in different animals infected with material from Creutzfeldt–Jakob disease and Kuru (Gibbs *et al.* 1979), and many strains of agent responsible for these diseases apparently exist. Traub *et al.* (1977) report a number of cases of transmissible virus dementia or non-transmissible Creutzfeldt–Jakob disease in which plaques and tangles occurred at an age when their presence was not likely to be due to ageing. Their separation of the spongiform encephalopathies of man into transmissible spongiform encephalopathies and non-transmissible Creutzfeldt–Jakob disease may prove to be unnecessary if the disorders are due to different strains of an agent producing different results in inoculated animals (including extremely long incubation periods), as occurs in scrapie infected mice. Attempts to transmit Alzheimer's disease to experimental animals have failed, except from two cases of familial Alzheimer's disease (Gibbs *et al.* 1979), and there is no direct evidence for infectivity of slow agent type in Alzheimer's disease and no firm evidence of transmission of Creutzfeldt–Jakob disease from one human to another except by direct inoculation. Nevertheless, the possibility from the variations in histology in Creutzfeldt–Jakob disease, with neuritic plaques produced in a small number of cases, clearly tempts the speculation that transmissible agents, producing a wide spectrum of human disorder, may exist.

Recently, De Boni & Crapper (1978) and Crapper-McLachlan & De Boni (1980) have reported the successful stimulation of paired helical filaments, not absolutely identical to the human variety, in the processes of a small proportion of human foetal neurons in culture exposed to high dilutions of a cell-free saline extract of cerebral cortex taken from cases of Alzheimer's disease. The agent has also been detected by a similar technique in the CSF in three cases of clinically diagnosed Alzheimer's disease and in one control (Crapper-McLachlan & De Boni, 1980), the latter raising the possibility that PHF 'agent' may occur in normal brain. Clearly, the continued search for an infective agent and a susceptible host is justified at this time.

Whatever the significance ultimately assigned to plaques and tangles in the symptomatology, pathology, neurochemistry, pathogenesis and aetiology of Alzheimer's disease, continued investigation of these two changes remains a major challenge in all research into dementia and ageing in the human central nervous system. Until their role is precisely defined, knowledge of an important area of neuropathology and human ageing will be incomplete.

B. E. TOMLINSON

REFERENCES

Ball, M. J. (1976). Neurofibrillary tangles and the pathogenesis of dementia; a quantitative study. *Neuropathology and Applied Neurobiology* **2**, 395–410.

Blessed, G., Tomlinson, B. E. & Roth, M. (1968). The association between quantitative measures of dementia and of senile change in the cerebral grey matter of elderly subjects. *British Journal of Psychiatry* **114**, 797–811.

Brody, H. (1955). Organisation of the cerebral cortex. III: A study of ageing in the human cerebral cortex. *Journal of Comparative Neurology* **102**, 511–556.

Brody, H. (1970). Structural changes in ageing nervous system. *Interdisciplinary Topics in Gerontology* **7**, 9–21.

Brody, H. (1976). An examination of cerebral cortex and brain stem ageing. In *Neurobiology of Ageing*, vol. 3. (ed. R. D. Terry and S. Gershon), pp. 177–181. Raven Press: New York.

Bruce, M. E. & Fraser, A. H. (1975). Amyloid plaques in the brains of mice infected with scrapie: morphological variations and staining properties. *Neuropathology and Applied Neurobiology* **1**, 189–202.

Bruce, M. E., Dickinson, A. G. & Fraser, H. (1976). Cerebral amyloidosis in scrapie in the mouse: effect of agent strain and mouse genotype. *Neuropathology and Applied Neurobiology* **2**, 471–478.

Brun, A. & Gustafson, L. (1976). Distribution of cerebral degeneration in Alzheimer's disease. A clinico-pathological study. *Archiv für Psyhiatrie und Nervenkrankheiten* **223**, 15–133.

Brunmuhl, A. (1956). Kongophile Angiopathie und senile Plaques bei greisen Hunden. *Archiv für Psychiatrie und Nervenkrankhieten* **194**, 396–414.

Burger, P. C. & Vogel, F. S. (1973). The development of the pathological changes of Alzheimer's disease and senile dementia in patients with Down's syndrome. *American Journal of Pathology* **73**, 457–476.

Burkes, J. S., Huddlestone, J., Alfrey, A. C., Norenberg, M. D. S. & Lewin, E. (1976). A fatal encephalopathy in chronic haemodialysis patients. *Lancet* i, 764–768.

Christie, J. E., Glen, A. I. M., Yates, C. M., Blackburn, I. M., Shering, A., Jellinek, E. H. & Zeisel, S. (1969). Choline and lecithin effects on CSF choline levels and on cognitive function in Alzheimer pre-senile dementia. In *Alzheimer's Disease. Early Recognition of Potentially Reversible Deficits* (ed. A. I. M. Glen and L. J. Whalley), pp. 163–168. Churchill Livingstone: Edinburgh.

Colon, E. J. (1972). The elderly brain. A quantitative analysis of the cerebral cortex in two cases. *Psychiatrie, Neurologie Neurochirurgie* (*Amsterdam*) **75**, 261–270.

Constantinidis, J. (1978). Is Alzheimer's disease a major form of senile dementia? Clinical, anatomical and genetic data. In *Alzheimer's Disease, Senile Dementia and Related Disorder* (*Ageing*, vol. 7) (ed. R. Katzman, R. D. Terry and K. L. Bick), pp. 15–25. Raven Press: New York.

Constatinidis, J., Richard, J. & de Ajuriaguerra, J. (1978) Dementia with senile plaques and neurofibrillary tangles. In *Studies in Geriatric Psychiatry* (ed. A. D. Isaacs and F. Post), pp. 119–152. Wiley: New York.

Cornwell, G. G. & Westermark, P. (1980). Senile amyloidosis: a protean manifestation of the ageing process. *Journal of Clinical Pathology* **33**, 1146–1152.

Corsellis, J. A. N. (1962). *Mental Illness and the Ageing Brain.* Oxford University Press: London.

Corsellis, J. A. N. (1976*a*) Ageing and the dementias. In *Greenfield's Neuropathology* (3rd edn) (ed. W. Blackwood and J. A. N. Corsellis), pp. 796–848. Edward Arnold: London.

Corsellis, J. A. N. (1976*b*). Some observations on the Purkinje cell population and on brain volume in human ageing. In *Neurobiology of Ageing*, vol. 3. (ed. R. D. Terry and S. Gershon), pp. 205–209. Raven Press: New York.

Corsellis, J. A. N., Bruton, C. J. & Freeman-Browne, D. (1973). The aftermath of boxing. *Psychological Medicine* **3**, 270–303.

Crapper, D. R. (1973). Experimental neurofibrillary degeneration and altered electrical activity. *Electroencephalography and Clinical Neurophysiology* **35**, 575–588.

Crapper, D. R. (1976). Functional consequences of neurofibrillary degeneration. In *Neurobiology of Ageing*, vol. 3. (ed. R. D. Terry and S. Gershon), pp. 405–432. Raven Press: New York.

Crapper, D. R. & Dalton, A. J. (1973*a*). Aluminium induced neurofibrillary degeneration, brain electrical activity and alterations in acquisition and retention. *Physiology and Behaviour* **10**, 935–945.

Crapper, D. R. & Dalton, A. J. (1973*b*). Alterations in short term retention, conditioned avoidance response acquisition and motivation following aluminium induced neurofibrillary degeneration. *Physiology and Behaviour* **10**, 925–933.

Crapper, D. R. & Tomko, G. J. (1975). Neuronal correlates of an encephalopathy induced by aluminium neurofibrillary degeneration. *Brain Research* **97**, 253–264.

Crapper, D. R., Krishnan, S. S. & Quittkat, S. (1976). Aluminium, neurofibrillary degeneration and Alzheimer's disease. *Brain* **99**, 67–80.

Crapper-McLachlan, D. R. & De Boni, U. (1980). Aetiologic factors in senile dementia of Alzheimer type. In *Ageing of the Brain and*

Dementia (*Aging*, vol. 13) (ed. L. Amaducci, A. N. Davison and P. Antuono), pp. 173–181. Raven Press: New York.

Davies, P. & Maloney, A. F. (1976). Selective loss of cholinergic neurons in Alzheimer's disease. *Lancet* ii, 1403.

Davies, P. & Verth, A. H. (1978). Regional distribution of muscarinic acetylcholine receptor in normal and Alzheimer-type dementia brains. *Brain Research* **138**, 385–392.

Dayan, A. D. & Ball, M. J. (1973). Histometric observations on the metabolism of tangle-bearing neurons. *Journal of Neurological Science* **19**, 422–426.

De Boni, U. & Crapper, R. D. (1978). Paired helical filaments of the Alzheimer type in cultured neurons. *Nature* **271**, 566–568.

De Boni, U., Otoos, S., Scott, J. W. & Crapper, D. R. (1976). Neurofibrillary degeneration induced by systemic aluminium. *Acta Neuropathologica* (*Berlin*) **35**, 285–294.

De Fendis, F. V. (1974). *Central Cholinergic Systems and Behaviour*. Academic Press: New York.

Dickinson, A. G., Meikel, V. M. & Fraser, H. (1968). Identification of a gene which controls the incubation period of some strains of scrapie in mice. *Journal of Comparative Pathology* **78**, 293–299.

Dickinson, A. G., Meikel, V. M. & Fraser, H. (1969). Genetic control of the concentration of ME7 scrapie agent in the brain of mice. *Journal of Comparative Pathology* **79**, 15–22.

Duckett, S. & Galle, P. (1980). Electron–microprobe studies of aluminium in the brains of cases of Alzheimer's disease and ageing patients. *Journal of Neuropathology and Experimental Neurology* **39**, 350.

Erlich, S. S. & Davis, R. L. (1980). Alzheimer's disease in the very aged. *Journal of Neuropathology and Experimental Neurology* **39**, 352.

Etienne, P., Gauthier, S., Dastoor, D., Collier, B. & Ratner, J. (1979). Alzheimer's disease: clinical effect of lecithin treatment. In *Alzheimer's Disease. Early Recognition of Potentially Reversible Deficits* (ed. A. I. M. Glen and L. J. Whalley), pp. 173–178. Churchill Livingstone: Edinburgh.

Gambetti, P., Velasco, M. E., Dahl, D., Bignami, A., Roessmann, U. & Sindely, S. D. (1980). Alzheimer's neurofibrillary tangles: an immunohistochemical study. In *Aging of the Brain and Dementia* (*Aging*, vol. 13) (ed. L. Amaducci, A. N. Davison and P. Antuono), pp. 55–63. Raven Press: New York.

Gambetti, P., Autilio-Gambetti, L. & Shecket, G. (1981). Immunological and silver staining characteristics of neurofibrillary tangles of Alzheimer type (NFT-AT). *Journal of Neuropathology and Experimental Neurology* **30**, 317.

Ghetti, B. (1980). Experimental studies on neurofibrillary degeneration. In *Ageing of the Brain and Dementia* (*Aging*, vol. 13) (ed. L. Amaducci, A. N. Davison and P. Antuono), pp. 183–198. Raven Press: New York.

Gibbs, C. J., Gadjusek, D. C. & Amyer, H. (1979). Strain variations in the viruses of Creutzfeldt–Jakob disease and Kuru. In *Slow Transmissible Diseases of the Nervous System*, vol. 2. (ed. S. B. Prusiner and W. J. Hadlow), pp. 87–110. Academic Press: New York.

Gibson, P. H., Stones, M. & Tomlinson, B. E. (1976). Senile changes in the human neocortex and hippocampus compared by the use of the electron and light microscopes. *Journal of Neurological Science* **27**, 389–405.

Glenner, G. G., Terry, W. & Isersky, C. (1973). Amyloidosis: its nature and pathogenesis. *Seminal Haematology* **10**, 65–86.

Gonatas, N. K. & Gambetti, P. (1970). The pathology of the synapse in Alzheimer's disease. In *Ciba Foundation Synposium on Alzheimer's Disease and Related Conditions* (ed. G. E. W. Wolstenholme and M. O'Connor), pp. 169–183. Churchill Livingstone: London.

Gonatas, N. K., Anderson, W. & Evangelista, I. (1967). The contribution of altered synapses in the senile plaque: an electronmicroscopic study in Alzheimer's dementia. *Journal of Neuropathology and Experimental Neurology* **26**, 25–39.

Grundke-Iqbal, I., Johnson, A. B., Terry, R. D., Wisniewski, H. M. & Iqbal, K. (1979). Alzheimer neurofibrillary tangles: antiserum and immunohistological staining. *Annals of Neurology* **6**, 532–539.

Henderson, G., Tomlinson, B. E. & Gibson, P. H. (1980). Cell counts in human cerebral cortex in normal adults throughout life using an image analysing computer. *Journal of Neurological Science* **46**, 113–136.

Hirano, A. (1974). Parkinsonism-dementia complex on Guam: current status of the problem. In *Proceedings of the 10th International Congress of Neurology, Barcelona 1973* (ed. A. Subirana and J. M. Espadaler), p. 348. Excerpta Medica: Amsterdam.

Hirano, A., Malamud, N. & Kurland, L. T. (1961). Parkinsonism-dementia complex, an endemic disease on the Island of Guam. II: Pathological features. *Brain* **84**, 662–679.

Hubbard, B. M. & Anderson, J. M. (1981). A quantitative study of cerebral atrophy in old age and senile dementia. *Journal of Neurological Science* **50**, 135–145.

Iqbal, K., Wisniewski, H. M., Shelanski, M. L., Brostoff, S., Liwnicz, B. H. & Terry, R. D. (1974). Protein changes in senile dementia. *Brain Research* **77**, 337–343.

Iqbal, K., Wisniewski, H. M., Grundke-Iqbal, I., Koothals, J. K. & Terry, R. D. (1975). Chemical pathology of neurofibrils: neurofibrillary tangles of Alzheimer's pre-senile dementia. *Journal of Histochemistry and Cytochemistry* **23**, 563–569.

Iqbal, K., Grundke-Iqbal, I., Wisniewski, H. M. & Terry, R. D. (1978). Chemical relationship of the paired helical filaments of Alzheimer's dementia to human normal neurofilaments and neurotubules. *Brain Research* **142**, 321–332.

Ishii, T. (1976). On various ultrastructural types of distended processes and degenerated synapses in senile brain, particularly those in senile plaques. *Advances in Neurological Science* **20**, 373–384.

Ishii, T. & Haga, S. (1976). Immunoelectronmicroscopic localisation of immunoglobulins in amyloid fibrils of senile plaques. *Acta Neuropathologica* (*Berlin*) **36**, 243–249.

Jervis, G. A. (1948). Early senile dementia in mongoloid idiocy. *American Journal of Psychiatry* **105**, 102–106.

Johnson, A. B., Cohen, S. A., Said, S. I. & Terry, R. D. (1981). Neuritic plaque amyloid, microangiopathy and Alzheimer neurofibrillary tangles: do they share a common antigen? *Journal of Neuropathology and Experimental Neurology* **40**, 310.

Karczmar, A. G. (1975). Cholinergic influences on behaviour. In *Cholinergic Mechanisms* (ed. P. G. Waser), pp. 501–529. Raven Press: New York.

Kidd, M. (1963). Paired helical filaments in electronmicroscopy in Alzheimer's disease. *Nature* (*London*) **197**, 192–193.

Kidd, M. (1964). Alzheimer's disease – an electron microscopic study. *Brain* **87**, 307–321.

Klatzo, I., Wisniewski, H. & Streicher, E. (1965). Experimental production of neurofibrillary degeneration. I. Light microscopic observations. *Journal of Neuropathology and Experimental Neurology* **24**, 187–199.

Krigman, M. R., Feldman, R. G. & Bensch, K. (1965). Alzheimer's presenile dementia. A histochemical and electronmicroscopic study. *Laboratory Investigation* **14**, 381–396.

Liwnicz, B. H., Kristensson, K., Wisniewski, H. M., Shelanski, M. L. & Terry, R. D. (1974). Observations on axoplasmic transport in rabbits with aluminium induced neurofibrillary tangles. *Brain Research* **80**, 413–420.

Loew, D. M. (1980). Pharmacological approaches to the treatment of senile dementia. In *Aging of the Brain and Dementia* (*Aging*, vol. 13) (ed. L. Amaducci, A. N. Davison and P. Antuono), pp. 287–304. Raven Press: New York.

Malamud, N., Hirano, A. & Kurland, L. T. (1961). Pathoanatomic changes in amyotrophic lateral sclerosis on Guam. *Archives of Neurology* (*Chicago*) **5**, 401–415.

Mandybur, T. I. (1975). The incidence of cerebral amyloid angiopathy in Alzheimer's disease. *Neurology* (*Minneapolis*) **25**, 120–126.

Mandybur, T. I., Nagpaul, A. S., Pappas, Z. & Niklowitz, W. J. (1977). Alzheimer's neurofibrillary change in subacute sclerosing panencephalitis. *Annals of Neurology* **1**, 103–107.

Matsuyama, H. & Nakamura, S. (1978). Senile changes in the brain in the Japanese: incidence of Alzheimer's neurofibrillary change and senile plaques. In *Alzheimer's Disease, Senile Dementia and Related Diseases* (*Aging*, vol. 7) (ed. R. Katzman, R. D. Terry and K. L. Bick), pp. 287–297. Raven Press: New York.

McDermott, J. R., Smith, A. I., Iqbal, K. & Wisniewski, H. M. (1977). Aluminium and Alzheimer's disease. *Lancet* ii, 710–711.

McDermott, J. R., Ward, M. K., Smith, A. I., Parkinson, I. S. & Kerr, D. N. S. (1978). Brain aluminium concentrations in dialysis encephalopathy. *Lancet* i, 901–903.

Mehraein, P., Yamada, M. & Tarnowska-Dzidusko, E. (1975). Quantitation studies on dendrites in Alzheimer's disease and senile dementia. In *Physiology and Pathology of Dendrites* (ed. G. W. Kreutzberg), pp. 453–458. Raven Press: New York.

Morimatsu, M., Hirai, S., Murimatsu, A. & Yoshikawa, M. (1975). Senile degenerative brain lesions and dementia. *Journal of the American Geriatric Society* **23**, 390–406.

Mountjoy, C. Q., Tomlinson, B. E. & Gibson, P. H. (1982). Amyloid and senile plaques and cerebral blood vessels. A semi-quatitative investigation of a possible relationship. (To be published).

Olson, M. I. & Shaw, C. (1969). Pre-senile dementia and Alzheimer's disease in mongolism. *Brain* **92**, 147.

Oyanagi, S. (1979). Aging of the central nervous system and its fine structure. Neurofibrillary change and senile plaques. *Seishin Iqatu* **21**, 834–846. (In Japanese – quoted by Yagashita *et al.* 1981.)

Paula-Barbosa, M. N., Brito, R., Silva, C. A., Farin, R. & Cruz, C. (1979). Neurofibrillary changes in the cerebral cortex of a patient with S.S.P.E. *Acta Neuropathologica* **48**, 157–160.

Pauli, B. & Luginbühl, G. (1971). Fluorescenzmikrokopische Untersuchungen der cerebralen Amyloidose bei alten Hunden und senilen Menschen. *Acta neuropathologica* (*Berlin*) **19**, 121–128.

Peri, D. P. & Brody, A. R. (1980). Alzheimer's disease: X-ray spectrometric evidence of aluminium accumulation in neurofibrillary tangle-bearing neurons. *Science* **208**, 297–298.

Perry, E. K. & Perry, R. H. (1980). The cholinergic system in Alzheimer's disease. In *Biochemistry of Dementia* (ed. P. J. Roberts), pp. 135–183. John Wiley & Sons: Chichester.

Perry, E. K., Perry, R. H., Blessed, G. & Tomlinson, B. E. (1977). Necropsy evidence of central cholinergic deficits in senile dementia. *Lancet* i, 189.

Perry, E. K., Tomlinson, B. E., Blessed, G., Bergmann, K. & Perry, R. H. (1978). Correlation of cholinergic abnormalities with senile plaques and ventral test scores in senile dementia. *British Medical Journal* ii, 1457–1459.

Perry, E. K., Oakley, A. E., Candy, J. M. & Perry, R. H. (1981). Properties and possible significance of substance P and insulin fibrils. *Neuroscience Letters* **25**, 321–325.

Powers, J. M. & Spicer, S. S. (1977). Histochemical similarity of senile plaque amyloid to apudamyloid. *Virchows Archiv für pathologische Anatomie und Physiologie und für klinische Medizin* **376**, 107–115.

Powers, J. M. & Skeen, J. T. (1980). An immunoperoxidase study of senile plaques. *Journal of Neuropathology and Experimental Neurology* **39**, 385.

Roth, M., Tomlinson, B. E. & Blessed, G. (1966). Correlation between scores for dementia and counts of 'senile plaques' in cerebral grey matter of elderly subjects. *Nature* (*London*) **209**, 109.

Scheibel, A. B. (1978). Structural aspects of the ageing brain: spine systems and the dendritic arbor. In *Alzheimer's Disease, Senile Dementia and Related Disorders* (*Aging*, vol. 7) (ed. R. Katzman, R. D. Terry and K. L. Bick), pp. 353–373. Raven Press: New York.

Scheibel, M. E., Lindsay, R. D., Tomiyasu, U. & Scheibel, A. B. (1975). Progessive dendritic changes in the ageing human cortex. *Journal of Neuropathology and Experimental Neurology* **47**, 392–403.

Schlaepfer, W. W. (1978). Deformation of isolated neurofilaments and the pathogenesis of neurofibrillary pathology. *Journal. of Neuropathology and Experimental Neurology* **37**, 244–254.

Schochet, S. S. Jr, Lampert, P. W. & Earle, K. M. (1968). Neuronal changes induced by intrathecal vincristine sulfate. *Journal of Neuropathology and Experimental Neurology* **27**, 645–658.

Schwartz, P. (1970). *Amyloidosis: Cause and Manifestations of Senile Deterioration.* C. C. Thomas: Springfield, Ill.

Shefer, V. G. (1973). Absolute number of neurons and thickness of the cerebral cortex during aging, senile vascular dementia and Pick's and Alzheimer's disease. *Neuroscience and Behavioural Physiology* **6**, 319–324.

Shibayama, H. & Kitoh, J. (1978). Electronmicroscopic structure of the Alzheimer's neruofibrillary changes in a case of atypical senile dementia. *Acta Neuropathologica* (*Berlin*) **41**, 229–234.

Solitare, G. B. & Lamarche, J. B. (1966). Alzheimer's disease and senile dementia as seen in mongoloids. *American Journal of Mental Deficiency* **70**, 840–848.

Spillane, J. A., White, P., Goodhardt, M. J., Flack, R. H. A., Bowen, D. M. & Davison, A. N. (1977). Selective vulnerability of neurons in organic dementia. *Nature* (*London*) **266**, 558–559.

Terry, R. D. (1963). The fine structure of neurofibrillary tangles in Alzheimer's disease. *Journal of Neuropathology and Experimental Neurology* **22**, 269–292.

Terry, R. D. & Pena, C. (1965). Experimental production of neurofibrillary degeneration. 2. Electronmicroscopy, phosphatase histochemistry and electron probe analysis. *Journal of Neuropathology and Experimental Neurology* **24**, 200–210.

Terry, R. D. & Wisniewski, H. (1970). The ultrastructure of the neurofibrillary tangle and the senile plaque. In *Ciba Foundation Symposium on Alzheimer's Disease and Related Conditions* (ed. G. E. Wolstenholme and M. O'Connor), pp. 145–168. Churchill Livingstone: London.

Terry, R. D., Gonatas, N. K. & Weiss, M. (1964). Ultrastructural studies in Alzheimer's presenile dementia. *American Journal of Pathology* **44**, 269–297.

Terry, R. D., Peck, A., Deteresa, R., Schechter, R. & Horoupian, D. S. (1980). Some morphometric aspects of the brain in senile dementia of the Alzheimer type. *Journal of Neuropathology and Experimental Neurology* **39**, 314.

Tomko, G. J. & Crapper, D. R. (1974). Neuronal variability: non-stationary responses to identical visual stimuli. *Brain Research* **79**, 405–418.

Tomlinson, B. E. (1972). Morphological brain changes in non-demented old people. In *Aging of the Central Nervous System* (ed. H. M. Van Praag and A. F. Kalverboer), pp. 38–57. Bohn: Haarlem.

Tomlison, B. E. (1977). The pathology of dementia. In *Dementia* (2nd edn) (ed. C. E. Wells), pp. 113–180. F. A. Davis: Philadelphia.

Tomlinson, B. E. (1979). The ageing brain. In *Recent Advances in Neuropathology* (ed. W. T. Smith and J. B. Cavanagh), pp. 129–159. Churchill Livingstone: Edinburgh.

Tomlinson, B. E. & Henderson, G. (1976). Some quantitative cerebral findings in normal and demented old people. In *Neurobiology of Aging*, vol. 3 (ed. R. D. Terry and S. Gershon), pp. 183–204. Raven Press: New York.

Tomlinson, B. E. & Irving, D. (1977). The numbers of limb motor neurons in the human lumbosacral cord throughout life. *Journal of Neurological Science* **34**, 213–219.

Tomlinson, B. E. & Kitchener, D. (1972). Granulovacuolar degeneration of the hippocampal pyramidal cells. *Journal of Pathology* **106**, 165–185.

Tomlinson, B. E., Blessed, G. & Roth, M. (1968). Observations on the brains of non-demented old people. *Journal of Neurological Science* **7**, 331–356.

Tomlinson, B. E., Blessed, G. & Roth, M. (1970). Observations on the brains of demented old people. *Journal of Neurological Science* **11**, 205–242.

Tomlinson, B. E., Irving, D. & Blessed, G. (1981). Cell loss in the locus coeruleus in senile dementia of Alzheimer type. *Journal of Neurological Science* **49**, 419–428.

Torack, R. M. & Lynch, R. G. (1981). Cytochemistry of brain amyloid in adult dementia. *Acta neuropathologica* **53**, 189–196.

Traub, R., Gajdusek, D. C. & Gibbs, C. J. Jr (1977). Transmissible virus dementia: The relation of transmissible spongiform encephalopathy to Creutzfeldtz–Jakob disease. In *Aging and Dementia* (ed. W. L. Smith and M. Kinsbourne), pp. 91–152. Spectrum Publications: New York.

White, P., Hiley, C. R., Goodhardt, M. J., Carrasco, L. H., Keet,

J. P., Williams, I. E. I. & Bowen, D. M. (1977). Neocortical cholinergic neurons in elderly people. *Lancet* i, 668–670.
Wisniewski, H. M. & Terry, R. D. (1967). Experimental colchicine encephalopathy. 1. Introduction of neurofibrillary degeneration. *Laboratory Investigation* **17**, 577–587.
Wisniewski, H. M., Shelanski, M. L. & Terry, R. D. (1968). Effects of mitotic spindle inhibitors on neurotubules and neurofilaments in anterior horn cells. *Journal of Cell Biology* **38**, 224–229.
Wisniewski, H. M., Terry, R. D. & Hirano, A. (1970*a*). Neurofibrillary pathology. *Journal of Neuropathology and Experimental Neurology* **29**, 163–176.
Wisniewski, H. M., Johnson, A. B., Raine, C. S., Kay, W. J. & Terry, R. D. (1970*b*). Senile plaques and cerebral amyloidosis in aged dogs. A histochemical study. *Laboratory Investigation* **23**, 287–296.
Wisniewski, H. M., Ghetti, B. & Terry, R. D. (1973). Neuritic (senile) plaques and filamentous changes in aged rhesus monkeys. *Journal of Neuropathology and Experimental Neurology* **32**, 566–584.
Wisniewski, H. M., Bruce, M. E. & Fraser, H. (1975). Infectious aetiology of neuritic (senile) plaques in mice. *Science* **190**, 1108–1110.
Wisniewski, H. M., Narang, H. K. & Terry, R. D. (1976*a*). Neurofibrillary tangles of paired helical filaments. *Journal of Neurological Science* **27**, 173–181.
Wisniewski, H. M., Narang, H. K., Corsellis, J. A. N. & Terry, R. D. (1976*b*). Ultrastructural studies of the neuropil and neurofibrillary tangles in Alzheimer's disease and post-traumatic dementia. *Journal of Neuropathology and Experimental Neurology* **35**, 367.
Woodard, J. S. (1962). Clinico-pathological significance of granulovacuolar degeneration in Alzheimer's disease. *Journal of Neuropathology and Experimental Neurology* **21**, 85–91.
Woodard, J. S. (1966). Alzheimer's disease in late adult life. *American Journal of Pathology* **49**, 1157–1169.
Wright, J. R., Calkins, E., Breen, W. T., Stolte, G. & Schultz, R. T. (1969). Relationship of amyloid to aging. Review of the literature and a systematic study of 83 patients derived from a general hospital population. *Medicine* **48**, 39–60.
Yagashita, S., Itah, Y., Wang, N. & Amano, N. (1981). Reappraisal of the fine structure of Alzheimer's neurofibrillary tangles. *Acta Neuropathologica (Berlin)* **54**, 239–246.

Psychological Medicine, 1982, **12**, 695–700

The neuropathology of schizophrenia[1]

The distinguished American neurologist, Plum (1972), once called schizophrenia 'the graveyard of neuropathologists'. Certainly the topic of neuropathological change in schizophrenia has been nearly as silent as a tomb for almost three decades. Interest in the neuropathology of schizophrenia was still high in 1952 when leading neuropathologists of the world, meeting at the First International Congress of Neuropathology in Rome, devoted many hours to formal presentations and discussions of pathological material from schizophrenic patients who died in mental hospitals on both sides of the Atlantic. Although more than 250 published papers had already appeared concerning the pathology of schizophrenia or dementia praecox prior to this Congress, neither the previous work nor the new material presented led to a consensus of opinion as to the neuropathological characteristics of this common disorder. On the contrary, perusal of the Congress Proceedings suggests that a dichotomy of views emerged, with most of the central European investigators, maintaining, as they had in earlier reports, that rather specific changes occurred in basal ganglia (Hopf, 1952; Vanderhorst, 1952; Fungfeld, 1952), basal forebrain (Buttlar-Brentano, 1952), or cerebral cortex (Josephy, 1930; Buscaino, 1924; Fungfeld, 1952; Hyden, 1952). Their colleagues from England and America, on the other hand, generally reported non-specific alterations which they attributed to convulsive treatments, surgical, agonal or post-mortem changes (Meyer, 1952; Rowland & Mettler, 1949).

NEURONE PATHOLOGY IN SCHIZOPHRENIA

An exception was Bruetsch (1952) of Indianapolis, who maintained that a subgroup of approximately 9% of schizophrenics displayed minute acellular areas in the cortex secondary to rheumatic occlusive endarteritis. A similar observation was reported earlier by Winkelman & Book (1949) and was confirmed by the Vogts (1952). Earlier findings included grape-like metachromatic globules in basal ganglia and white matter (Buscaino, 1924) and focal areas of demyelination (Ferraro, 1943). Josephy (1930) described lipoid accumulations in pyramidal neurones of layer II in pre-frontal cortex and hippocampus similar to those described by Spielmeyer (1931), as well as calcifications in globus pallidus and glial nodules in the basal ganglia, thalamus and brain stem.

Cecil and Oscar Vogt (1952), in a monumental series of studies commencing at the turn of the century, were the first to compare serial sections of whole brain specimens from schizophrenic patients and normal control subjects. Together with their collaborators they described numerous alterations in schizophrenic brains, including cell loss in cingulate and inferior temporal cortex, 'dwarf' cells (*Schwarzellen*) in basal ganglia and dorsal medial thalamus, apparently preceded by peculiar vacuolization and lipoid inclusions in clusters of neurones. From the same institute, Hopf (1952) reported 'dwarf cells' in basal ganglia of nine of ten patients with catatonic schizophrenia; Buttlar-Brentano (1952) described similar changes, i.e. progressive vacuolization, balloon cells, shrinkage and disappearance of cytoplasm in neurones in the nucleus basalis of substantia innominata, bed nucleus of stria terminalis, and periventricular, supraoptic, tuber and mammillary nuclei. Similar neuronal alterations and glial proliferation had been previously reported in hypothalamus, especially tuber cinereum by Dide (1934) and Morgan & Gregory (1935).

Most neuropathologists of Great Britain and the United States remained sceptical, however, and in 1957 David, in an extensive review of the reported pathology of schizophrenia, dismissed

[1] Address for correspondence: Dr Janice R. Stevens, Intramural Research Program, National Institute of Mental Health, Saint Elizabeths Hospital, Washington, D.C., USA.

Buttlar-Brentano's observation of 'dwarf' cells in substantia innominata, commenting 'It is difficult to envisage how an alteration of as unspecific a region as this could have the systemic effects presumably required to induce schizophrenic behaviour.'

David suggested that only quantitative cell counts in schizophrenic and matched control material could confirm or deny the reports of focal neuronal degeneration. Negative results of such an undertaking had been previously reported for cerebral cortex by Dunlap (1929). Colon (1972) reached an opposite conclusion, finding a 70% reduction of neurones in cortical layers IV and V in selected areas of the frontal cortex of schizophrenic brains compared with controls. More recently, Dom *et al.* (1981) reported that cell counts on serial sections of basal ganglia and thalamus showed a 50% decrease in small neurones in pulvinar and large neurones in nucleus accumbens in brains of schizophrenics studied at the Vogt Institute. The difficulty of such studies are well known, and it is not surprising that psychiatrists turned with relief to the more easily quantified new technologies of gas–liquid chromatography, mass-spectrography and 'grinding and binding' for the measurement of biochemical constituents and receptor sites in schizophrenic and control brains.

The first International Congress of Neuropathology coincided with, but was too early to profit from, MacLean's (1952) heuristic introduction of limbic system anatomy pathology and physiology to psychiatry or David might not have dismissed Buttlar-Brentano's report of pathology in nucleus basalis so lightly. Assuming that the profound disturbances in higher nervous functions must involve cerebral cortex, a majority of studies of schizophrenic neuropathology has concerned cerebral cortex. Moreover, with few exceptions, the pathological material was generally stained only with conventional neuropathological techniques for myelin, Nissl substance and occasionally axis cylinders and lipoids.

GLIAL CHANGES

Employing the lithium carbonate stain for glia, Scharenberg (1952) reported a marked astrocyctic proliferation in cases of fatal catatonia. Five years later, Nieto, also using the lithium carbonate method, reported a pathological increase of fibrillary gliosis in periventricular and periaqueductal regions of the diencephalon and mesencephalon in a majority of schizophrenic brains. In a subsequent publication Nieto & Escobar (1972), emphasized that the same sections of the brain displaying intense fibrillary gliosis with the lithium carbonate method were quite unremarkable in Nissl or myelin preparations. More recently, Fisman (1975) reported glial nodules in brain stem, especially the medial reticular area and trigeminal nucleus, in six of eight schizophrenic brains, noting a resemblance to viral, in particular herpes zoster, encephalitis. Both of these studies may be criticized as patients were generally of advanced age, the criteria for diagnosis were not specified, and material from 'blind' controls was not included.

Using stringent criteria for diagnosis of schizophrenia and restricting the specimens examined to patients under 54 years of age, we recently compared histological material from the brains of 28 patients meeting International Classification of Disease criteria for schizophrenia with similar material from age-matched non-schizophrenic control patients who died in the same hospital during the same period with a variety of neuropsychiatric disorders and with neuropathological material from age-matched patients deceased in a general hospital of medical or surgical causes (Stevens, 1982*a*, *b*). Nissl, myelin or hematoxylin-eosin stains of this material revealed striking pathology in a few of the schizophrenic patients. A marked dropout of large neurones in the globus pallidus was apparent in three cases, and there was bilateral infarction in the inner or outer segment of pallidum in two cases. All five of these patients had admission diagnoses of catatonic schizophrenia and followed a course typical of chronic schizophrenia. Heavy deposits of iron–calcium concretions in globus pallidus, infiltration of the basal forebrain with corpora amylacea and abundant ependymal granulations, all common during middle and advanced age in normal controls' brains, were present in the brains of schizophrenic patients who died in their 20s and 30s.

The most prominent and ubiquitous pathology, however, appeared only with the Holzer stain for glial fibrils. With this method, 70% of schizophrenic patients demonstrated increased fibrillary gliosis affecting primarily the periventricular regions and the anterior and inferior horns of the lateral ventricle, third ventricle, periaqueductal gray or basal forebrain. The gliosis was similar in distribution to that reported by Nieto (1957) and Nieto & Escobar (1972). Although gliosis in mesencephalic tegmentum was also common, the discrete glial nodules described by Fisman (1975) were seldom seen. The location of gliosis varied greatly from case to case, being more pronounced in basal forebrain (substantia innominata, lateral hypothalamus, bed nucleus of stria terminalis) in certain cases, while in others periaqueductal, interpeduncular, dorsal medial thalamus or hypothalamic regions were principally affected. An attempt to correlate the subtype of schizophrenia with the pathological findings was entirely unsuccessful. This was not surprising, as a review of the clinical charts indicated that the patients diagnosed as catatonic schizophrenia on admission (as a majority were) generally proceeded during subsequent years of hospitalization to manifest flattened affect, isolation, delusions, ideas of reference, or pathological suspiciousness typical of paranoid schizophrenia. Subsequently, a majority progressed to states of abulic amotivational incoherent or hebephrenic behaviour or autistic preoccupation, with auditory hallucinations occasionally interrupted by episodes of severe agitation or assaultiveness. A correlation between location of the pathology and specific clinical phenomenology was sometimes suggestive – for example, sleep and feeding disturbances with hypothalamic gliosis, speech disturbance with pallidal pathology.

VENTRICULAR ENLARGEMENT IN SCHIZOPHRENIA

The introduction of computed tomography into psychiatric research (Johnstone *et al.* 1976) has led to a rediscovery of the ventricular dilatation so consistently reported in schizophrenic patients studied by pneumoencephalography more than half a century ago (Jacobi & Winkler, 1927). The new evidence of ventricular enlargement must now direct attention once again to the long disputed neuropathological studies of schizophrenia. If the ventricles are enlarged, something must have disappeared. Although Weinberger *et al.* (1979) observed no correlation between lateral ventricular size and length of illness, Tanaka *et al.* (1981) reported a positive correlation between the size of the third ventricle and the duration of schizophrenia. If confirmed in serial studies of individual patients, this observation indicates that a progressive destructive process occurs in this disease. These radiological findings alone are sufficient reason to return to the study of the neuropathology of schizophrenia.

SIGNIFICANCE OF MORPHOLOGICAL, ELECTROPHYSIOLOGICAL AND BIOCHEMICAL CHANGES FOR THE CONCEPT OF 'FUNCTIONAL PSYCHOSIS'

As Yatsu, Professor of Neurology at the University of Oregon likes to say, 'Gliosis is a tombstone'. So, of course, are lipoid degeneration, cell dropout, mineral deposits, ependymal granulations and, probably, corpora amylacea. These neuropathological gravestones spur the search for aetiology. Such studies should now include techniques which have developed since the pioneering, but long neglected, studies of Alzheimer (1897), Dide (1934), the Vogts (1952), and so many others. Evidence for biological antecedents of schizophrenia has grown appreciably in the past decade with the explosion of growth in neurobiomedical technologies. Increased dopamine binding sites (Lee *et al.* 1978; Owen *et al.* 1978), increased norepinephrine in schizophrenic basal forebrain (Farley *et al.* 1980; Kleinman *et al.* 1982), abnormal EEG spectra (Stevens, 1976; Stevens *et al.* 1979; Fenton *et al.* 1980), enlarged cerebral ventricles (Johnstone *et al.* 1976; Weinberger *et al.* 1979), atrophy of cerebellar vermis (Weinberger *et al.* 1980), and evidence of immunological incompetence (Liederman & Prilipko, 1976), autoimmunity (Semenov *et al.* 1961; Baron *et al.* 1977; Pandey *et al.* 1981) or viral residence in brain (Tyrell *et al.* 1979; Albrecht *et al.* 1980; Stevens, 1982*a*; Torrey *et al.* 1982) all challenge long cherished notions of psychogenesis.

Chemical and morphological abnormalities in schizophrenia also raise questions about the increasingly obsolete concept of 'functional psychosis' and research diagnostic criteria which demand the exclusion of cases with evidence of organic brain disease from the schizophrenias.

Ferraro at the International Neuropathological Congress of 1952 enquired:

What should our attitude be in the presence of organic cerebral changes found in cases clinically diagnosed as functional psychosis?...Must we adhere to the concept that a diagnosis of schizophrenia is incompatible with the presence of cerebral pathology? Must we every time that organic changes are found in the brain of a supposedly schizophrenic patient change our diagnosis into one of organic psychosis simulating dementia praecox? Must we talk in such cases of schizophrenia-like condition?

Clearly, a new definition is required, encompassing new findings disclosed by new technologies. This is even more likely to be the case as the revolutionary changes in neuropathology which have followed the introduction of immunohistochemistry are applied to the study of receptors, enzymes, peptides, viruses, and immunological reactions in schizophrenic brains.

EVIDENCE FOR UNITY AS WELL AS DIVERSITY OF THE SCHIZOPHRENIC SYNDROME: THE DOPAMINE HYPOTHESIS

If the increased neuroleptic binding found in the basal ganglia and forebrain of schizophrenic brains is not related to neuroleptic treatment, this finding is the most consistent contribution to the pathology of schizophrenia in the last decade (Lee *et al.* 1978; Owen *et al.* 1978). How can an increase in putative dopamine binding sites in the striatum be integrated with the gliosis, cell metamorphosis or loss and ventricular enlargement which, up to now, have been the principal neuropathological findings of schizophrenia?

There are a number of clues that schizophrenia is due to an encephalopathy resulting from activation of a latent infectious agent. The seasonal peak of births in early spring of future schizophrenics (Torrey & Torrey, 1979), the pockets of high incidence of schizophrenia in certain geographical areas (Torrey, 1980), and recent immunological findings in cerebrospinal fluid (Tyrell *et al.* 1979; Albrecht *et al.* 1980; Torrey *et al.* 1982) are consistent with repeated reactivation of a viral infection or immunological process in this disorder. Viruses and neurotransmitters bind to specific, apparently related, sites on neuronal membranes (Munzel & Koschel, 1981; Lentz *et al.* 1982). Viruses may alter binding of other substances to the cell membrane and, following entry of the cell, can direct the metabolic machinery without necessarily destroying the host cell (Glasgow, 1979). Reportedly abnormal *T* cell response to mitogens (Liederman & Prilipko, 1976) and antibrain antibodies in serum (Semenov *et al.* 1961; Heath & Krupp, 1967; Pandey *et al.* 1981) may also relate to the chronic residence of virus in brain.

The discovery of a viral aetiology for schizophrenia need not contradict the considerable evidence for hereditary factors in this disorder. Viral genome, incorporated in cell nucleus, can be transmitted with the genetic material of the host cell. If, as several studies suggest, cytomegalovirus, or varicella zoster virus, both members of the herpes family are associated with schizophrenia (Albrecht *et al.* 1980; Torrey *et al.* 1982; Stevens, 1982*a*), the reported amelioration of herpes zoster by treatment with L-dopa raises the possibility that virus and dopamine may compete for the same, or closely related, binding sites on neural membranes. The favourable effect of neuroleptics in schizophrenia could thus be only indirectly related to dopamine receptor blockade, but directly related to preventing viral binding and entry to the cell, to synaptosomes or to interference with replication of viral DNA within the cell (Hahn, 1979).

NEEDED: A NEW SPECIALTY OF NEUROPSYCHIATRY OR PSYCHONEUROLOGY

Neurologists have taken a long holiday from the study of psychiatry in general and from schizophrenia in particular. Equally remiss, an entire generation of psychiatrists has been trained with a curriculum often devoid of neuroanatomy, neuropathology and neurology, not to mention the explosion of new information and technology in neurochemistry, immunology, virology, and neuroradiology. In partial recognition of the growing similarity of both clinical problems and technologies in neurological and psychiatric research, American neurologists have recently given birth to the new subspecialty of *behavioural neurology*, deliberately avoiding the uncomfortable possibility that this concept might be better called *psychiatry* or, at the very least, *neuropsychiatry*. *Pari passu*, psychiatrists, at least those not exclusively enamoured of the psychotherapies (increasingly the province of non-medical professionals), have rediscovered the importance and excitement of the study of the brain. Few psychiatric training programmes provide adequate preparation for such work. Psychiatry's new horizons require retreading of practitioners as well as research physicians in the basic neurological sciences in order that the changes in these disciplines can be applied to the baffling clinical problems posed by the major psychoses. Clearly, neuropsychiatry (or psycho-neurology) like its enormously successful young parents, the neurosciences, is a specialty whose time has come, and for which appropriate training programmes are urgently needed by both psychiatrists and neurologists.

JANICE R. STEVENS

REFERENCES

Albrecht, F., Torrey, E. F., Boone, E., Hicks, J. T. & Daniel, N. (1980). Raised cytomegalovirus-antibody level in cerebrospinal fluid of schizophrenic patients. *Lancet* ii, 769–772.

Alzheimer, A. (1897). Beiträge zur pathologischen Anatomie der Hirnrinde und zur anatomischen Grundlage einiger Psychosen. *Monatschrift für Psychiatrie und Neurologie* **2**, 82–119.

Baron, M., Stern, M., Anavi, R. & Witz, J. P. (1977). Tissue binding factor in schizophrenic sera: a clinical and genetic study. *Biological Psychiatry* **12**, 199–219.

Bruetsch, W. L. (1952). Specific structural neuropathology of the central nervous system (rheumatic, demyelinating, vasofunctional, etc.) in schizophrenia. In *Proceedings of the First International Congress of Neuropathology*, Vol. 3, pp. 487–499. Rosenberg & Sellier: Torino, Italy.

Buscaino, V. M. (1924). Histologic pathology and pathogenesis of dementia praecox, amentia, and extrapyramidal syndromes. *Encephale* **19**, 217–224.

Buttlar-Brentano, K. (1952). Pathohistologische Feststellungen am basalkern Schizophrener. *Journal of Nervous and Mental Disease* **116**, 646–653.

Colon, E. J. (1972). Quantitative cytoarchitectonics of the human cerebral cortex in schizophrenic dementia. *Acta Neuropathology* **20**, 1–9.

David, G. B. (1957). The pathological anatomy of the schizophrenias. In *Schizophrenia: Somatic Aspects* (ed. D. Richler), pp. 93–130. Pergamon Press: Oxford.

Dide, M. M. (1934). Les syndromes hypothalamiques et la dyspsychogenese. *Revue Neurologique* **6**, 941–943.

Dom, R., de Saedleer, J., Bogerts, J. & Hopf, A. (1981). Quantitational cytometric analyses of basal ganglia in catatonic schizophrenia. In *Biological Psychiatry* (ed. C. Perris, G. Struwe and B. Jansson), pp. 723–726. Elsevier: Amsterdam.

Dunlap, C. G. (1929). The pathology of the brain in schizophrenia. In *Proceedings of the Association for Research in Nervous and Mental Disease. A Series of Research Publications*, Vol. 8, pp. 371–377. Hoeber: New York.

Farley, I. J., Shannak, K. S. & Hornykiewicz, O. (1980). Brain monoamine changes in chronic paranoid schizophrenia and their possible relation to increased dopamine receptor sensitivity. In *Receptors for Neurotransmitters and Peptide Hormones* (ed. G. Pepeu, M. J. Kuhar and S. J. Enna), pp. 427–433. Raven Press: New York.

Fenton, G. W., Fenwick, P. B. C., Dollimore, J. L., Dunn, T. L. & Hirsch, S. R. (1980). EEG spectral analysis in schizophrenia. *British Journal of Psychiatry* **136**, 445–455.

Ferraro, A. (1943). Histopathological findings in two cases clinically diagnosed dementia praecox. *Journal of Nervous Disease and Experimental Neurology* **2**, 84–94.

Ferraro, A. (1952). Discussion. In *Proceedings of the First International Congress of Neuropathology*, Vol. 3, pp. 631–634. Rosenberg & Sellier: Torino, Italy.

Fisman, M. (1975). The brain stem in psychosis. *British Journal of Psychiatry* **126**, 414–422.

Fungfeld, E. W. (1952). Pathologisch-anatomische Untersuchungen im nucleus anterior thalami bei Schizophrenie. In *Proceedings of the First International Congress of Neuropathology*, Vol. 3, pp. 648–659. Rosenberg & Sellier: Torino, Italy.

Glasgow, L. A. (1979). Biology and pathogenesis of viral infections. In *Viral Agents and Viral Diseases of Man* (ed. G. J. Galasso, T. C. Merigan and R. A. Buchanan), pp. 39–76. Raven Press: New York.

Hahn, F. E. (1979). Anti-plasmid and antiviral effect of chlorpromazine. *Naturwissenschaften* **66**, 467.

Heath, R. G. & Krupp, I. M. (1967). Schizophrenia as an immunologic disorder. I. Demonstration of antibrain globulins by fluorescent antibody techniques. *Archives of General Psychiatry* **16**, 1–9.

Hopf, A. (1952). Über histopathologische Veränderungen im pallidum and striatum bei Schizophrenie. In *Proceedings of the First International Congress of Neuropathology*, Vol. 3, pp. 629–635. Rosenberg & Sellier: Torino, Italy.

Hyden, H. (1952). Nerve cell chemistry and neuropathological problems studied by means of quantitative methods. In *Proceedings of the First International Congress of Neuropathology*, Vol. 3, pp. 570–594. Rosenberg & Sellier: Torino, Italy.

Jacobi, W. & Winkler, H. (1927). Encephalographische Studien au chronisch Schizophrenen. *Archiv für Psychiatrie und Nervenkrankheiten* **81**, 299–332.

Johnstone, E. C., Crow, T. J., Frith, C. D., Husband, J. & Kreel, L. (1976). Cerebral ventricular size and cognitive impairment in chronic schizophrenia. *Lancet* ii, 924–926.

Josephy, H. (1930). Dementia praecox (Schizophrenie). In *Die Anatomie der Psychosen* (ed. O. Bumke), pp. 763–778. Springer: Berlin.

Kleinman, J. E., Karoum, F., Rosenblatt, J. E., Gillin, J. C., Hong, J., Bridge, T. P., Zalcman, S., Storch, F., del Carmen, R. & Wyatt, R. J. (1982). Postmortem neurochemical studies in chronic schizophrenia. In *Biological Markers in Psychiatry and Neurology* (ed. I. Hanin and E. Usdin), pp. 67–76. Pergamon Press: Oxford.

Lee, T., Seeman, P., Tourtelotte, W. W., Farley, I. J. & Hornykiewicz, O. (1978). Binding of ^{3}H neuroleptics and ^{3}H apomorphine in schizophrenic brains. *Nature* **274**, 897–900.

Lentz, T. L., Burrage, T. G., Smith, A. L., Crick, J. & Tignor, G. H. (1982). Is the acetylcholine receptor a rabies virus receptor? *Science* **215**, 182–184.

Liederman, R. R. & Prilipko, L. L. (1976). The behavior of *T* lymphocytes in schizophrenia. In *Neurochemical and Immunologic*

Components in Schizophrenia (ed. D. Bergsma and A. Goldstein), pp. 365–377. Alan R. Liss: New York.

MacLean, P. D. (1952). Some psychiatric implications of physiological studies on fronto-temporal portion of the limbic system (visceral brain). *Electroencephalography and Clinical Neurophysiology* **4**, 407–418.

Meyer, A. (1952). Critical evaluation of histopathological findings in schizophrenia. In *Proceedings of the First International Congress of Neuropathology*, Vol. 1, pp. 649–666. Rosenberg & Sellier: Torino, Italy.

Morgan, L. O. & Gregory, H. S. (1935). Pathological changes in the tuber cinereum in a group of psychoses. *Journal of Nervous and Mental Disease* **82**, 286–298.

Munzel, P. & Koschel, K. (1981). Rabies virus decreases agonist binding to opiate receptors of mouse neuroblastoma-rat glioma hybrid cells 108-CC-15. *Biochemical and Biophysical Research Communications* **101**, 1241–1250.

Nieto, D. (1957). Cerebral lesions in schizophrenia. Their neuroanatomical and neurophysiological significance. In *Proceedings of the Second International Congress for Psychiatry*, Vol. 2, pp. 131–134.

Nieto, D. & Escobar, A. (1972). Major psychoses. In *Pathology of the Nervous System* (ed. J. Minckler), pp. 2654–2665. McGraw-Hill: New York.

Owen, F., Crow, T. J., Poulter, M., Cross, A. J., Longden, A. & Riley, G. J. (1978). Increased dopamine receptor sensitivity in schizophrenia. *Lancet* ii, 223–225.

Pandey, S., Gupta, A. K. & Shaturvedi, U. C. (1981). Autoimmune model of schizophrenia with special reference to antibrain antibodies. *Biological Psychiatry* **16**, 1123–1136.

Plum, F. (1972). Prospects for research on schizophrenia. 3. Neurophysiology. Neuropathological findings. *Neurosciences Research Program Bulletin* **10**, 384–388.

Rowland, L. P. & Mettler, F. A. (1949). Cell concentration and laminar thickness in the frontal cortex of psychotic patients. *Journal of Comparative Neurology* **90**, 255–265.

Scharenberg, K. (1952). Discussion. In *Proceedings of the First International Congress of Neuropathology*, Vol. 3, pp. 610–623. Rosenberg & Sellier: Torino, Italy.

Semenov, S. F., Morozov, G. V. & Kuznetzova, N. I. (1961). Evaluation of the clinical significance of antibrain antibodies in the serum of patients with schizophrenic and other neuropsychiatric disorders. *Zhurnal Nevropatologii i Psikhiatrii imeni S. S. Korsakova (Moskva)* **61**, 1210–1214.

Spielmeyer, W. (1931). The problem of the anatomy of schizophrenia. In *Schizophrenia (Dementia Praecox). An Investigation of the Most Recent Advances. Research Publications*, Vol. 10. Williams & Wilkins: Baltimore.

Stevens, J. R. (1976). Computer analysis of the telemetered EEG in the study of epilepsy and schizophrenia. *Acta neurochirurgica* (Suppl.) **23**, 71–84.

Stevens, J. R. (1982*a*). Neuropathologic changes in schizophrenia: search for a virus. In *Proceedings of the Psychobiology of Schizophrenia* (ed. M. Namba & H. Kaiya). Japan (in the press).

Stevens, J. R. (1982*b*). Neuropathologic changes in schizophrenia. *Archives of General Psychiatry* (in the press).

Stevens, J. R., Bigelow, L., Denney, D., Lipkin, J., Livermore, A. Jr, Rauscher, F. & Wyatt, R. J. (1979). Telemetered EEG–EOG during psychotic behaviors of schizophrenia. *Archives of General Psychiatry* **36**, 251–262.

Tanaka, T., Hazama, H., Kawakara, R. & Kobayuslu, K. (1981). Computerized tomography of the brain in schizophrenic patients. *Acta psychiatrica scandinavica* **63**, 191–197.

Torrey, E. F. (1980). *Schizophrenia and Civilization*. Jason Aronson: New York.

Torrey, E. F. & Torrey, B. B. (1979). A shifting seasonality of schizophrenic births. *British Journal of Psychiatry* **134**, 183–186.

Torrey, E. F., Yolken, R. H. & Winfrey, C. J. (1982). Cytomegalovirus antibody in cerebrospinal fluid of schizophrenic patients. *Science* **216**, 892–893.

Tyrell, D. A. J., Crow, T. J., Parry, R. P., Johnstone, E. & Ferrier, I. N. (1979). Possible virus in schizophrenia and some neurological disorders. *Lancet* ii, 839–841.

Vanderhorst, L. (1952). Histopathology of clinically diagnosed schizophrenic psychosis or schizophrenia-like psychoses of unknown origin. In *Proceedings of the First International Congress of Neuropathology*, Vol. 3, pp. 648–659. Rosenberg & Sellier: Torino, Italy.

Vogt, C. & Vogt, O. (1952). Alterations anatomiques de la schizophrénie et d'autres psychoses dites fonctionelles. In *Proceedings of the First International Congress of Neuropathology*, Vol. 1, pp. 516–532. Rosenberg & Sellier: Torino, Italy.

Weinberger, D. R., Torrey, E. F., Neophytides, A. N. & Wyatt, R. J. (1979). Lateral cerebral ventricular enlargement in chronic schizophrenia. *Archives of General Psychiatry* **36**, 735–739.

Weinberger, D. R., Kleinman, J. E., Luchins, D. J., Bigelow, L. B. & Wyatt, R. J. (1980). Cerebellar pathology in schizophrenia: A controlled post-mortem study. *American Journal of Psychiatry* **137**, 359–361.

Winkelman, N. W. & Book, M. H. (1949). Observations on the histopathology of schizophrenia. I. The cortex. *American Journal of Psychiatry* **105**, 889–896.

GENETICS

Psychological Medicine, 1977, **7**, 7–10

High risk for schizophrenia: genetic considerations[1]

Being the identical twin of a schizophrenic, as Meehl (1962) pointed out, is the best single predictor of schizophrenia, but such twins are hardly appropriate subjects for prospective high-risk studies. Some monozygotic co-twins of schizophrenics will already be affected when the case is discovered. Unless ascertained soon after the onset of the first twin's illness, the discordant partners are likely to be no longer at high risk, since most pairs that become concordant do so within a few years. They would not be of much help in detecting early signs of disorder or making predictions about their response to environmental changes. Furthermore, some pairs may be discordant because the illness in the proband was a symptomatic schizophrenia. Studied retrospectively, however, they remain of value in the search for stable constitutional traits predisposing to schizophrenia, as exemplified in the approach of Wyatt *et al.* (1973). Such a trait should in general distinguish schizophrenics from non-schizophrenics but should occur in both affected and unaffected members of discordant MZ pairs.

The offspring of two schizophrenic parents also incur a risk of developing schizophrenia – usually taken to be around 40% – which places them, like MZ co-twins, within the high risk range of 25% or over, using the term in the sense in which it is generally employed by geneticists when speaking of recurrence risks in genetic disease. In their risk study Erlenmeyer-Kimling (1975) and her colleagues have been able to include a group of 13 such children, aged 7–12 at first contact, together with 9 of their siblings.

The great majority of the high-risk studies which have burgeoned recently (Garmezy, 1974) examine children with one schizophrenic parent, since they are more accessible. On average they have only a moderately high risk of around 10% of becoming affected if they live long enough. Up till recently, the range varied from 7% to 17% in different studies, and the risk depends to some extent on the type of schizophrenia in the proband and the characteristics of the spouse. Though schizophrenia cannot be called a genetic disease in the same sense as Huntington's chorea or cystic fibrosis, it has been argued from the results in family, twin and adoption studies that genetic factors are the most uniformly potent cause (Gottesman & Shields, 1972). No environmental indicator predicts a raised risk of schizophrenia in small or moderate-sized samples of persons not already known to be genetically related to a schizophrenic. What, then, can we hope to learn from prospective high-risk work about the developmental genetic aspects of schizophrenia and about gene–environment interaction that cannot be discovered by other, simpler methods?

The children of schizophrenics are not uniformly at risk. Whichever model of inheritance is preferred, they will be genetically heterogeneous, with some of them at much higher risk for schizophrenia than others. On a simple monogenic theory half of them should be at no increased risk at all. Prospective studies might offer a better chance of recognizing different phenotypic expressions of various genotypes than retrospective studies where it is difficult or impossible to assess reliably the premorbid condition of an active or remitted schizophrenic. This is most obviously so as regards developmental characteristics and psychophysiological, attentional and other experimental psychological measures. A combination of suspect characteristics in the same person would be suggestive. Hanson *et al.* (1976) made use of longitudinal data collected in a study of child development. They found that the 30 children of schizophrenic parents from Minneapolis were remarkably normal on a host of perinatal, neurological and psychometric variables. However, of the 116 experimental and control children all 5 who had a combination of poor motor skills, large intra-individual variance on

[1] Address for correspondence: Dr James Shields, Institute of Psychiatry, De Crespigny Park, Denmark Hill, London SE5 8AF.

intelligence tests, and ratings of 'schizoid' behaviour at the ages of 4 and 7 were the children of schizophrenic parents. It was predicted that these 5 are especially vulnerable to future schizophrenia.

Besides any information which might accrue concerning early or modifiable signs of the developing illness, there is the possibility of leads to fundamental disturbances of psychological functioning that might be thought to be closer to what was inherited in schizophrenia than the psychosis itself. By looking at characteristics which resemble those of schizophrenics and studying them in the relatives of schizophrenics and in control groups, some of the risk studies should be maximizing their chances of finding any such behavioural characteristics of *schizoidia* – if they exist (Shields *et al.* 1975).

To find out whether any such characteristics are more clearly inherited than schizophrenia, one would need to carry out genetic studies of them in schizophrenics' families and in the general population. The incidence of schizophrenia in the families of persons from the general population found to be deviant in such characteristics would also be needed in order to see whether they have any general bearing on the predisposition to schizophrenia. For example, if it were discovered that fidgetiness in childhood was a good predictor or early manifestation of Huntington's chorea in Huntington families, this would not imply that fidgety children in other families were at risk for this rare disease. There is no special reason to suppose that a style of thinking, a perceptual anomaly or a physiological measure will be any more simply inherited or less heterogeneous in its aetiology than schizophrenia itself. One might, however, be fortunate enough to identify a normal behavioural variable which at one of its extremes contributed to some extent to the predisposition to schizophrenia along with other perhaps more specific factors (Smith & Mendell, 1974). Shorter-term longitudinal studies and cross-sectional studies at different ages should shed light on which characteristics are age-dependent and which remain stable indicators of high risk. Stable traits are clearly of greater value for genetic investigations than state-dependent ones, and prospective studies may help identify them.

On the environmental side the hope is that a variable of one kind or another may be identified to which those genetically at risk for schizophrenia are particularly sensitive and which offers scope for preventive intervention. Perinatal factors and the nature of the final precipitating events are as easily investigated retrospectively as prospectively, but it would be interesting to have premorbidly made assessments of the quality of family life and social adjustment.

Follow-up information is the ultimate test of any claim to have identified individuals at highest risk genetically, or a genetic trait in the population which is correlated with the predisposition to schizophrenia, or an interacting environmental factor which offers scope for prevention. One of the studies described by Garmezy (1974), that of McNeil & Kaij, starts as early as the eighth month of pregnancy with recordings of the foetal heart beat for orienting response and habituation. Obviously it will not be feasible to follow such subjects through to the final life event before the onset in those who become schizophrenic, and then on to an age where the healthy offspring are all too old to be any longer at risk.

An inevitable drawback from the genetic point of view of studying the children of schizophrenics prospectively is that only a minority of schizophrenics have schizophrenic parents, in particular parents who were already schizophrenic when the children were born. The earlier the age at which the high risk children are ascertained, the greater the proportion exposed from an early age to environmental circumstances not experienced by most schizophrenics. Rearing by psychotic and other sick parents (Rutter, 1966) can lead to behaviour disturbances in children for environmental reasons.[2] Childhood differences found between high-risk and low-risk groups may therefore not reflect an increased schizophrenia risk but relate to the quality or lack of family life which is hard to match experimentally. Furthermore, not all schizophrenics have marked childhood or adolescent problems. Many of the experimental variables studied which are thought to indicate increased schizophrenia risk, such as unstable psychophysiology or disordered attention, may be non-specific for schizo-

[2] Younger sibs of schizophrenics do not suffer this particular disadvantage but have other limitations as subjects for prospective studies. They are more often used as controls than as persons with a moderately high risk themselves.

phrenia and in addition present the all too common problem of unreliable measurement. It is therefore particularly desirable to discover which offspring have schizophrenic outcomes. On investigation at successive ages one might expect the composition of the sick group among high-risk offspring to change, some subjects with behaviour disorders dropping out or showing themselves to be non-schizophrenic, and others, including definite schizophrenics, being added.

The current enthusiasm for high-risk studies is due more than anything to the imaginative and productive work of Mednick and Schulsinger in Copenhagen. Thanks to the facilities for and attitudes towards genetic and epidemiological research in the Scandinavian countries, these workers would appear to be the first who might come near to approaching these seemingly unrealistic follow-up requirements. This is not the place to describe their projects in detail. Many of their earlier papers are republished in Mednick *et al.* (1974) and are succinctly described by Schulsinger & Jacobsen (1975). Currently their hypothesis is that potential schizophrenics have an autonomic nervous system that responds too quickly and too much to 'unkind environments'; an abnormally fast electrodermal recovery rate, which 'may be an important part of the genetic pattern transmitted from parent to child'; and a particular sensitivity to certain types of perinatal stress. Their psychophysiological findings have apparently not been confirmed by van Dyke *et al.* (1974) on the adopted-away children of schizophrenics or by Erlenmeyer-Kimling (1975) even when both parents were schizophrenic. This may be partly due to considerations such as age, diagnosis and other characteristics of the sample or to testing procedures. From their later work (Mirdal *et al.* 1974) and the careful work of McNeil & Kaij (1973, 1974) in Sweden, the association with perinatal factors, if it exists, may be much more slender than was originally thought. Their extensive data have only been partly analysed; and many of their conclusions – and further studies – have been largely based on the results of the first 20 sick children in their high-risk group identified in 1967. Their prospective study of 3-year-old Mauritian children with abnormal psychophysiology, some attending special nursery schools and others not (Schulsinger *et al.* 1975), should be interesting for what it can tell us about the stability of psychophysiology and its relation to behaviour problems and environment, but it would be premature to suppose that it has much specific bearing on the prevention of schizophrenia.

Nevertheless, the Mednick–Schulsinger team (Hanne Schulsinger, 1976) have followed up and, in 1972, succeeded in interviewing and testing a high proportion of their 207 high-risk and 104 low-risk subjects originally studied in 1962. At follow-up they were aged between 20 and 30 (mean approaching 24). The investigators themselves admit to 'a low threshold for diagnostic labelling', since they 'did not want to exclude even minimal psychopathological manifestations' in either group. However, in the high-risk group the number of definite schizophrenics identified blindly by procedures which included the PSE (10 according to CATEGO, 15 according to a consensus diagnosis) was not unexpectedly high; and there was only one schizophrenic among the low-risk controls.

It is therefore with great interest that one waits the detailed report of the extensive social, psychological and psychophysiological information collected in 1962 and 1972, to see how it relates to clinical state at an age when the group has survived nearly half the risk period for schizophrenia. But in view of the inherent difficulties and the rather slender relation found in earlier longitudinal studies (e.g. Hagnell, 1966) between previous personality assessments and subsequent breakdown, it may be unwise to set expectations very high. Schizophrenia is likely to be too diverse in aetiology for the recognition of a premorbid schizophrenic personality or a single biological characteristic that could be equated with the genotype. Yet one hopes the efforts of the Mednick and Schulsinger and other high risk studies will at least succeed in identifying and relating to one another some of the multiple causes in the development of many schizophrenias.

JAMES SHIELDS

REFERENCES

Erlenmeyer-Kimling, L. (1975). A prospective study of children at risk for schizophrenia: methodological considerations and some preliminary findings. In *Life History Research in Psychopathology*, vol. 4 (ed. R. D. Wirt, G. Winokur & M. Roff). University of Minnesota Press: Minneapolis.

Garmezy, N. (1974). Children at risk: The search for the antecedents of schizophrenia. *Schizophrenia Bulletin* **8**, 14–90; **9**, 55–125.

Gottesman, I. I. & Shields, J. (1972). *Schizophrenia and Genetics: a Twin Study Vantage Point*. Academic Press: New York.

Hagnell, O. (1966). *A Prospective Study of the Incidence of Mental Disorder*. Scandinavian University Books: Stockholm.

Hanson, D. R., Gottesman, I. I. & Heston, L. L. (1976). Some possible childhood indicators of adult schizophrenia inferred from children of schizophrenics. *British Journal of Psychiatry* **129**, 142–154.

McNeil, T. F. & Kaij, L. (1973). Obstetric complications and physical size of offspring of schizophrenic, schizophrenic-like, and control mothers. *British Journal of Psychiatry* **123**, 341–348.

McNeil, T. F. & Kaij, L. (1974). Reproduction among female mental patients: obstetric complications and physical size of offspring. *Acta Psychiatrica Scandinavica* **50**, 3–15.

Mednick, S. A., Schulsinger, F., Higgins, J. & Bell, B. (eds.) (1974). *Genetics, Environment and Psychopathology*. North-Holland: Amsterdam.

Meehl, P. E. (1962). Schizotaxia, schizotypy, schizophrenia. *American Psychologist* **17**, 827–838.

Mirdal, G. K. M., Mednick, S. A., Schulsinger, F. & Fuchs, F. (1974). Perinatal complications in children of schizophrenic mothers. *Acta Psychiatrica Scandinavica* **50**, 553–568.

Rutter, M. (1966). *Children of Sick Parents: an Environmental and Psychiatric Study*. Maudsley Monograph no. 16. Oxford University Press: London.

Schulsinger, F. & Jacobsen, B. (1975). The heredity–environment issue in psychiatry. Perspectives from research at the Psykologisk Institut, Department of Psychiatry, Kommunehospitalet. *Acta Psychiatrica Scandinavica* Supplement 261, pp. 44–58.

Schulsinger, F., Mednick, S. A., Venables, P. H., Raman, A. C. & Bell, B. (1975). Early detection and prevention of mental illness: the Mauritius project. *Neuropsychobiology* **1**, 166–179.

Schulsinger, H. (1976). A ten-year follow-up of children of schizophrenic mothers: clinical assessment. *Acta Psychiatrica Scandinavica* **53**, 371–386.

Shields, J., Heston, L. L. & Gottesman, I. I. (1975). Schizophrenia and the schizoid: the problem for genetic analysis. In *Genetic Research in Psychiatry* (ed. R. R. Fieve, D. Rosenthal & H. Brill). Johns Hopkins University Press: Baltimore and London.

Smith, C. & Mendell, N. R. (1974). Recurrence risks from family history and metric traits. *Annals of Human Genetics, London* **37**, 275–286.

van Dyke, J. L., Rosenthal, D. & Rasmussen, P. V. (1974). Electrodermal functioning in adopted-away offspring of schizophrenics. *Journal of Psychiatric Research* **10**, 199–215.

Wyatt, R. J., Murphy, D. L., Belmaker, R., Cohen, S., Donnelly, C. H. & Pollin, W. (1973). Reduced monoamine oxidase activity in platelets: a possible genetic marker for vulnerability to schizophrenia. *Science* **179**, 916–918.

Psychological Medicine, 1981, **11**, 441–447

Immunogenetics and schizophrenia[1]

There is overwhelming evidence for a major contribution of genetic elements to the aetiology of schizophrenia (Slater & Cowie, 1971), but the principal problems remain; what is the nature of the hereditary contribution, and what is the path by which genetic information is translated into a frank behavioural disorder?

The genetic evidence comes not only from the well-known family studies (Ødegaard, 1963; Elsässer, 1952; Schulz, 1932; Hallgren & Sjögren, 1959; Kay *et al.* 1975) and twin studies (Luxenburger, 1930; Essen-Möller, 1941; Kallmann, 1946; Slater, 1953; Tienari, 1968; Kringlen, 1968; Fischer *et al.* 1969; Gottesman & Shields, 1972), but also from the convincing cross-fostering and adoption studies (Heston, 1966; Kety *et al.* 1968; Mednick *et al.* 1974). From the latter, it seems clear that children with an affected biological parent have the same elevated chance of becoming ill, irrespective of whether they are reared by the natural parent or an adoptive or foster parent. That adoptive or foster homes are not themselves 'schizophrenogenic' is confirmed by the findings (Wender *et al.* 1971, 1974; Karlsson, 1974) that there is no increased incidence of schizophrenia in adopting parents or their other adopted children. In summary,

> the evidence indicates that the psychosis risk is already fixed at birth, and since the rates are the same in offspring in schizophrenic fathers and mothers one may conclude that the risk is actually set at the time of conception. The family environment seems to be excluded as a significant cause of schizophrenic illness. No family-connected factors have been identified that are not fully accounted for by the hereditary contribution (Karlsson, 1974).

The fact that the genetic element is not simple, however, is indicated by the discordance, varying in magnitude from study to study, found in identical twins. Twin studies are notoriously difficult to interpret except where they form part of fuller family analyses; the concordance in dizygotic twins depends on the population frequency of the disease as well as on its severity (Childs, 1976) and inheritance and, where heritability is not absolute, a concordance rate in identical twins may be quite low. However, there are data (Kety, 1978) suggesting that the children of an unaffected discordant twin do develop the illness in the expected proportions. Again, some life-event studies (Brown & Birley, 1968; Uhlenhuth & Paykel, 1972; Eisler & Polak, 1971) purport to demonstrate that the stress of adverse experiences can initiate the illness (psychogenic psychosis). However, other similar studies do not (Morrison *et al.* 1968; Murphy *et al.* 1962; Hudgens *et al.* 1973). Moreover, closer analysis of some of the positive studies shows serious methodological weaknesses; for example, one showed an increase in antecedent life events only by excluding the classical insidious onset cases characteristic of the nuclear condition (Brown & Birley, 1968). This does not mean, of course, that adverse life events are unimportant in precipitating relapse; they are, indeed, crucial in destabilizing (Leff *et al.* 1973) the contained patient. Certainly a role for physical stress factors in the pathogenesis cannot at present be ruled out, as for example in puerperal schizophrenia (Hays, 1978), while likewise ingestion of lysergic acid diethylamide may produce the same effect in a predisposed subject (Anastasopoulos & Photiades, 1962) or at least accelerate the onset of the disorder.

In the light of such evidence for both genetic and environmental elements in the aetiology, several inheritance models of schizophrenia have been proffered but remain unverified. There is good, but not yet conclusive, evidence for the monogenic (dominant) thesis (Slater, 1972). Thus Heston's (1970) work and data from Karlsson (1973) argue cogently for the presence of a dominant principal

[1] Address for correspondence: Professor D. F. Roberts, Department of Human Genetics, The University, 19 Claremont Place, Newcastle upon Tyne NE2 4AA.

gene, while Kety (1978), in his family study of half-sibs, found a very high incidence (50 % risk) in half-sibs where the common parent was schizophrenic. But the argument for a polygenic mode of inheritance, which allows for the combined effect of environmental and hereditary elements, is just as acceptable, and suggests that the genetic contribution predominates, with a heritability of upwards of 60 % (Gottesman & Shields, 1968). This dispute, however, is of secondary importance to discovery of the mechanism by which the genetic error is implemented.

IMMUNOGENETICS

In the last decade there has been a remarkable development of immunogenetics as applied to man. Genetic factors have been shown to be implicated at a number of points in both the humoral and cellular immune responses. In the humoral response, following the definition of the molecular structure of the immunoglobulins, the number of genes controlling the regions of their several chains has been indicated, and also how they act (Milstein & Munro, 1973). The marker allotypes, the Gm, Inv and Am groups, have been shown to be due to single amino acid substitutions which are point mutations in the sequences coding for the chains of immunoglobulins (Grubb, 1970). Besides these qualitative differences, some genetic influence on the level of immunoglobulins in apparently healthy individuals has been demonstrated (Billewicz *et al.* 1974), and though many deficiencies are non-genetic, the inherited bases of several, especially of IgA and IgM, have been established (Grundbacher, 1972*a*, *b*; Kelch *et al.* 1971; Waldmann *et al.* 1976; Tomkin *et al.* 1971). In the complement system, similarly, there are polymorphisms – different alleles at the same locus producing slightly different substances – in each of the components of complement except C5, and again there are genes responsible for deficiency of specific components (Day *et al.* 1972; Klemperer *et al.* 1966; Polley, 1968; Leddy *et al.* 1974; Boyer *et al.* 1975). The existence of genetically controlled circulating antibodies has long been known.

At the cellular level, blood-group antigens on the red cells were the earliest to be discovered (Landsteiner, 1901). Lymphocytes have provided a particularly vigorous development, notably in the exploration of the human chromosome major histocompatibility region (Bodmer *et al.* 1978; WHO, 1975), the identification of a large number of alleles at the loci controlling the HLA-A and B antigens, and rather smaller numbers at the HLA-C and D loci. The differentiation of B and T cells by rosetting and immunofluorescence has led to the identification of B cell types and T cell types, again under genetic control, and indeed another major polymorphic system of cell surface antigens (reminiscent of mouse Ia antigens) has been established in man.

These developments have had a profound effect in various fields of somatic medicine. Yet the application of immunogenetic concepts to schizophrenia appears to have lagged somewhat, despite the facts that an auto-immune hypothesis of schizophrenia was put forward as long ago as 1967 (Heath & Krupp, 1967) and that there is good evidence for a weak association with the red cell surface antigens. For schizophrenia, there have been some 40 studies of ABO associations, covering over 12000 patients (Mourant *et al.* 1978). Though the results differ among themselves, there is a strong suggestion of an elevated incidence of bloodgroup B. Schizophrenia is the only one of the psychoses to show such an association, and of the several classical genetic markers examined in schizophrenia only the B bloodgroup demonstrates an association. It is possible that further exploration in an immunogenetic context would provide the clue for the next stage of advance in the understanding of the disorder.

One area of immunogenetics in which there has been recent interest in schizophrenia is the HLA association. The HLA (human leukocyte antigen) histocompatibility system is controlled by several loci situated close together on the short arm of human chromosome 6. There is great polymorphism in this system, in that at each locus there are many different alleles available, so that millions of distinguishable antigenic configurations can be derived – a veritable demonstration of the individuality of the human genotype. Other genes also are thought to occur in this region analogous to the immune response (Ir) genes that are known in animals. The demonstration of associations between histocompatibility antigens and disease has been particularly useful. First, it has caused reconsideration of aetiologies, has demonstrated relationships between a number of diseases, and has shown what a wide range of disorders stems from immunopathology. Secondly, it has suggested mechanisms by which the disorders are brought about. Thirdly, associations, where close, may aid in diagnosis, as with B27 in ankylosing spondylitis. None of the disease associations is absolute. Even in the case of ankylosing spondylitis, the disorder with the strongest HLA association, only a minority of B27 positive persons actually develop it; this genetic factor alone is thus not a sufficient condition for the production of the disorder, and obviously some trigger is necessary to convert a predisposition to a manifestation of disease.

There have now been some 20 studies of HLA types in schizophrenia. There is little concordance in results, either between studies or between subgroups of patients within a study. Overall, the most consistent increase in frequency appears for antigens A28, Cw4, B18, B9 and B5, though each of these is visible in only a minority of studies. Several groups of workers have tried to delineate the paranoid and hebephrenic subtypes – a dubious exercise – and here increased frequencies of A1 in hebephrenic and A9 in paranoid are the most consistent; of critical relevance, the diagnostic criteria of these subtypes differ in the different studies. Practically all such studies refer to analyses of patient populations, and while they are useful in providing pointers, the interpretation of their results is often ambivalent. Sample size is all too frequently small, so that an apparent association may be a sampling artefact, even assuming that techniques are reliable. If an antigen association is validated, it may indicate that the antigen itself contributes to the aetiology, perhaps because of its antigenic similarity to some virus or as part of a polygenic system making for liability to the disorder. One major criticism lies in the diagnostic criteria. Only when the patients for inclusion in such studies are accepted on the basis of rigorous criteria would it be meaningful to attempt comparison between series. In this respect, it is interesting that the elevation of A1 was found in one study in 57 patients with Schneiderian first-rank criteria (McGuffin *et al.* 1978). Another criticism is the absence of family studies, for these supply essential information that population surveys cannot. They are crucial to the establishment of the correctness of the interpretations suggested by population studies. Only they can elucidate the relationship of the HLA (or indeed any other) genotype to the disease-conferring genes: whether it is the HLA antigen itself, whether it is some other linked gene, whether the association represents a multifactorial or monogenic inheritance and, if the former, whether it is the antigen itself that is involved or whether it reflects the susceptibility of particular families with their particular genetic constitution quite independent of the antigen. Family studies are at present in progress in at least two centres in Britain (Newcastle upon Tyne and London).

Future studies of HLA in schizophrenia should, therefore, involve (*a*) larger numbers of *propositi* so that pooling of data from different series from different localities becomes unnecessary, and subdivision by clinical or other details is possible; (*b*) the use of criteria for clinical diagnosis that are as clear and as standardized as possible; (*c*) a rigorous statistical approach, and the incorporation of actuarial data (which may well be more predictive of the outcome than clinical symptoms) rather than the more subjective attempts at categorization; (*d*) the incorporation of family studies.

MECHANISMS

For an immunogenetic hypothesis to be acceptable, there requires to be a mechanism, either some identifiable defect in the immune system or some substance evoking the specific immune response. For the first there is relatively little evidence, and more could be done following up by modern techniques some of the early suggestions (Heath & Krupp, 1967). The presence of abnormal leukocytes has been claimed (Fessel & Hirata-Hibi, 1963); so has a reduction in the number of DNA-synthesizing lymphocytes (Babayan *et al.* 1976), while elevation of autoantibodies (Ismailov, 1972), of globulin plasma factor, of serum IgA, and of CSF Ig or measles antibody (Fuller-Torrey, 1978) are reported, though some at least of these findings may reflect the effect of extrinsic factors. The second implies some structural, biochemical, or inflicted change in patients to which their immune system can respond, acting perhaps against imbalance or breakdown products, or an infecting organism.

There is a veritable mountain of data – *neurological* (Quotkin *et al.* 1976; Larsen, 1964; Hertzig & Birch, 1966), *psychophysiological* (Tucker *et al.* 1975; Myers *et al.* 1973; Ornitz, 1970; Saarma, 1974; Cowen, 1973; Shagass *et al.* 1974; Brezinova & Kendell, 1977; Gruzelier & Venables, 1972), *encephalographic* (Davis, 1942; Jasper *et al.* 1939; Sem-Jacobsen *et al.* 1955; Kennard & Levy, 1952), *anatomical* (Weinberger *et al.* 1979; Jellinek, 1976; Johnstone *et al.* 1978; Marsden, 1976), *biochemical* (Perry *et al.* 1979; Bird *et al.* 1977; Arreevi *et al.* 1979) – suggesting an organic basis. Kraepelin himself held that brain pathology would one day prove to be the key, though he cited (wrongly) Alzheimer morphology as characteristic. There is little doubt that subtle yet severe brain dysfunction, involving defective cognitive filtering or disturbed neurochemical processes, is fundamental. The confirmation of an HLA association would direct attention to the most promising paths to follow in exploring that mountain.

Functionally, the HLA gene complex controls both the inner and outer structures of cellular membranes via their topochemistry. All nervous system functions are very dependent on the properties of cellular membrane, and many of the biological investigations of schizophrenia have been concerned with the pathology of such structures. Thus disturbances in permeability (e.g. for neurotransmitters), receptor properties (e.g. toxins, viruses, drugs), and antigenicity conditions (e.g. for auto-immunity development) have all been suggested.

In support of the biochemical involvement in schizophrenia, acting via neurohumoral function, there is the exacerbation of symptoms in patients, and their induction in normals, by drugs such as the amphetamines (Kornetsky, 1976), probably associated with dopaminergic activity, and the reduction of symptoms by neuroleptic drugs (Crow & Gillbe, 1974). There is evidence from studies of post-mortem material and of dopamine turnover, not that dopamine neurones are overactive in schizophrenia, but that the number of dopamine receptors is increased in the brain of the majority of schizophrenic patients (Owen *et al.* 1978). While such an increase, or the capacity for it, may be intrinsic, there may well be an element of induction, presumably over a period, suggesting a triggering effect of, say, a slow-acting virus. For this there is some recent evidence (Tyrrell *et al.* 1979; Crow *et al.* 1979) and this would conceivably be one mechanism for an HLA association; for example, if the configuration of the virus resembles that of an HLA antigen, it would not be recognized as foreign by those carrying that antigen; or the product of the locus might affect some stage in the viral replication cycle, or determine an abnormal response to an otherwise common virus.

A direct attack on humoral and cellular immunity in schizophrenia in Russia embraces the two mechanisms (Vartanian *et al.* 1978; Liedeman & Prilipko, 1978). One area of enquiry concerns the identification of brain tissue antigens to which antibodies are detectable in sera from schizophrenic patients. These occur at an elevated frequency over that from normals, and appear to be directed against alpha^2 glycoprotein. Another area concerns the functional activity of lymphocytes of schizophrenic patients. Response to phytohaemaglutanin and concanavlin A is reduced, there is an increased proportion of B lymphocytes and reduction of active T lymphocytes, and it appears that the serum from most (81%) schizophrenic patients contains substances which reduce the number of DNA synthesizing cells in the mitogen-stimulated culture. It is unlikely that the total number of T lymphocytes is reduced, but instead that there exists a population of silent T lymphocytes in schizophrenic patients, that is, the cells do not respond to T mitogens. Antibodies to T lymphocytes appear to be one of the substances which produce such an inhibiting effect, and it seems that the same holds for antibodies to brain antigens since the human brain possesses antigenic determinants very similar to those of human thymocytes. Indeed, antithymic activity in the serum of schizophrenic patients tends to be higher than in normals. It is, moreover, intermediate in relatives of schizophrenic patients though the distributions overlap, and this suggestion of some genetic control is supported by the significance of the correlation of the quantitative levels among biological relatives and its absence between spouses, and by the different frequencies of antibodies against brain tissue in relatives of patients with and without such antibodies. Unfortunately, this index is not specific to schizophrenics, for similar levels are found in manic depressives and patients with thyrotoxic goitre.

These and other studies, if confirmed, would suggest that there exist factors in the serum of schizophrenic patients that somehow change the physiological and functional state of the peripheral blood lymphocytes, and that there is an appreciable genetic element governing the presence of such factors. A logical next step would be to isolate individual lymphocyte subpopulations, to discover which of them may be producing suppressive factors.

The idea that schizophrenia may be an immunogenetic problem is a sapling with many branches. If it is still too early to decide which should be pruned out and which nurtured to provide the mature tree of understanding, the young plant itself appears vigorous.

D. F. ROBERTS AND H. G. KINNELL

REFERENCES

Anastasopoulos, G. & Photiades, H. (1962). Effect of LSD-25 on relatives of schizophrenic patients. *Journal of Mental Science* **108**, 95–98.

Arreevi, A., Mackay, A. V., Iversen, L. L. & Spokes, E. G. (1979). Reduction of angiotensin-converting enzyme in substantia nigra in early onset schizophrenia. *New England Journal of Medicine* **300**, 502–503.

Babayan, N. G., Sekoyan, R. V. & Prilipko, L. L. (1976). The effect of serum of schizophrenic patients and of normal donors on the NA synthesis of lymphocytes. *Byulleten eksperimentalnoi biologii i meditsiny* **81** (4), 430–432.

Billewicz, W. Z., McGregor, I. A., Roberts, D. F., Rowe, D. S. & Wilson, R. J. M. (1974). Family studies in immunoglobulin levels. *Clinical and Experimental Immunology* **16**, 13–22.

Bird, E. D., Spokes, E. G., Barnes, J., Mackay, A. V., Iversen, L. L. & Shepherd, M. (1977). Brain norepinephrine and dopamine in schizophrenia. *Lancet* ii, 1157–1159.

Bodmer, W. F., Bodmer, J. G., Batchelor, J. R., Festenstein, H. & Morris, P. (eds.) (1978). *Histocompatibility Testing* 1977. Munksgaard: Copenhagen.

Boyer, J. T., Gall, E. P., Norman, M. E., Nilsson, U. R. & Zimmerman, T. S. (1975). Hereditary deficiency of the seventh component of complement. *Journal of Clinical Investigation* **56**, 905–913.

Brezinova, V. & Kendell, R. E. (1977). Smooth pursuit eye movements of schizophrenics and normal people under stress. *British Journal of Psychiatry* **130**, 59–63.

Brown, G. W. & Birley, J. L. T. (1968). Crisis and life changes and the onset of schizophrenia. *Journal of Health and Social Behaviour* **9**, 203–214.

Childs, B. (1976). Human behavioural genetics. In *Aspects of Genetics in Paediatrics* (ed. D. Barltrop), pp. 45–53. Fellowship of Postgraduate Medicine: London.

Cowen, M. A. (1973). Electrophysiological phenomena associated with the S-protein system in normal and schizophrenic subjects. *Biological Psychiatry* **7**, 113–127.

Crow, T. J. & Gillbe, C. (1974). Brain dopamine and behaviour. A critical analysis of the relationship between dopamine antagonism and therapeutic efficacy of neuroleptic drugs. *Journal of Psychiatric Research* **11**, 163–172.

Crow, T. J., Ferrier, I. N. & Johnstone, E. C. (1979). Characteristics of patients with schizophrenia or neurological disorder and virus-like agent in cerebrospinal fluid. *Lancet* i, 842–844.

Davis, P. A. (1942). Comparative study of the EEGs of schizophrenic and manic depressive patients. *American Journal of Psychiatry* **99**, 210–217.

Day, N. K., Geiger, H., Stroud, R., de Bracco, M., Mancado, B., Windhorst, D. B. & Good, R. A. (1972). Clr deficiency: an inborn error associated with cutaneous and renal disease. *Journal of Clinical Investigation* **51**, 1102–1108.

Eisler, M. & Polak, P. R. (1971). Social stress and psychiatric disorder. *Journal of Nervous and Mental Disease* **153**, 227–233.

Elsässer, G. (1952). *Die Nachkommen Geisteskranker Eltempaare*. Thieme: Stuttgart.

Essen-Möller, E. (1941). Psychiatrische Untersuchungen an einer Serie von Zwillingen. *Acta psychiatrica scandinavica* Suppl. 23.

Fessel, W. J. & Hirata-Hibi, M. (1963). Abnormal leukocytes in schizophrenia. *Archives of General Psychiatry* **9**, 601–613.

Fischer, M., Harvald, B. & Hauge, M. (1969). A Danish twin study of schizophrenia. *British Journal of Psychiatry* **115**, 981–990.

Fuller-Torrey, E. (1978). Immunoglobulins and viral antibodies in psychiatric patients. *British Journal of Psychiatry* **132**, 342–348.

Gottesman, I. I. & Shields, J. (1968). In pursuit of the schizophrenic genotype. In *Progress in Human Behaviour Genetics* (ed. S. G. Vandenberg), pp. 67–103. Johns Hopkins Press: Baltimore.

Gottesman, I. I. & Shields, J. (1972). *Schizophrenia and Genetics: a Twin Study Vantage Point*. Academic Press: New York.

Grubb, R. (1970). *The Genetic Markers of Human Immunoglobulins*. Chapman & Hall: London.

Grundbacher, F. J. (1972*a*). Genetic aspects of selective immunoglobulin A deficiency. *Journal of Medical Genetics* **9**, 344–347.

Grundbacher, F. J. (1972*b*). Human X chromosome carries quantitative genes for immunoglobulin M. *Science* **178**, 311–312.

Gruzelier, J. H. & Venables, P. H. (1972). Skin conductance and orienting activity in a heterogeneous sample of schizophrenics: possible evidence of limbic dysfunction. *Journal of Nervous and Mental Disease* **155**, 277–287.

Hallgren, B. & Sjögren, T. (1959). A clinical and genetico-statistical study of schizophrenia and low-grade mental deficiency in a large Swedish rural population. *Acta psychiatrica scandinavica* Suppl. 140.

Hays, P. (1978). Taxonomic map of the schizophrenics, with special reference to puerperal psychosis. *British Medical Journal* ii, 755–757.

Heath, R. G. & Krupp, I. M. (1967). Schizophrenia as an immunologic disorder. *Archives of General Psychiatry* **16**, 1–33.

Hertzig, M. E. & Birch, H. G. (1966). Neurologic organisation in psychiatrically disturbed adolescent girls. *Archives of General Psychiatry* **15**, 590–598.

Heston, L. L. (1966). Psychiatric disorders in foster-home reared children of schizophrenic mothers. *British Journal of Psychiatry* **112**, 819–825.

Heston, L. L. (1970). The genetics of schizophrenia and schizoid disease. *Science* **167**, 249–256.

Hudgens, R. W., Morrison, J. R. & Barchka, R. G. (1973). Personal catastrophe and depression: a consideration of the subject with respect to medically-ill adolescents, and a requiem for retrospective 'life event' studies. Presented at the Conference on Stressful Life Events at City University of New York, 5 June 1973.

Ismailov, T. I. (1972). A study of autoantibodies to DNA in schizophrenics and other neuropsychiatric disorders. *Zhurnal neuropatologii i psikhiatrii imeni S.S. Korsakova* **72** (8), 1188–1191.

Jasper, H. H., Fitzpatrick, C. P. & Solomon, P. (1939). Analogues and opposites in schizophrenia and epilepsy. *American Journal of Psychiatry* **95**, 835–851.

Jellinek, E. H. (1976). Cerebral atrophy and cognitive impairment in chronic schizophrenia. *Lancet* ii, 1202–1203.

Johnstone, E. C., Crow, T. J., Frith, C. D., Stevens, M., Kreel, L. & Husband, J. A. (1978). The dementia of dementia praecox. *Acta psychiatrica scandinavica* **57**, 305–324.

Kallmann, F. J. (1938). *The Genetics of Schizophrenia*. Augustin: New York.

Kallmann, F. J. (1946). The genetic theory of schizophrenia: an analysis of 691 schizophrenic twin index families. *American Journal of Psychiatry* **103**, 309–322.

Karlsson, J. L. (1973). An Icelandic family study of schizophrenia. *British Journal of Psychiatry* **123**, 549–554.

Karlsson, J. L. (1974). Inheritance of schizophrenia. *Acta psychiatrica scandinavica* Suppl. 247, p. 103.

Kay, D. W. K., Roth, M. & Atkinson, M. W. (1975). Genetic hypotheses and environmental factors in the light of psychiatric morbidity in the families of schizophrenics. *British Journal of Psychiatry* **127**, 109–118.

Kennard, M. A. & Levy, S. (1952). The meaning of the abnormal EEG in schizophrenia. *Journal of Nervous and Mental Disease* **116**, 413–423.

Kelch, R. P., Franklin, M. & Schmickel, R. D. (1971). Group D deletion syndrome. *Journal of Medical Genetics* **8**, 341–345.

Kety, S. (1978). The syndrome of schizophrenia. The Maudsley Lecture, 17 November 1978, given to the Royal College of Psychiatrists, London. Reprinted (1980) in *British Journal of Pschiatry* **136**, 421–436.

Kety, S. S., Rosenthal, D., Wender, P. & Schulsinger, F. (1968). The types and prevalence of mental illness in the biological and adoptive families of adopted schizophrenics. In *The Transmission of Schizophrenia* (ed. D. Rosenthal and S. S. Kety). Pergamon Press: Oxford.

Klemperer, M. R., Woodworth, H. C., Rosen, F. S. & Austen, K. F. (1966). Hereditary deficiency of 2nd component of complement in man. *Journal of Clinical Investigation* **45**, 880–890.

Kornetsky, C. (1976). Hyporesponsivity of chronic schizophrenic patients to dextroamphetamine. *Archives of General Psychiatry* **33**, 1425–1428.

Kringlen, E. (1968). An epidemiological-clinical twin study on schizophrenia. In *The Transmission of Schizophrenia* (ed. D. Rosenthal and S. S. Kety). Oxford University Press: London.

Landsteiner, K. (1901). Über Agglutinationserscheinungen normalen menschlichen Blutes. *Wiener Klinische Wochenschrift* **14**, 1132–1134.

Larsen, V. L. (1964). Physical characteristics of disturbed adolescents. *Archives of General Psychiatry* **10**, 55–88.

Leddy, J. P., Frank, M. M., Gaither, T., Baum, J. & Klemperer, M. R. (1974). Hereditary deficiency of the 6th component of complement in man, I. *Journal of Clinical Investigation* **53**, 544–553.

Leff, J. P., Hirsch, S. R., Gaind, R., Rohde, P. D. & Stevens, B. C. (1973). Life events and maintenance therapy in schizophrenic relapse. *British Journal of Psychiatry* **123**, 659–660.

Liedeman, R. R. & Prilipko, L. L. (1978). The behaviour of *T* lymphocytes in schizophrenia. *Birth Defects: Original Article Series*, **14**, 365–377.

Luxenburger, H. (1930). Heredität und Familientypus der Zwangsneurotiker. *Archiv für Psychiatrie* **91**, 590–594.

Marsden, C. D. (1976). Cerebral atrophy and cognitive impairment in chronic schizophrenia. *Lancet* ii, 1079.

McGuffin, P., Farmer, A. E. & Rajah, S. M. (1978). Histocompatibility antigens and schizophrenia. *British Journal of Psychiatry* **132**, 149–151.

Mednick, S. A., Schulsinger, F., Higgins, J. & Bell, B. (1974). *Genetics, Environment and Psychopathology*. North-Holland: Amsterdam.

Milstein, C. & Munro, A. J. (1973). Genetics of immunoglobulins and of the immune response. In *Defence and Recognition* (ed. R. R. Porter), pp. 199–228. Butterworth: London.

Morrison, J. R., Hudgens, R. W. & Barchka, R. G. (1968). Life events and psychiatric illness. *British Journal of Psychiatry* **114**, 423–432.

Mourant, A. E., Kopec, A. C. & Domaniewska-Sobczak, K. (1978). *Blood Groups and Diseases*. Oxford University Press: London.

Murphy, G. E., Robins, E., Kulin, N. O. & Christensen, R. F. (1962). Stress, sickness and psychiatric disorder in a 'normal' population: a study of 101 young women. *Journal of Nervous and Mental Disease* **134**, 228–236.

Myers, S., Caldwell, D. & Purcell, G. (1973). Vestibular dysfunction in schizophrenia. *Biological Psychiatry* **7**, 255–261.

Ødegaard, Ø. (1963). The psychiatric disease entities in the light of a genetic investigation. *Acta psychiatrica scandinavica* **39**, Suppl. 169, 94–104.

Ornitz, E. M. (1970). Vestibular dysfunction in schizophrenia and childhood autism. *Comprehensive Psychiatry* **11**, 159–173.

Owen, F., Cross, A. J., Crow, T. J., Longden, A., Poulter, M. & Riley, G. J. (1978). Increased dopamine-receptor sensitivity in schizophrenia. *Lancet* ii, 223–225.

Perry, T. L., Buchanan, J., Kish, S. J. & Hansen, S. (1979). Gamma-aminobutyric-acid deficiency in brains of schizophrenic patients. *Lancet* i, 237–239.

Polley, M. J. (1968). Inherited C'3 deficiency in man. *Science* **161**, 1149–1151.

Quotkin, F., Rifkin, A. & Klein, D. F. (1976). Neurologic soft signs in schizophrenia and character disorders. *Archives of General Psychiatry* **33**, 845–853.

Saarma, J. (1974). Autonomic component of the orienting reflex in schizophrenics. *Biological Psychiatry* **9**, 55–60.

Schulz, B. (1932). Zur Erb pathologie der Schizophrenie. *Zeitschrift für die gesamte Neurologie und Psychiatrie* **143**, 175–293.

Sem-Jacobsen, C. W., Petersen, M. C., Lazarte, J. A., Dodge, H. W. Jr & Holman, C. B. (1955). Intracerebral electrographic recordings from psychotic patients during hallucinations and agitation. *American Journal of Psychiatry* **112**, 278–288.

Shagass, C., Amadeo, M. & Overton, D. A. (1974). Eye-tracking performance in psychiatric patients. *Biological Psychiatry* **9**, 245–260.

Slater, E. (1953). *Psychotic and Neurotic Illnesses in Twins*. MRC Special Report Series no. 278. HMSO: London.

Slater, E. (1972). The case for a major partially dominant gene, In *Genetic Factors in Schizophrenia* (ed. A. Sorsby and N. E. Morton), pp. 173–180. C. C. Thomas: Springfield, Ill.

Slater, E. & Cowie, V. (1971). *The Genetics of Mental Disorders*. Oxford University Press: London.

Tienari, P. (1968). Schizophrenia in monozygotic male twins. In *The Transmission of Schizophrenia* (ed. D. Rosenthal and S. S. Kety). Oxford University Press: London.

Tomkin, G. H., Mawhinney, M. & Nevin, N. C. (1971). Isolated absence of IgA with autosomal dominant inheritance. *Lancet* ii, 124–125.

Tucker, G. J., Campion, E. W. & Silberfarb, P. M. (1975). Sensorimotor functions and cognitive disturbance in psychiatric patients. *American Journal of Psychiatry* **132**, 17–21.

Tyrrell, D. A. J., Parry, R. P., Crow, T. J., Johnstone, E. & Ferrier, I. N. (1979). Possible virus in schizophrenia and some neurological disorders. *Lancet* i, 839–841.

Uhlenhuth, E. H. & Paykel, E. S. (1972). Symptom intensity and life events. *Archives of General Psychiatry* **28**, 473–477.

Vartanian, M. E., Kolyaskina, G. I., Lozovsky, D. V., Burbaeva, G. S. & Ignatov, S. A. (1978). Aspects of humoral and cellular immunity in schizophrenia. In *Neurochemical and Immunologic Components in Schizophrenia* (ed. D. Bergsma and A. L. Goldstein), pp. 339–364. Alan Liss: New York.

Waldmann, T. A., Broder, S., Krakauer, R., Durm, M., Meade, B. & Goldman, C. (1976). Defects in immunoglobulin A secretion and in immunoglobulin A specific suppressor cells in patients with isolated immunoglobulin A deficiency. *Clinical Research* **24**, 483A.

Weinberger, D. R., Torrey, E. F. & Wyatt, R. J. (1979). Cerebellar atrophy in chronic schizophrenia. *Lancet* i, 718–719.

Wender, P. H., Rosenthal, D., Zahn, T. P. & Kety, S. S. (1971). The psychiatric adjustment of the adopting parents of schizophrenics. *American Journal of Psychiatry* **127**, 1013–1018.

Wender, P. H., Rosenthal, D., Kety, S. S., Schulsinger, F. & Welner, J. (1974). Crossfostering. A research strategy for clarifying the role of genetic and experimental factors in the etiology of schizophrenia. *Archives of General Psychiatry* **30**, 121–128.

World Health Organization Bulletin (1975). Nomenclature for factors of the HLA system; **52**, 261–265.

Psychological Medicine, 1982, **12**, 471–473

X-linked mental retardation[1]

More males than females are intellectually handicapped. This male excess is approximately 25%. In 1971 Lehrke, an educational psychologist, was the first to put forward the hypothesis that the male excess might result from genes on the X chromosome. Prior to that there had been a few isolated case reports of families where intellectual handicap showed an X-linked pattern of inheritance. In diseases inherited on the X chromosome the female is a carrier; she having two X chromosomes will be partially or completely protected, because one of her X chromosomes is inactive in every cell. Half of her sons will receive the X chromosome carrying the abnormal gene and will therefore be affected; half of her daughters will be carriers. If X-linked conditions are important as a cause of intellectual handicap, then it would be anticipated that many more families would have two intellectually handicapped sons than two intellectually handicapped daughters. In a survey of moderately retarded school-age children in New South Wales, Australia (Turner & Turner, 1974), it was found that there were three times as many families with two affected sons than families with two affected daughters. A similar excess of male sibships was reported by Davison (1973) in a survey in Oxfordshire and, more recently, by Herbst (1980) in British Columbia. Calculations from the survey in New South Wales suggested that a prevalance figure of X-linked genes associated with mental handicap among the moderately retarded was 5·8/10000; in British Columbia a prevalance figure of 18/10000 was found from a survey involving both the moderately and mildly intellectually handicapped. This means that approximately 20% of intellectual handicap in the male is caused by genes on the X chromosome.

There are a number of clinical conditions associated with intellectual handicap which are coded on the X chromosome. These include the Coffin Lowry Syndrome, Hunter's Syndrome, Lesch Nyhan Syndrome and the intellectual handicap associated with a proportion of boys with Duchenne Muscular Dystrophy. These are all relatively rare conditions. In the majority, the affected males have no detectable metabolic abnormality and no obvious clinical stigmata; in fact, this lack of physical stigmata may be diagnostic of X-linked mental retardation (Turner *et al.* 1971). In a moderately retarded population the majority of affected individuals have microcephaly, neurological signs or a dysgenic appearance.

THE DISCOVERY OF THE MARKER X CHROMOSOME

In 1969 Lubs described an X-linked family in which the affected males had a marker which was visible on the end of the long arm of the X chromosome in approximately 30% of the metaphases. A proportion of the carrier females also showed the marker, but in a more variable proportion of metaphases. In 1977 Harvey *et al.* described four families showing the marker. Sutherland (1977) showed that the demonstration of the marker in lymphocyte culture was dependent on characteristics of the media in which the cells were growing. It was consistently visible in culture mediums deficient in folic acid. In 1975 Turner *et al.* described two families with X-linked mental retardation in which the affected males had unexplained testicular enlargement post-pubertally. On a re-examination of twenty-three X-linked families looking for the presence of the marker (Turner *et al.* 1978), this was found in the affected males of seven families and all these males were also found to have testicular enlargement. The marker X chromosome is nearly always found associated with testicular enlargement, although some families have now been described with testicular enlargement not showing the marker and the reverse is also recorded in one family (Jennings *et al.* 1980).

[1] Address for correspondence: Dr Gillian Turner, The Prince of Wales Children's Hospital, High Street, Randwick, NSW 2031, Australia.

Table 1. *Fragile X-linked mental retardation: clinical features*

Intelligence	IQ range 30–65, rarely borderline normal Occasional picture of hyperactivity or autism in childhood Generally friendly, shy, non-aggressive as teenagers Repetitive speech
Growth	Birth weight normal; usually bigger than normal sibs Height above 50th percentile in infancy and childhood Head circumference above 50th percentile, occasionally above 97th percentile
Facies	Prominent forehead, jaw and big ears
Testes	May be 3–4 ml in childhood (normal 2 ml) Post pubertal boys 30–60 ml (normal below 25 ml)
Occasional features	Epilepsy; increased reflexes in lower limbs Gynaecomastia striae, fine skin Thickening of scrotal sac

CLINICAL FEATURES

The clinical features of the male with the marker X is shown in Table 1.

CARRIER FEMALES OF X-LINKED MENTAL RETARDATION

The intelligence of the carrier female is usually normal, but one-third have learning difficulties. This is probably related to the random inactivation of one of the X chromosomes in each cell which may affect the CNS function in a proportion of cells. In the past some of these families have been erroneously classified as cultural–familial retardation due to the normal appearance of the affected males and the mild retardation of the carrier mother. The mild intellectual handicap of some of the carriers of X-linked mental retardation stimulated us into surveying for the marker one hundred and twenty-eight mildly retarded schoolgirls. The marker was found in five, and in four there were moderately retarded males in the family history. Assuming that heterozygous expression also occurs in X-linked mental retardation without the marker, X-linked genes may account for 10% of mild retardation in the female (Turner *et al.* 1980).

GENETIC COUNSELLING

Any family with an intellectually handicapped son with no physical stigmata should be assumed to have X-linked mental retardation. If the family history is positive for other affected males on the maternal side the diagnosis is confirmed, and further offspring will then be at 50–50 risk of the sons being intellectually handicapped or the daughters being carriers. If there is no family history of other affected males, then it is reasonable to consider a recurrence risk rate of at least 1 in 10 for subsequent children being affected. The families in which the affected males show the marker enable the diagnosis to be confirmed in the singleton, but the problem then is that only a proportion of the carrier females show the marker in adult life. In childhood and adolescence the carrier female can usually be identified in that the sisters of affected males are found to have the marker in 50%, which is the expected proportion. As yet, there have been no longitudinal studies confirming that the marker may actually disappear with age. At present, all that can be offered in terms of antenatal diagnosis is foetal sexing and termination of the male foetus. There has been difficulty in reliably demonstrating the marker in fibroblast culture, but this problem is likely to be solved in the near future.[1] Once this is available then, in families with the marker X, any female at risk of being a carrier can have her pregnancy monitored by amniocentesis.

The recognition of X-linked mental retardation with and without the marker is a big step forward.

[1] Successful demonstration of the marker, both by amniocentesis and by foetal blood sampling, has recently been reported in correspondence in the *Lancet*.

It means that another large chip has been taken off the block of undiagnosed intellectual handicap. It opens up new possibilities for reducing the prevalence of intellectual handicap by genetic counselling and by antenatal diagnosis. The families themselves are relieved at long last to have a diagnosis, even though this has implications that the mother may be a carrier. We are still only at the descriptive phase of this disease or diseases, and other subgroups may well be defined. The next awaited breakthrough is the delineation of the biochemical defect underlying this intellectual handicap. This will provide us with considerable insight into the nature of the learning process and the biochemical background behind conceptual thought. Future developments in this field should be exciting.

GILLIAN TURNER

REFERENCES

Davison, B. C. (1973). *Genetic Studies in Mental Retardation. Journal of Psychiatry* Special Publication No. 8. Headley Bros.: Ashford.

Harvey, J., Judge, C. & Weiner, S. (1977). Familial X-linked mental retardation with an X chromosome abnormality. *Journal of Medical Genetics* **14**, 46–50.

Herbst, D. S. (1980). Nonspecific X-linked mental retardation. II: The frequency in British Columbia. *American Journal of Medical Genetics* **7**, 461–469.

Jennings, M., Hall, J. G. & Hoehn, H. (1980). Significance of phenotypic and chromosomal abnormalities in X-linked mental retardation (Matin–Bell or Renpenning Syndrome). *American Journal of Medical Genetics* **7**, 417–432.

Lehrke, R. (1971–2). A theory of X-linkage of major intellectual traits. *American Journal of Mental Deficiency* **76**, 611–619.

Lubs, H. A. (1969). A marker X chromosome. *American Journal of Human Genetics* **21**, 231–244.

Sutherland, G. R. (1977). Fragile sites on human chromsomes. Demonstration of their dependence on type of tissue culture medium. *Science* **197**, 265–266.

Turner, G. & Turner, B. (1974). X-linked mental retardation. *Journal of Medical Genetics* **11**, 109–113.

Turner, G., Turner, B. & Collins, E. (1971). X-linked mental retardation without physical abnormality. Renpenning's Syndrome. *Developmental Medicine and Child Neurology* **13**, 71–78.

Turner, G., Eastman, C., Casey, J., McLeay, A., Procopis, P. & Turner, B. (1975). X-linked mental retardation associated with macro-orchidism. *Journal of Medical Genetics* **12**, 367–371.

Turner, G., Gill, R. & Daniel, A. (1978). Marker X chromosome, mental retardation and macro-orchidism. *New England Journal of Medicine* **299**, 1472.

Turner, G., Daniel, A. & Frost, M. (1980). X-linked mental retardation, macro-orchidism and the Xq27 fragile site. *Journal of Pediatrics* **96**, 837–841.

Psychological Medicine, 1982, **12**, 231–233

Chromosome loss and senescence[1]

In most cytogenetic laboratories routine chromosome analyses are carried out on cultured, human lymphocytes. In the majority of individuals a number of these cells are aneuploid, i.e. they are missing, or have gained, one or more chromosomes. A correlation between the percentage of aneuploid cells and age was first shown by Jacobs *et al.* (1961).

Since then, a relationship between increased hypodiploidy (chromosome loss) and age in females has been confirmed by several laboratories (Jacobs *et al.* 1963; Hamerton *et al.* 1965; Sandberg *et al.* 1967; Cadotte & Fraser, 1970; Jarvik & Kato, 1970; Nielsen, 1970; Jarvik *et al.* 1974*b*; Martin *et al.* 1980). The evidence for a similar phenomenon occurring in males is less conclusive, although Martin *et al.* (1980) found that it does occur to a significant extent. The incidence of hyperdiploid cells (where extra chromosomes are present) is very low in both aged and young subjects but does increase slightly with age.

The human chromosome complement can be divided into 7 groups, based on the size and morphology of the chromosomes. Many workers in this field observed that, in females, an excessive number of cells were missing a chromosome from the C/X group and, in males, from the G/Y group. It was suggested that it was the sex chromosomes that were being lost. Although this has not been confirmed in males, the use of Giesma banding has established that one of the X-chromosomes is lost in females (Fitzgerald, 1975; Martin *et al.* 1980).

It appears that there is an overall increase in chromosome loss with age in females and possibly in males. In addition, there appears to be a second process operating in females involving one of the X-chromosomes. Jacobs *et al.* (1963) and Hamerton *et al.* (1965) observed that the incidence of hypodiploidy increased gradually with age in males. In females the pattern was similar until middle age, when the increase in hypodiploid cells underwent a sudden jump. The rate of increase levelled out again at 65–70 years. Martin *et al.* (1980) found that not only had hypodiploidy increased significantly in both sexes when compared with young subjects, but that the incidence in elderly females was also significantly greater than in elderly males. They suggested that this difference could be due to the excessive number of cells missing an X-chromosome in the ageing females.

Before ascertaining how age can cause an increase in hypodiploidy, the factors contributing to the existence of such cells in young subjects must be considered. The incidence of chromosome loss must depend, first, on the frequency of non-disjunction and, secondly, on the ability of the resulting abnormal cells to survive. Jarvik *et al.* (1974*b*) and Nicholls *et al.* (1978) observed that chromosome loss by group in young subjects does not follow a purely random pattern. Both authors also took into consideration the factor of chromosome size on the basis that the smaller the chromosome, the more likely it is to be lost during cell division. Two other factors could promote non-disjunction. Premature centromeric division (PCD) is a process which causes early separation of the centromere during mitosis. The chromatids orientate independently on the spindle; if both move to the same pole a hypodiploid and a hyperdiploid cell will result. A similar outcome will occur if, as suggested by Stadler *et al.* (1965), the presence of heterochromatic 'stickiness' physically delays chromatid separation during mitosis. Once non-disjunction has occurred, the continued existence of the aneuploid cells depends on their ability to survive.

Yunis (1965) considered that survival was dependent on the genetic importance of a chromosome to the cell as a whole. Thus a chromosome with a large amount of late-replicating DNA (which Yunis thought could be an expression of metabolic gene inactivation) would not affect cell survival if it were lost or present in excess. Hoehn (1975) used a similar concept in his construction of an

[1] Address for correspondence: Judith M. Martin, Department of Neuropathology, Institute of Psychiatry, De Crespigny Park, Denmark Hill, London SE5 8AF.

ideogram showing the relative genetic lengths of the chromosomes. The genetic length is the proportion of a chromosome that is genetically active: the greater the genetic length, the more important is the chromosome to cell survival. Nicholls *et al.* (1978) incorporated genetic length (as well as chromosome size) into their model for chromosome loss in young males and females. While the pattern of loss in these subjects conformed very well to the expected values calculated from this model, that of aged subjects was significantly different.

The next problem is how does ageing cause changes in the frequency of non-disjunction and cell survival. Orgel's error theory of ageing (Orgel, 1963, 1970) proposed that an accumulation of abnormal proteins could be caused by specific mutations in structural genes. Martin *et al.* (1980) suggested that such an accumulation of mutations in the appropriate genes could result in inaccurate control of mitosis and an increase in the frequency of non-disjunction – for example by PCD. Stadler *et al.* (1965) postulated that the heterochromatinization of autosomal segments could be under genetic control. A change in the distribution of heterochromatin may cause an increase in delayed chromatid separation and therefore in non-disjunction. In addition, since heterochromatin is generally considered to be genetically inactive, a change in the genetic length of a particular chromosome may decrease its influence on cell survival.

A mechanism for excessive sex chromosome loss was suggested by Hamerton *et al.* (1965). Since the Y-chromosome and one of the X-chromosomes are relatively genetically inactive, aneuploid cells associated with these chromosomes would be more likely to survive than if an autosome were involved. However, they give no explanation as to why this does not occur in young subjects. Fitzgerald (1975) did give such an explanation, at least in females. He found a higher incidence of PCD in women over 60 years than in young subjects. Using Giemsa banding he showed that the chromosome involved was an X-chromosome. The resulting cells had a chromosome complement of 45,X (72%), 47,XXX or with X-'fragments'. This led him to suggest that non-disjunction caused by PCD for some reason results mainly in hypodiploid cells.

Jarvik (1965) suggested the possibility that hypodiploidy may be more frequent in subjects with senile dementia than in aged controls. This was tested by Nielsen (1968, 1970). His results were negative in the males; however, in the females the senile dements (10 subjects) had a significantly greater frequency of chromosome loss than aged controls (10 subjects). Jarvik *et al.* (1971) tested 15 female controls and 8 senile dements with similar results. However, Jarvik *et al.* (1974*a*), using a larger number of subjects (42 controls and 36 senile dements), found that the difference in chromosome loss between the two groups failed to reach significance. They thought a possible reason for this was that, whereas their first group had been resident in the community, the second was taken from old peoples' homes. They also consider that the control group could have included subjects undergoing subtle mental changes, although they appeared physically and mentally normal. This, it was argued, would tend to increase artificially the frequency of hypodiploidy in the control group. However, Martin *et al.* (1981) could find no difference in hypodiploidy between 55 elderly female controls and 46 senile dements. The source of subjects in this survey was similar to that of Nielsen's (long-stay geriatric, surgical and neurological wards and an old peoples' home). Both Jarvik *et al.* (1974*a*) and Martin *et al.* (1981) noted a high degree of individual variation in hypodiploidy, an observation that would make it essential for a suitably large sample to be used in such a survey.

Chromosome loss appears to be influenced only by ageing in general. However, a fruitful line of research could be an investigation into hypodiploidy in patients with pre-senile dementia who are still in their middle age. Two recent papers have been published which show encouraging results with patients with Alzheimer's disease. Both Ward *et al.* (1979) and Nordenson *et al.* (1980) found that most of their Alzheimer patients had a higher degree of hypodiploidy than age- and sex-matched controls.

In conclusion, let us consider some of the implications of increased chromosome loss and ageing. Jarvik *et al.* (1974*a*) suggested that increased hypodiploidy could serve a beneficial purpose: those who have a high frequency of these cells in early life are somehow selected for survival. However, what must be borne in mind is that all the studies on chromosome loss and ageing mentioned in this review have utilized lymphocytes. This would suggest that hypodiploidy could have a detrimental effect on the immune response of an individual. There is evidence that both the immune response and the ability to respond to mitogenic agents (such as phytohaemagglutinin) does decrease with age (Pisciotta *et al.* 1967; Roberts-Thomson *et al.* 1974). The reason for excessive X-chromosome loss in females remains a problem. Jacobs *et al.* (1963) suggested that, as they observed this increased loss to begin between 45 and 65 years, it was in some way associated with hormonal changes occurring at this time.

Obviously, although much progress has been made in the problem of chromosome loss and ageing, many questions still remain unanswered, relating both to the causes of hypodiploidy and its implications to the persons in which it occurs. It is hoped that future research – cytogenetic, biochemical and physiological – will answer these questions.

JUDITH M. MARTIN

REFERENCES

Cadotte, M. & Fraser, D. (1970). Étude de l'aneuploidie observée dans les cultures de sang et de moelle en fonction du nombre et de longeur des chromosomes de chaque groupe et de l'âge et du sexe des sujets. *L'Union Medicale du Canada* **99**, 2003–2007.

Fitzgerald, P. H. (1975). A mechanism of X-chromosome aneuploidy in lymphocytes of ageing women. *Human Genetics* **28**, 153–158.

Hamerton, J. L., Taylor, A. I., Angell, R. & McGuire, V. M. (1965). Chromosome investigations of a small human population: chromosome abnormalities and chromosome counts according to age and sex among the population of Tristan da Cunha. *Nature* (*London*) **206**, 1232–1234.

Hoehn, H. (1975). Functional implications of differential chromosome banding. *American Journal of Human Genetics* **27**, 676–686.

Jacobs, P. A., Court Brown, W. M. & Doll, R. (1961). Distribution of human chromosome counts in relationship to age. *Nature* (*London*) **191**, 1178–1180.

Jacobs, P. A., Brunton, M., Court Brown, W. M., Doll, R. & Goldstein, H. (1963). Change of human chromosome count distributions with age: evidence for a sex difference. *Nature* (*London*) **197**, 1080–1081.

Jarvik, L. F. (1965). Chromosomal changes and ageing. In *Contributions to the Psychology of Ageing* (ed. R. Kastenbaum), pp. 87–88. Springer: New York.

Jarvik, L. F. & Kato, T. (1970). Chromosome examinations in aged twins. *American Journal of Human Genetics* **22**, 562–573.

Jarvik, L. F., Altschuler, K. Z., Kato, T. & Blummer, B. (1971). Organic brain syndrome and chromosome loss in aged twins. *Diseases of the Nervous System* **32**, 159–170.

Jarvik, L. F., Yen, R. S. & Goldstein, F. (1974*a*). Chromosomes and mental status. *Archives of General Psychiatry* **30**, 186–190.

Jarvik, L. F., Yen, R. S. & Moralishvili, E. (1974*b*). Chromosome examinations in ageing institutionalised women. *Journal of Gerontology* **29**, 269–276.

Martin, J. M., Kellett, J. M. & Kahn, J. (1980). Aneuploidy in cultured human lymphocytes: I. Age and sex differences. *Age and Ageing* **9**, 147–153.

Martin, J. M., Kellett, J. M. & Kahn, J. (1981). Aneuploidy in cultured human lymphocytes: II. A comparison between senescence and dementia. *Age and Ageing* **10**, 24–28.

Nicholls, P., Martin, J. M. & Kahn, J. (1978). A mathematical model predicting chromosome loss in cultured cells of young adults. *Journal of Theoretical Biology* **73**, 237–245.

Nielsen, J. (1968). Chromosomes in senile dementia. *British Journal of Psychiatry* **114**, 303–309.

Nielsen, J. (1970). Chromosomes in senile, presenile and arteriosclerotic dementia. *Journal of Gerontology* **25**, 312–315.

Nordenson, I., Adolfsson, R., Beckman, G., Bucht, G. & Winblad, B. (1980). Chromosal abnormality in dementia of Alzheimer type. *Lancet* i, 481–482.

Orgel, L. E. (1963). The maintenance of the accuracy of protein synthesis and its relevance to ageing. *Proceedings of the National Academy of Sciences USA* **49**, 517–521.

Orgel, L. E. (1970). The maintenance of the accuracy of protein synthesis and its relevance to ageing. *Proceedings of the National Academy of Sciences USA* **67**, 1476.

Pisciotta, A. V., Westring, D. W., Deprey, C. & Walsh, B. (1967). Mitogenic effect of phytohaemagglutinin at different ages (human). *Nature* (*London*) **215**, 193–194.

Roberts-Thomson, I. C., Whittingham, S., Youngchaiyud, U. & Mackay, J. R. (1974). Ageing, immune response, and mortality. *Lancet* ii, 368–370.

Sandberg, A. A., Cohen, M. M., Rimm, A. A. & Levine, M. L. (1967). Aneuploidy and age in a population survey. *American Journal of Human Genetics* **19**, 633–643.

Stadler, G. R., Bühler, E. M. & Bühler, U. K. (1965). Possible role of heterochromatin in human aneuploidy. An hypothesis. *Human Genetics* **1**, 307–310.

Ward, B. E., Cook, R. H., Robinson, A. & Austin, J. H. (1979). Increased aneuploidy in Alzheimer disease. *American Journal of Human Genetics* **3**, 137–144.

Yunis, J. J. (1965). Interphase deoxyribonucleic acid condensation, late deoxyribonucleic acid replication and gene inactivation. *Nature* (*London*) **205**, 311–312.

PSYCHOPHARMACOLOGY

Psychological Medicine, 1974, **4**, 353–359

Animal models for evaluating psychotropic drugs

There is still no sure way of determining in animals any elements, precursors, or equivalents of human intrapsychic events and hence much of the pertinent evidence from studies of animal behaviour is at best circumstantial. In the context of 'aberrance' such information is doubly unsatisfactory since the aetiology of most psychiatric conditions is obscure and very little is known about naturally occurring behaviour disorders in animals. In spite of these uneasy foundations, the demands upon workers in this broad field of research continue to increase—the preclinical evaluation of psychotropic drugs is a notable example. The experimenter can find himself trying to identify or reproduce features of human syndromes in animals, but without the necessary basic information and without adequate means of checking the validity of his assumptions. On the one hand, he risks being admonished for trying to mimic epiphenomena, and, on the other, for oversimplifying his constructs to such a degree that applications to man are highly questionable. It is not surprising, therefore, that extrapolations from animal experimental data to the psychiatric clinic are closely hedged with *caveats*.

The basic issues involved have not changed over the years and the central problem has always been that of determining homology—that is, are the behaviour patterns being compared in different species alike both in origin and fundamental structure? It seemed sensible to adopt this criterion from comparative anatomy, but the position has not changed greatly since Russell and his colleagues (National Institute of Mental Health, 1962) noted . . . 'at the present stage of the development of the behavioural sciences it is difficult to establish that apparently similar behavioural patterns are truly homologous'. A broad strategy for research was therefore recommended—in particular, for evaluating psychotropic drugs in animals, but it is of general interest.

It contained a series of steps: (1) the analysis of a human aberrant behaviour pattern for its basic characteristics; (2) the selection of aspects of animal behaviour as similar as possible to these characteristics; (3) a search for chemical agents which might affect these characteristics in animals; (4) tests of the effects of these agents on the human behaviour patterns originally analysed.

These guidelines appear worthwhile and practical but they are not generally followed in the pharmaceutical industry, where the emphasis is on comparisons of empirically derived profiles of new substances with those of established drugs. The shortcomings of this latter strategy, sometimes described as a criterion drug approach, are well known, the most important being the production of 'me-too' relatives at the expense of excluding drugs with novel and unexpected actions. The output of 'new' drugs in the past few years, with one or two exceptions, amply justifies these criticisms.

The reasons behind adopting the criterion drug—as opposed to the criterion behaviour—approach which was embodied in the proposals of Russell and his colleagues (National Institute of Mental Health, 1962) must in part reflect commercial pressures but an important pragmatic factor may be that the behaviourally oriented method is inherently unworkable. The search for behavioural homology, or approximations to it, was implicit in the first two steps of the strategy outlined above. In order to be meaningful, the process of selection of *basic* characteristics from a given human syndrome can hardly ignore questions of origin and of fundamental structure. Knowledge of these matters would make recourse to animal models of academic interest and its lack underlines the fallacy of trying to seek homologies along unspecified parameters. The only way left, then, is to construct parallels based upon associated physiological and gross behavioural symptoms, with the theoretical bias of the experimenter determining the degree to which *a priori* assumptions are made about underlying unitary lesions or disease processes. With these limitations in mind, it is hardly surprising that nearly all the major therapeutic discoveries have been 'in large measure due to chance, the prepared mind and serendipity' (Lasagna, 1964). Occasionally, when drugs have been introduced on purportedly rational grounds they have made little therapeutic impact, and the prospect of having to wait for future inspired clinical observations in unexpected settings is a gloomy one. It is also possible that, as in the past, incorrect hypotheses will sometimes lead to major advances; the logic behind the very first attempts to introduce into psychiatry treatments such as ECT, lithium, and the benzodiazepines can be criticized, while in no way diminishing the importance of the discoveries themselves.

Progress in psychopharmacology has been likened to a process of successive approximations (Steinberg, 1964) in which the two main research tools, drugs and behaviour, are progressively refined with varying emphasis placed upon them in differing studies. The problem, as always, lies in interpreting the data and a natural trend has been to seek for some system and coherence in the increasingly credible neurochemical and physiological substrates of behaviour. The most strikingly successful example of this is provided by the introduction of L-dopa for the treatment of Parkinson's disease. The induction of 'turning' behaviour in rats by lesions in, and/or chemical and electrical stimulation of, the nigrostriatal pathways has provided a most valuable technique (Ungerstedt, 1971a, b). Nevertheless, turning behaviour is not a model of Parkinson's disease; it is a test in rats for studying the effects of specific neuronal disturbances of dopamine. Successful extrapolations to man have depended upon the results of research into the distribution and levels of dopamine and its metabolites in normal and affected human subjects.

MODELS OF SOME PSYCHIATRIC DISORDERS

The elusiveness of structural and other lesions in psychiatric conditions such as schizophrenia and affective disorders has handicapped attempts to develop rationally derived treatments for these states. There have, however, been some recent interesting and provocative developments which illustrate very well the present state of the art of extrapolating between species.

SCHIZOPHRENIA

There are several clues which suggest that disorders of dopamine may underlie aspects of schizophrenic illnesses. The evidence is derived from the possible relationship between the therapeutic potency of neuroleptic drugs and the induction of extrapyramidal effects through some common central action such as blockade of dopamine receptors (Van Rossum, 1966; Randrup and Munkvad, 1972; however, for contrary evidence see Crow and Gillbe, 1973, 1974). Animal studies suggesting that amphetamine-induced stereotyped behaviour is mediated by dopamine (Randrup and Munkvad, 1972) are linked with observations of similar patterns of behaviour in amphetamine psychosis. Similarities between the relative potencies of the stereoisomers of amphetamine in producing stereotypy in animals (Snyder, 1972) and psychosis in human subjects have led Angrist *et al.* (1971) to suggest that 'animal stereotypy . . . should be utilized as an animal model for the human stimulant psychoses', and to point to 'the striking clinical similarity of amphetamine psychosis to paranoid schizophrenia'. The observer is left to ponder the question of common underlying disturbances (Snyder, 1973) in these two conditions which are by no means identical.

Carlsson *et al.* (1973) have reported that concurrent treatment with the tyrosine hydroxylase inhibitor, α-methyl-p-tryosine, potentiates the antipsychotic effects of phenothiazine and butyrophenone drugs. They suggest that, when neuroleptic drugs block central catecholamine receptors, this then induces a compensatory increase in the presynaptic synthesis and release of these amines. Partially inhibiting catecholamine synthesis with α-methyl-p-tyrosine might overcome this putative feedback mechanism and thus enhance the therapeutic effects of these drugs. Both the clinical observations and the suggested underlying mechanisms need further evaluation, but this work illustrates how, at one level, a neurochemical hypothesis can be studied in intact animals without recourse to approximations of the human pathological state. In a behavioural test of the interactions between the two treatments, one sensitive measure was found to be operant responding for food by rats (Ahlenius and Engel, 1971).

Another model for schizophrenia has been proposed (Stein and Wise, 1971) in which it is suggested that an endogenous (abnormal) accumulation of 6-hydroxydopamine results in the deterioration of noradrenergic pathways that mediate reward in the brain; the experiments were done in rats responding for electrical stimulation of such pathways. There is, however, some difficulty in reconciling this intriguing hypothesis with the clinical complexities of schizophrenic states; the authors select as two primary symptoms of schizophrenia the deficit in goal-directed thinking and the capacity to experience pleasure, both of which are assumed to reflect impairment of noradrenergic reinforcement pathways. Detailed studies of the ways in which both dopaminergic and noradrenergic fibres can sustain electrical self-stimulation behaviour (Crow, 1972; 1973) and also of interactions between different fibre systems do not provide unqualified support for formulations in terms of unitary neurophysiological 'lesions', in this particular case resulting in 'a regression to primitive and less goal-directed modes of behaviour regulation' (Stein *et al.*, 1972).

MANIC-DEPRESSIVE DISORDERS

Recently, Ashcroft and his colleagues (M.R.C. Brain Metabolism Unit, 1972) have presented a modified amine hypothesis for the aetiology of affective illness. They emphasize attempts to differentiate sub-groups of patients on both behavioural and metabolic measures and then to link these with observations of the behaviour of animals treated in such ways as to affect the functioning of central transmitter systems. These authors make the point that 'the feeling state and cognitive aspects can only be examined in man . . . It seems however that certain of the behavioural and autonomic changes may have much in common in man and other species'. The methods for inducing such changes in animals do pose a problem, for if surgical or chemical lesions are required to demonstrate these concomitants of 'mood' then their validity is somewhat suspect. Ashcroft and his colleagues (M.R.C. Brain Metabolism Unit, 1972) were obliged to refer to anatomical and functional similarities of higher mammalian nervous systems, disturbances of which result in fragments of behaviour 'which may be the building blocks of more complex adaptive reactions'. A parallel is drawn between chemically induced stereotypies in animals and in man, and apparently purposeless, repetitive behaviour patterns that are sometimes seen clinically—for example, in hypomanic patients or in agitated depression. If such a crucial emphasis is to be placed upon changes in exploratory and stereotyped behaviour patterns in depression and in hypomania, rather careful *clinical* evaluations will be needed of endogenous and chemically induced patterns of stereotypy in man. Would the occurrence and degree of these types of behaviour in the premorbid state have any predictive validity? In animal tests—for example, in rats—the possible value of measures of exploration and stereotypy can lead one to overlook how relatively unsubtle they may be as indices of central transmitter events (Norton, 1973). Measures of apparent purposive locomotor activity, sometimes in novel situations, are generally taken to reflect exploration but there is evidence that amphetamine in low doses actually reduces investigatory behaviour while increasing ambulation. At higher doses stereotypy occurs, but, since purposive locomotion and stereotypy are mutually exclusive components of a rat's repertory of expressed behaviour, this must complicate inferences about dynamic changes in transmitter systems.

ANXIETY STATES AND BEHAVIOUR MODIFICATION

The history of systematic attempts to create animal models of human neurosis dates from the celebrated studies in dogs in Pavlov's laboratory and many reasons have been advanced why these and subsequent experiments have failed to improve substantially our understanding of human neurotic disorders. A prominent feature of such experiments has been the artificiality (for the animal) of the test situation. Nowadays this can be exceedingly complex: lights wink, buzzers sound, electric shocks may be delivered and can be delayed if the animal presses a lever which sometimes also produces food or water. This can result in an exceptional tendency in the subject to suppress its normal responses to such happenings, and in the experimenter, to record only what he set out to measure. Thus when Davis (1968) wrote,

'although it is tempting to discuss the effects of reserpine on "fear" or on "anxiety", it is more productive to discuss the effects of reserpine (i.p.) at 1 mg/kg on conditioned suppression, or more accurately, on conditioned suppression of bar pressing in male Sprague-Dawley rats under a variable interval schedule ($\bar{X} = 30$ sec, range = 5–90 sec) of 45 mg dry food reinforcement, during the presentation of a 1250 cps tone for 60 sec at 92 db upon which the grid delivery of a 2-sec ·8 mA electrical shock was contingent',

he diminished one source of ambiguity but screwed on the lid of the black box even more firmly. There is no denying the place of such experiments in furthering our understanding of how animals learn, for example, to avoid traumatic events such as shocks and to respond to cues which signal food, but questions do arise about the general value of the information so obtained, even within the species and strain being studied. To take one example, signalled electric shocks are widely used to influence animal behaviour, but it is permissible to ask (Bolles, 1970) whether owls normally hoot a few seconds before pouncing on a rat. Similarly, a rat's behaviour is very different when it has to learn to run and jump to avoid shocks than when it has to press a lever. Psychiatrists and psychologists have begun to look carefully at concepts such as 'preparedness' (Marks, 1969; Seligman, 1970) and at species–specific patterns of responding (Bolles, 1970); these radically challenge the premises of general learning theories which hold that all events are equally associable.

In contrast with the immense literature on avoidance of electric shocks by animals there seems only recently to have been an interest in avoidance of other sorts of aversive stimuli. Following on the studies of Garcia and his colleagues (see reviews by Revusky and Garcia, 1970; Seligman, 1970; Rozin and Kalat, 1971), it has become clear that animals can learn to avoid taste cues often after a single pairing with an internal aversive state—for example, nausea after poisoning or irradiation—and that such associations can be formed with great facility. This is in marked contrast with attempts to demonstrate avoidance of noises or lights which have been repeatedly paired with nausea, or tastes paired with electric shocks; there appears, therefore, to be some specificity in this regard. In the light of such observations, there has been a perceptible shift among psychologists towards the recognition of some sort of continuum between instinctive and acquired behaviour. There are also other findings which may be of interest to psychiatrists: the avoidance of taste cues for poisons can develop even if there is a delay of several hours between the presentation of the conditioned stimulus and the onset of the internal, aversive, unconditioned stimulus. It seems unlikely that intermediate cues, such as aftertastes, function as mediators for such learning. One can speculate whether analogous processes may not be involved in the genesis of phobic behaviour. For example, are there particular types of aversive states which link readily with certain conditioned stimuli and not with others; would direct contiguity be unnecessary for the subsequent development of avoidance responses? If some specificity of conditioned and unconditioned stimuli could be identified in this rapid learning paradigm, would not similar considerations be relevant to the modification of such behaviour once it had been acquired?

Techniques of aversion therapy frequently employ discrete episodes of externally applied punishment which are made contiguous with, or consequent on, the behaviour to be changed (Rachman and Teasdale, 1969). Their limited value may partly derive from the fact that behaviour which is acquired in the rather special way discussed above, is less likely to be affected than behaviour that develops gradually over repeated trials. Furthermore, the aversive states engendered by experimentally contrived episodic punishment—for example, electric shocks—may not be biologically relevant to all kinds of maladaptive behaviour patterns and attempts to treat overeating by pairing favourite foods with highly unpleasant odours (Foreyt and Kennedy, 1971) are especially interesting in this context. There are difficulties, however, even when such therapeutic models are made more specific. For example, one might predict that aversion treatment of alcoholism with disulfiram would be more potent than aversion with electric shocks. Yet one must acknowledge that in this case severe nausea and sickness are relatively poor at inducing 'poison' avoidance of alcohol in physically dependent heavy drinkers. But it should be possible to test whether *abstinent*, hospitalized alcoholics given controlled exposures to alcohol and disulfiram would subsequently show a diminished tendeny to relapse.

The efficacy of response prevention in modifying human and animal avoidance behaviour is partly due to the fact that prolongation of the conditioned stimulus renders it ineffective as a cue (Katzev, 1967). However, relatively few trials are needed and an equally important aspect of these procedures may be that the intensely unpleasant emotional state which arises during 'flooding' serves to punish and hence inhibit the subsequent expression of avoidance responses. Critical features of the aversive state must be its intensity and duration and also, especially, its qualitative relevance. This formulation, which focuses primarily on behaviour, is necessarily restricted in its scope and it ignores, for example, questions of meaning, gain, and manipulation.

In animal studies shocks are almost exclusively used as unconditioned stimuli in experiments on the conditioned suppression of appetitive behaviour. It may be that other types of aversive stimuli cannot easily be paired with neutral cues in order reliably to induce conditioned emotional reactions. More detailed explorations of such questions (for example, Best *et al.*, 1973) must increase the validity of animal indices of conditioned fear while perhaps restricting their range. There is one essential proviso: the animal tests cannot be expected to produce plausible models of anxiety states while so little is known *in man* about relationships between 'normal' fear and morbid anxiety. If extrapolations from animals are to have any substance at all in this context, it must at least be demonstrated that a number of 'known' drugs for treating morbid anxiety have consistent effects on analogous tests of experimentally contrived fear in both animals and in man. Drugs such as the benzodiazepines and barbiturates have palliative effects in anxiety states and withholding these drugs typically results in a return of symptoms. Experimental observations in animals (Kumar, 1971a, b) are consistent with clinical findings. This type of drug-induced 'symptom relief' is sometimes confused with the rare phenomenon of state-dependent learning, which is also a function of the presence or absence of a drug in the system. The critical difference is that a drug must first be shown to modify learning or extinction before there is any question of assessing whether the persistence of such newly acquired changes depends upon the maintenance of the drug state of the subject.

DRUG DEPENDENCE

There is one field of research in which there has been surprisingly good agreement between human and animal findings: this is the self-administration of drugs and the development of behavioural and physiological dependence. The great majority of the relevant animal studies have been done in rodents and in primates. Screening methods in animals for drugs with dependence-inducing properties now play an important part in drug evaluation programmes. Data from biochemical and physiological research therefore can be linked with behavioural observations in intact animals and, allowing for interspecific variations, such work provides a coherent framework for clinical investigations of addiction. The very considerable value of such laboratory data might lead one to overlook an apparent paradox—anecdotal reports of drug-seeking behaviour by unconstrained animals in their natural habitats (Forsyth, 1968; Siegel, 1973) do not adequately counter the impression that the repeated voluntary ingestion of centrally acting substances is by and large a peculiarly human pastime.

SOME GENERAL CONSIDERATIONS

Advances in pharmacokinetics have done much to increase the predictive value of tests of drug-behaviour interactions in animals. The discussion here has been around a perhaps more fundamental source of interspecific variation. In the context of drug studies this is described as pharmacodynamic variation, and it is due to inherent differences between the organization and function of integrated systems in intact animals, including limitations of their capabilities. As a practical illustration, studies of antiemetic drugs in rats and mice would be unproductive, since these animals cannot vomit. In the examples of recent research discussed earlier, it was tacitly assumed that, since behavioural and physiological indices covaried with disturbances of feeling, thinking, and perceiving in man, analogous indices in animals could serve as useful tools provided that certain criteria were met. A number of interesting speculations automatically arise, the two poles of which are either that human mental disturbances are more complex but nevertheless homologous versions of more primitive (unknown) mammalian disorders or, alternatively, that they are a new penalty, in an evolutionary sense, for having higher mental development—for example, the ability to think and talk, of itself generates the possibility of disorders of these faculties. This statement could equally well be made in terms of novel central transmitter system interactions and it incorporates the possibility of either reactive or endogenous disorganization.

The underlying issues are sometimes confused, although the implications for research are crucially important. There is no validity to the concept of a phylogenetic continuum with man at the top of a mammalian hierarchy, yet the very process of searching for animal models of human disorders induces a tendency to anthropomorphize and *vice versa*. A naked ape may more easily ignore Scott's (1967) warning not to think of monkeys as small people with fur coats. The search for valid animal models and for structural and functional 'common denominators' must therefore take into account the divergent lines of the phylogenetic tree. In the light of this it seems wishful to expect, for example, that *analogous* behavioural studies in a variety of species will necessarily illuminate subtle motivational changes that may be induced by centrally acting drugs. Apart from purely empirical evaluations, it is difficult to see how batteries of tests of operant responding applied to monkeys, rats, and pigeons can be meaningfully interpreted. Indeed, the outcome tends to be an emphasis on the reinforcement schedules employed with, consequently, a diminished appreciation of species differences and independent lines of development. Attempts to take account of such factors are hindered, as Hodos and Campbell (1969) have pointed out, by the fact that evolutionary insights cannot be derived in the usual way, since there are no behavioural fossils.

In spite of, or perhaps because of, all these hazards, the comparative approach to behaviour is both challenging and exciting and it allows little room for fixed opinions and expectations. There is no *a priori* reason why even if homologous patterns of normal or aberrant behaviour are adequately characterized, they should necessarily resemble each other any more than a bat's wing does a hand. Alternatively, through ecological convergence, analogous forms may in fact represent the end points of quite different lines of development. Thus it is extremely difficult to interpret the few recorded instances of self-mutilative behaviour in animals (Lester, 1972); the apparent resemblance between 'superstitious' behaviour in animals and obsessive-compulsive behaviour in man poses similar problems. In the same vein, Roth and Kerr (1970) have commented that both depression and suicide are unknown quantities in animals, and this could apply to any psychiatric disorder. The definition of a behavioural event such as suicide in man is of little help; how would one know whether an animal had committed suicide?

The main need, in the first instance, seems to be for a closer dialogue between the clinic and the laboratory and recent developments in formulating and studying behavioural analogies of depressive disorders are good examples of this. Studies of learned helplessness (Seligman *et al.*, 1971), of disturbances of dominance hierarchies (Price, 1967), or of lasting consequences of mother–infant separations (Hinde and Spencer Booth, 1971) all attempts to tackle different aspects of the problem under controlled conditions in laboratory animals. The extent to which the findings are meaningful in terms of man can be established only by further research to which such studies themselves serve as pointers. The data cannot, however, provide more than a basis for speculation until matching clinical information has been gathered in man to check the validity of the assumptions being tested; this is a recurring need throughout the whole field. A telling point was made by Tinbergen (1968) in a slightly different context: 'Psychiatrists, at least many of them, show a disturbing tendency to apply the *results* rather than the *methods* of ethology to man'.

R. KUMAR

REFERENCES

Ahlenius, S., and Engel, J. (1971). Behavioral effects of haloperidol after tryosine hydroxylase inhibition. *European Journal of Pharmacology*, **15**, 187–192,

Angrist, B. M., Shopsin, B., and Gershon, S. (1971). Comparative psychotomimetic effects of stereoisomers of amphetamine. *Nature*, **234**, 152–153.

Best, P. J., Best, M. R., and Mickley, G. A. (1973). Conditioned aversion to distinct environmental stimuli resulting from gastrointestinal distress. *Journal of Comparative and Physiological Psychology*, **85**, 250–257.

Bolles, R. C. (1970). Species-specific defense reactions and avoidance learning. *Psychological Review*, **77**, 32–48.

Carlsson, A., Roos, B.-E., Wålinder, J., and Skott, A. (1973). Further studies on the mechanism of antipsychotic action: potentiation by α-methyltyrosine of Thiordazine effects in chronic schizophrenics. *Journal of Neural Transmission*, **34**, 125–132.

Crow, T. J. (1972). Catecholamine-containing neurones and electrical self-stimulation: 1. a review of some data. *Psychological Medicine*, **2**, 414–421.

Crow, T. J. (1973). Catecholamine-containing neurones and electrical self-stimulation: 2. a theoretical interpretation and some psychiatric implications. *Psychological Medicine*, **3**, 66–73.

Crow, T. J., and Gillbe, C. (1973). Dopamine antagonism and antischizophrenic potency of neuroleptic drugs. *Nature*, **245**, 27–28.

Crow, T. J., and Gillbe, C. (1974). Brain dopamine and behaviour: a critical analysis of the relationship between dopamine antagonism and the therapeutic efficacy of neuroleptic drugs. *Journal of Psychiatric Research*. (In press.)

Davis, H. (1968). Conditioned suppression: a survey of the literature. *Psychonomic Monograph*, Suppl. **2**, 283–291.

Foreyt, J. P., and Kennedy, W. A. (1971). Treatment of overweight by aversion therapy. *Behaviour Research and Therapy*, **9**, 29–34.

Forsyth, A. A. (1968). *British Poisonous Plants*. 2nd edn. Bulletin No. 161. Ministry of Agriculture, Fisheries and Food. H.M.S.O.: London.

Hinde, R. A., and Spencer-Booth, Y. (1971). Effects of brief separation from mother on rhesus monkeys. *Science*, **173**, 111–118.

Hodos, W., and Campbell, C. B. G. (1969). *Scala naturae*: why there is no theory in comparative psychology. *Psychological Review*, **76**, 337–350.

Katzev, R. (1967). Extinguishing avoidance responses as a function of delayed warning signal termination. *Journal of Experimental Psychology*, **75**, 339–344.

Kumar, R. (1971a). Extinction of fear. 1. Effects of amylobarbitone and dexamphetamine given separately and in combination on fear and exploratory behaviour in rats. *Psychopharmacologia*, **19**, 163–187.

Kumar, R. (1971b). Extinction of fear. 2. Effects of chlordiazepoxide and chlorpromazine on fear and exploratory behaviour in rats. *Psychopharmacologia*, **19**, 297–312.

Lasagna, L. (1964). On evaluating drug therapy: the nature of the evidence. In *Drugs in our Society*, Edited by P. Talalay. Johns Hopkins Press: Baltimore.

Lester, D. (1972). Self-mutilating behavior. *Psychological Bulletin*, **78**, 119–128.

Marks, I. M. (1969). *Fears and Phobias*. Heinemann: London.

Medical Research Council Brain Metabolism Unit (1972). Modified amine hypothesis for the aetiology of affective illness. *Lancet*, **2**, 573–577.

National Institute of Mental Health (1962). *Behavioral Research in Preclinical Psychopharmacology: Issues of Design and Techniques*. Prepared by The Pharmacology Unit, and The Committee on Preclinical Psychopharmacology, Psychopharmacology Service Center. U.S. Public Health Service Publication No. 968. Government Printing Office: Washington.

Norton, S. (1973). Amphetamine as a model for hyperactivity in the rat. *Physiology and Behavior*, **11**, 181–186.

Price, J. (1967). The dominance hierarchy and the evolution of mental illness. *Lancet*, **2**, 243–246.

Rachman, S., and Teasdale, J. (1969). *Aversion Therapy and Behaviour Disorders. An Analysis*. Routledge: London.

Randrup, A., and Munkvad, I. (1970). Biochemical, anatomical and physiological investigations of stereotyped behaviour induced by amphetamines. In *Symposium on Amphetamine and Related Drugs*, pp. 695–713. Edited by E. Costa and S. Garattini. Raven Press: New York.

Randrup, A., and Munkvad, I. (1972). Evidence indicating an association between schizophrenia and dopaminenergic hyperactivity in the brain. *Orthomolecular Psychiatry*, **1**, 2–7.

Revusky, S., and Garcia, J. (1970). Learned associations over long delays. In *Psychology of Learning and Motivation Advances in Research and Theory*. **4**, 1–84. Edited by G. H. Bower, Academic Press: New York.

Roth, M., and Kerr, T. A. (1970). Diagnosis of the reactive depressive illnesses. In *Modern Trends in Psychological Medicine. 2*, pp. 165–199. Edited by J. H. Price. Butterworths: London.

Rozin, P., and Kalat, J. W. (1971). Specific hungers and poison avoidance as adaptive specializations of learning. *Psychological Review*, **78**, 459–486.

Scott, J. P. (1967). Comparative psychology and ethology. *Annual Review of Psychology*, **18**, 65–86.

Seligman, M. E. P. (1970). On the generality of the laws of learning. *Psychological Review*, **77**, 406–418.

Seligman, M. E. P., Maier, S. F., and Solomon, R. L. (1971). Unpredictable and uncontrollable aversive events. In *Aversive Conditioning and Learning*, pp. 347–400. Edited by F. R. Brush. Academic Press: New York.

Siegel, R. K. (1973). An ethological search for self-administration of hallucinogens. *International Journal of the Addictions*, **8**, 373–393.

Snyder, S. H. (1972). Catecholamines in the brain as mediators of amphetamine psychosis. *Archives of General Psychiatry*, **27**, 169–179.

Snyder, S. H. (1973). Amphetamine psychosis: a model schizophrenia mediated by catecholamines. *American Journal of Psychiatry*, **130**, 61–67.

Stein, L., and Wise, C. D. (1971). Possible etiology of schizophrenia: progressive damage to the noradrenergic reward system by 6-hydroxydopamine. *Science*, **171**, 1032–1036.

Stein, L., Wise, C. D., and Berger, B. D. (1972). Noradrenergic reward mechanisms, recovery of function, and schizophrenia. In *The Chemistry of Mood, Motivation, and Memory*, pp. 81–103. Edited by J. L. McGaugh, Plenum Press: New York.

Steinberg, H. (1964). Drugs and animal behaviour. *British Medical Bulletin*, **20**, 75–80.

Tinbergen, N. (1968). On war and peace in animals and man. *Science*, **160**, 1411–1418.

Ungerstedt, U. (1971a). Striatal dopamine release after amphetamine or nerve degeneration revealed by rotational behaviour. *Acta Physiologica Scandinavica*, Suppl. 367, 49–68.

Ungerstedt, U. (1971b). Postsynaptic supersensitivity after 6-hydroxy-dopamine induced degeneration of the nigrostriatal dopamine system. *Acta Physiologica Scandinavica*, Suppl. **367**, 69–93.

Van Rossum, J. M. (1966). The significance of dopamine receptor blockade for the mechanism of action of neuroleptic drugs. *Archives Internationales de Pharmacodynamie et de Thérapie*, **160**, 492–494.

Psychological Medicine, 1974, **4**, 125–129

Pharmacogenetics and mental disease

As the array of potent behaviour-modifying drugs has grown, physicians employing these agents have become increasingly aware of the striking differences among individuals in therapeutic effectiveness and side-effects of the drugs (Omenn and Motulsky, 1973). These differences may be caused by different rates of biotransformation or elimination of the pharmacologically active species, different susceptibility to the drug action on specific cell receptors, or different mechanisms underlying a common psychiatric syndrome.

PHARMACOGENETICS OF SPECIFIC DRUGS

General discussion of the pharmacogenetics of specific drugs may be found in Kalow (1962), Motulsky (1964), Evans (1969), and Omenn and Motulsky (1973).

SUCCINYL CHOLINE (SUXAMETHONIUM) This depolarizing muscle relaxant is used widely in premedication for anaesthesia and for electroconvulsive therapy, because of its rapid onset and short duration of action. However, suxamethonium will paralyse breathing for several hours in the one in 2,500 Caucasians who has an abnormal form of the plasma enzyme pseudocholinesterase. A perfectly normal individual is genetically susceptible to a drug-induced catastrophe because the enzyme required to inactivate the drug does not function properly. In the absence of the drug, there are no known abnormalities. The psychiatrist or anaesthetist should inquire about personal or family history of sensitivity to suxamethonium; a simple screening test is available (Morrow and Motulsky, 1968). Equipment for sustained respiratory assistance should be at hand.

ACETYLATION IN THE LIVER The antituberculosis agent isoniazid (INH) and a number of other drugs are inactivated in the liver by an acetylating enzyme. Population screening shows that about 50% of Caucasians and Negroes and 15% of Orientals are 'slow acetylators', due to less activity of the enzyme; family studies prove that the trait is determined by a single gene. Since slow acetylators develop higher blood levels of drug on a standard dose, peripheral neuropathy from INH, CNS, and gastrointestinal symptoms from the antidepressant phenelzine (Nardil) (Evans *et al.*, 1965), and a lupus-like syndrome from hydralazine (Apresoline) occur in slow acetylators and not in rapid acetylators. Greater therapeutic effectiveness of phenelzine was reported for patients with neurotic depression who were slow acetylators (Johnstone and Marsh, 1973). Slow acetylators taking INH also are much more sensitive to toxicity from phenytoin (Dilantin), because INH in high concentrations inhibits metabolism of phenytoin and other drugs (Kutt, 1971).

OXIDANT DRUGS AND G6PD DEFICIENCY Glucose-6-phosphate dehydrogenase (G6PD) is the first enzyme of the energy-generating pentose-phosphate shunt pathway, essential to maintaining the integrity of the red blood cell. Deficiency of G6PD occurs with significant frequency in many population groups originating in subtropical and tropical countries, such as Africans, Southeast Asians, Indians, and Mediterraneans. Many drugs can precipitate acute haemolytic anaemia in these otherwise healthy but genetically predisposed individuals (Motulsky, 1972). The drug does not interact directly with the abnormal enzyme; rather, the red cells are more susceptible to drug injury. Several different mutations affecting G6PD cause enzyme deficiency. The Mediterranean-type G6PD deficiency is more severe than the Negro type, hence a larger number of drugs are a threat (Motulsky, 1972). Haemolytic anaemia caused by eating fava or broad beans (favism) occurs only in G6PD-deficient persons.

TRICYCLIC ANTIDEPRESSANTS: NORTRIPTYLINE The likelihood of side-effects from nortriptyline is correlated with the plasma concentration of the drug and not with the dose administered. Twin studies and family studies indicate a major role for genetic factors in the rate of elimination of nortriptyline, but the biochemical basis for individual differences is not yet known (Alexanderson and Sjöqvist, 1971).

PHARMACOGENETICS IN SPECIFIC MENTAL DISORDERS

DEPRESSION (AFFECTIVE DISORDERS) There is considerable evidence from twin and family studies that depressions (especially manic-depressive psychosis) are conditioned by genetic factors (Gershon *et al.*, 1971). According to the biogenic amine hypothesis (Schildkraut, 1969), depression appears to be associated with decreased action or turnover of noradrenaline (NE) and serotonin, while manic states are associated with increased biogenic amine turnover. Pharmacogenetic agents which deplete NE from nerve terminals (reserpine) or interfere with its biosynthesis (alpha-methyl tyrosine, alpha-methyl dopa) may precipitate depression. Drugs which enhance biosynthesis of NE (L-dopa) may induce hypomanic states, and agents which prolong the action of NE by inhibiting intraneuronal monoamine oxidase (MAO inhibitors) or the neuronal re-uptake of NE released into the synapse (tricyclics) are effective antidepressants. Electroconvulsive shock also acts to increase tyrosine hydroxylase activity and NE turnover (Musacchio *et al.*, 1969). Clinical observations suggest likely pharmacogenetic relationships among patients with depression. Thus, Pare *et al.* (1962) reported that two groups of patients could be differentiated by their response to either MAO inhibitors or tricyclic compounds (Pare *et al.*, 1962; Pare and Mack, 1971). In their experience, patients who responded to one class of antidepressant tended not to respond to the other. Patients showed the same pattern of pharmacological responsiveness during a subsequent episode of depression, which might have been precipitated by quite different life stresses. Also, relatives who had affective disorders shared the pattern of pharmacological responsiveness or unresponsiveness. Angst obtained comparable results with imipramine in family studies (Angst, 1964). While additional studies with placebo controls are required to substantiate these findings, it is easy to conceive of variations at each of the steps in biogenic amine biosynthesis and metabolism that would produce individual differences in the effectiveness of drugs in ameliorating or inducing affective disorders (Omenn, 1973a). About 10% of the patients treated with reserpine will develop depression (Harris, 1957). These patients have a history of affective disorder more often than do the 90% of reserpine-treated patients who do not develop depression. Reserpine depletes neuronal stores of NE and serotonin and induces increased activity of tyrosine hydroxylase, the rate-limiting step for biosynthesis of NE. Individuals may differ in their capacity to step up NE biosynthesis or individuals with low-normal stores of NE might be more severely depleted at similar doses of reserpine. Whatever the mechanism, reserpine unmasks a predisposition to depression. It should be emphasized that so general a phenotype as depression is likely to be predisposed to or mediated by multiple mechanisms, even if various alterations in biogenic amine metabolism serve as a common pathogenetic pathway. Differential responses to therapy and differential susceptibility to precipitation of attacks with reserpine or alpha methyl dopa or ACTH may provide insights and investigational 'handles' into the heterogeneous causes of the affective disorders.

SCHIZOPHRENIA Particular phenothiazines do not appear to be relatively better than others for different clinical subtypes of schizophrenic illness (Hollister, 1970). The extrapyramidal side effects of phenothiazines, however, do occur at a lower dose and with higher incidence in patients with a family history of spontaneous Parkinson's disease (Myrianthopoulos *et al.*, 1969). Given the evidence for genetic predisposition to schizophrenia (Rosenthal, 1970), one may wonder whether individuals who have a schizophrenic-like reaction to amphetamines or LSD are genetically predisposed to such psychotic reactions and would have been at a relatively high risk for development of 'spontaneous' schizophrenia. Pharmacological deductions have focused attention on dopamine as a possible neurotransmitter mediator of at least some types of schizophrenia. The active groups of potent antipsychotic phenothiazines, when viewed in a three-dimensional molecular model, appear to resemble the molecular conformation of dopamine (Horn and Snyder, 1971). The equivalence of D- and L-amphetamine in inducing psychosis also points to involvement of dopamine (Snyder *et al.*, 1970; Angrist *et al.*, 1971).

SEIZURE DISORDERS The normal pattern of electrical activity in the brain, as measured by the electroencephalogram (EEG), is determined almost entirely by multiple genetic factors (Vogel, 1970). Several single-gene mediated variants of the normal EEG have been described, affecting altogether about 15% of the general population (Vogel, 1970). The clinical significance of these variants is unknown. Studies are needed to determine whether individuals with different baseline EEG patterns have different responses to various psychopharmacological agents. The variety of anticonvulsive agents employed in clinical seizure disorders, for which biochemical mechanisms have yet to be elucidated, do not correlate very closely with clinical categories of seizure disorder. Family studies to explore pharmacogenetic relationships have not yet been performed.

DRUGS OF ABUSE AND ADDICTION SYNDROMES The most commonly abused agent, of course, is ethanol. Individuals differ markedly in tolerance for alcohol and in susceptibility to its effects. Recent studies with half siblings have shown that the excess familial incidence of alcoholism is among the biologically-related and not the adoptive family members, pointing to genetic rather than environmental influences (Schuckit, 1972). Genetic factors could play a role in variation of the acute intoxicating effects of alcohol, in the likelihood of chronic addiction, and in the risk of medical and behavioural complications (Omenn and Motulsky, 1972). Genetic factors are almost entirely responsible for individual differences in the rate of elimination of ethanol from the blood (Vesell *et al.*, 1971). Eskimos and Indians metabolize ethanol less rapidly than do Caucasians in western Canada (Fenna *et al.*, 1971). Most Oriental adults and infants show facial flushing and increased pulse pressure after doses of alcohol that have little or no effect on Caucasians (Wolff, 1972). The relationship between acute intoxication and chronic addiction is a central mystery in this field.

Among children born to mothers who were chronic alcoholics, a striking new syndrome has been recognized (Jones *et al.*, 1973). These children have retarded intrauterine and post-natal physical and mental development, microcephaly, decreased width to the palpebral fissure causing the eyes to appear rounded, and variable limb and cardiac malformations. The toxic mechanism and genetic variation in susceptibility have yet to be investigated. Caucasian, Negro, and American Indian children have been recognized to be affected.

MINIMAL BRAIN DYSFUNCTION—HYPERKINETIC YOUNGSTERS These children, usually boys, have motor hyperactivity, distractibility, impulsivity, and a learning performance below objective expectations. Some of them, but clearly not the majority, respond strikingly to such stimulant drugs as amphetamine and methylphenidate. The variation in responsiveness to these drugs may reflect differences in the metabolism of the drug, in the susceptibility to the drug action at the level of some cell enzyme or cell membrane, or in the underlying processes which lead to the behavioural problems. Studies are in progress to try to differentiate these possibilities (Omenn, 1973a).

SIMPLY-INHERITED BEHAVIOURAL DISORDERS WITH SPECIAL VULNERABILITY TO DRUGS Examples of autosomal dominant, autosomal recessive, and X-linked recessive diseases affecting the nervous system can be cited in which patients are usually susceptible to specific drugs (Cohen and Weber, 1972). Patients with Swedish or South African porphyria, in which there is a block in heme biosynthesis, may suffer their first attack when barbiturates, certian sulphonamides, the anti-fungal agent griseofulvin, and possibly anaesthetics, ethanol, or chloroquine are taken. The significance of preoperative or postoperative medications, especially 'routine sleeping pills', may be overlooked unless this diagnosis is considered in a patient with acute schizophrenic or paranoid psychosis. Acute porphyric attacks may remit with infusions of haematin (Watson *et al.*, 1973). Patients with Huntington's chorea develop increased choreiform movements on L-dopa; it is not clear whether the L-dopa affects their psychological or intellectual status. The proposal that administration of L-dopa be used to detect asymptomatic carriers of the gene for Huntington's disease (Klawans *et al.*, 1972) should be viewed with great caution, since the patient observes the test result, the rate of false positives or false negatives is unknown, and it is conceivable that L-dopa might even accelerate the degenerative process. The Lesch-Nyhan syndrome, an X-linked recessive condition, is characterized by choreoathetosis and a bizarre, compulsive behaviour with self-mutilation of lips, fingers, and eyes. There is deficiency of an enzyme of purine metabolism, leading to abnormal metabolism of such agents as 6-mercaptopurine, azathioprine (Imuran), and allopurinol. Finally, several of the inborn errors of metabolism that lead to mental retardation can be ameliorated by treatment with special dietary regimens, which might be considered a particular form of interaction between genotype and exogenous agent. Thus, diets restricted in phenylalanine or galactose are effective in preventing the development of mental retardation in patients with phenylketonuria and galactosemia, respectively. When an inherited enzyme abnormality causes decreased affinity for an essential coenzyme, exogenous administration of the coenzyme in massive doses may be effective. Examples are homocystinuria and methylmalonic aciduria. The finding of rare enzyme abnormalities in co-factor binding has refuelled the suggestion that individual variability in requirements for such dietary factors might lead to dietary deficiencies on the 'usual recommended daily dose' of these vitamins (Williams, 1956). Nevertheless, there is no evidence at this point that massive doses of nicotinic acid or vitamin C or other common vitamins will ameliorate schizophrenia or enhance intelligence.

The examples given here of genetically-determined variation in the metabolism of certain commonly used drugs or in the risk of side-effects probably represent only the tip of the iceberg in understanding the host-drug interaction in clinical medicine. From the point of view of investigating common psychiatric syndromes, the variation in patients' responses to commonly used pharmacological agents offers one of the most promising 'handles' on differentiating multiple causes of apparently similar clinical syndromes. We may hope that such pharmacogenetic investigation will lead to more rational therapy tailored to the needs of individual patients.

GILBERT S. OMENN AND ARNO G. MOTULSKY

The work was supported by grant GM 15253 and a Research Development Award (G.S.O.) from the U.S. Public Health Service.

REFERENCES

Alexanderson, B., and Sjöqvist, F. (1971). Individual differences in the pharmacokinetics of monomethylated tricyclic antidepressants: role of the genetic and environmental factors and clinical importance. *Annals of the New York Academy of Sciences*, **179**, 739–751.

Angrist, B. M., Shopsin, B., and Gershon, S. (1971). The comparative psychotomimetic effects of stereoisomers of amphetamine. *Nature*, **234**, 152–153.

Angst, J. (1964). Antidepressiver Effekt and genetische Faktoren. *Arzneimittelforschung*, **14**, Suppl. 496–500.

Cohen, S. N., and Weber, W. W. (1972). Pharmacogenetics. *Pediatric Clinics of North America*, **19**, 21–36.

Evans, D. A. P. (1969). Pharmacogenetics. In *Selected Topics in Medical Genetics*, pp. 69–109. Edited by C. A. Clarke. Oxford University Press: London.

Evans, D. A. P., Davison, K., and Pratt, R. T. C. (1965). The influence of acetylator phenotype on the effects of treating depression with phenelzine. *Clinical Pharmacology and Therapeutics*, **6**, 430–435.

Fenna, D., Mix, L., Schaefer, O., and Gilbert, J. A. L. (1971). Ethanol metabolism in various racial groups. *Canadian Medical Association Journal*, **105**, 472–475.

Gershon, E. S., Dunner, D. L., and Goodwin, F. K. (1971). Toward a biology of affective disorders. Genetic contributions. *Archives of General Psychiatry*, **25**, 1–15.

Harris, T. H. (1957). Depression induced by Rauwolfia compounds. *American Journal of Psychiatry*, **113**, 950.

Hollister, L. E. (1970). Choice of antipsychotic drugs. *American Journal of Psychiatry*, **127**, 186–190.

Horn, A. S., and Snyder, S. H. (1971). Chlorpromazine and dopamine: conformational similarities that correlate with the antischizophrenic activity of phenothiazine drugs. *Proceedings of the National Academy of Sciences*, **68**, 2325–2328.
Johnstone, E. C., and Marsh, W. (1973). Acetylator status and response to phenelzine in depressed patients. *Lancet*, **1**, 567–570.
Jones, K. L., Smith, D. W., Ulleland, C. N., and Streissguth, A. P. (1973). Pattern of malformation in offspring of chronic alcoholic mothers. *Lancet*, **1**, 1267–1271.
Kalow, W. (1962). *Pharmacogenetics: Heredity and the Response to Drugs*. Saunders: Philadelphia.
Klawans, H. L., Jr., Paulson, G. W., Ringel, S. P., and Barbeau, A. (1972). Use of L-dopa in the detection of presymptomatic Huntington's chorea. *New England Journal of Medicine*, **286**, 1332–1334.
Kutt, H. (1971). Biochemical and genetic factors regulating Dilantin metabolism in man. *Annals of the New York Academy of Sciences*, **179**, 705–722.
Morrow, A. C., and Motulsky, A. G. (1968). Rapid screening method for the common atypical pseudocholinesterase variant. *Journal of Laboratory and Clinical Medicine*, **71**, 350–356.
Motulsky, A. G. (1972). Hemolysis in glucose-6-phosphate dehydrogenase deficiency. *Federation Proceedings*, **31**, 1286–1292.
Motulsky, A. G. (1964). Pharmacogenetics. *Progress in Medical Genetics*, **3**, 49–74.
Musacchio, J. M., Julou, L., Kety, S. S., and Glowinski, S. S. (1969). Increase in rat brain tyrosine hydroxylase activity produced by electroconvulsive shock. *Proceedings of the National Academy of Sciences*, **63**, 1117–1119.
Myrianthopoulos, N. C., Waldrop, F. N., and Vincent, B. L. (1969). A repeat study of hereditary predisposition in drug-induced parkinsonism. In *Progress in Neuro-Genetics*. Edited by A. Barbeau and J.-R. Brunette. Excerpta Medica: Amsterdam. *International Congress Series No. 175*, 486–491.
Omenn, G. S. (1973a). Genetic issues in the syndrome of minimal brain dysfunction. *Seminars in Psychiatry*, **5**, 5–17.
Omenn, G. S. (1973b). A pharmacogenetic approach to depression, in Bruell, J. (ed.), *Prospects in Behavior Genetics*. Russell Sage Foundation: New York. (In press.)
Omenn, G. S., and Motulsky, A. G. (1972). A biochemical and genetic approach to alcoholism. *Annals of the New York Academy of Sciences*, **197**, 16–23.
Omenn, G. S., and Motulsky, A. G. (1973). Pharmacogenetics. *Year Book of Drug Therapy, 1973*, pp. 5–26. Year Book Medical Publishers: Chicago.
Pare, C. M. B., and Mack, J. W. (1971). Differentiation of two genetically specific types of depression by the response to antidepressant drugs. *Journal of Medical Genetics*, **8**, 306–309.
Pare, C. M. B., Rees, L., and Sainsbury, M. J. (1962). Differentiation of two genetically specific types of depression by the response to anti-depressants. *Lancet*, **2**, 1340–1343.
Rosenthal, D. (1970). *Genetic Theory and Abnormal Behavior*, pp. 92–200. McGraw-Hill: New York.
Schildkraut, J. J. (1969). Neuropsychopharmacology and the affective disorders. *New England Journal of Medicine*, **281**, 197–201, 248–255, 302–308.
Schuckit, M. A. (1972). Family history and half-sibling research in alcoholism. *Annals of the New York Academy of Sciences*, **197**, 121–125.
Snyder, S. H., Taylor, K. M., Coyle, J. T., and Meyerhoff, J. L. (1970). The role of brain dopamine in behavioral regulation and the actions of psychotropic drugs. *American Journal of Psychiatry*, **127**, 199–207.
Vesell, E. S., Page, J. G., and Passananti, G. T. (1971). Genetic and environmental factors affecting ethanol metabolism in man. *Clinical Pharmacology and Therapeutics*, **12**, 192–201.
Vogel, F. (1970). The genetic basis of the normal human electroencephalogram (EEG). *Humangenetik*, **10**, 91–114.
Watson, C. J., Dhar, G. J., Bossenmaier, I., Cardinal, R., and Petryka, Z. J. (1973). Effect of hematin in acute porphyric relapse. *Annals of Internal Medicine*, **79**, 80–83.
Williams, R. J. (1956). *Biochemical Individuality*. Wiley: New York.
Wolff, P. H. (1972). Ethnic differences in alcohol sensitivity. *Science*, **175**, 449–450.

Psychological Medicine, 1978, **8**, 177–180

Pharmacokinetics and psychotropic drugs[1]

The current wave of interest in pharmacokinetics of psychotropic drugs has its origins in the writings of Brodie in the years between 1960 and 1970 (for review see Brodie, 1967). Strictly speaking, the science of pharmacokinetics is concerned with rates of transfer of drug molecules within the body. Less strictly, it is the study of drug concentrations in plasma. A lifetime of research in drug analysis, and in the study of drug absorption, metabolism and excretion, had led Brodie to believe that many hitherto poorly controlled drug responses could be brought under control by changing the plasma levels of the drugs concerned. There seemed no reason why this idea should not apply equally to drugs acting on the central nervous system as to drugs affecting other systems, in spite of the blood–brain barrier, and so Brodie encouraged a number of workers to commence investigations of tranquillizers and antidepressants in this light (Curry & Brodie, 1967; Hammer & Brodie, 1967; Garattini *et al.* 1973). In the meantime, other workers were investigating lithium (Schou, 1969). However, in spite of more than 10 years of this work, and in spite of the fact that pharmacokinetic control has been a major factor in the use of lithium, fundamental misunderstandings remain. We are repeatedly asked: 'What should we measure, and with what methods?' 'What is the relation with effect?' 'Is there a clinically desirable concentration?'

Analytical methods are the oldest problem. Without good methods the work could not start. The major analytical achievements relevant to this work were the application of isotope derivative analysis to tricyclic antidepressants (Hammer & Brodie, 1967), and of gas-chromatography with electron capture detection to phenothiazines, and to benzodiazepines (Curry, 1968; Garattini *et al.* 1973). Later, combined gas-chromatography/mass spectrometry came prominently into the picture. In the hands of careful workers, these techniques now give reliable data. Provided reasonable precision and accuracy are demonstrated to have been achieved in any laboratory for a specific compound, the exact details of the method used in that laboratory are not important. For instance, at an absurd level, the shape of the test tubes does not matter if the method is proved adequate. However, authors have been able to claim significant modifications by doing obvious things, such as doubling the sample size to double sensitivity. Even so, the complexities are great. For example, chlorpromazine is partially converted to chlorpromazine *N*-oxide in the body. Reduction of the metabolite, present in plasma, back to chlorpromazine apparently occurs on storage of samples, and during analytical work-up. Unless strenuous efforts are made to prevent this reduction, inflated chlorpromazine data are obtained. So the chlorpromazine content of the sample may appear to increase on storage or, at best, appear to be erratic, Now, reduction in assay results on storage is all very well, but an increase? I cite this example to demonstrate the need for detailed knowledge of the chemistry involved in such work. Each group of workers should be asked for details of precision and accuracy of methods as used in its own laboratories.

Another point of relevance to the assays is that authors are not always specific regarding fluids measured. 'Blood levels' and 'plasma levels', to say nothing of 'serum levels', are still used as interchangeable terms. Additionally, centrifugation conditions for plasma are rarely checked to determine whether any haemolysis or cell contamination occurs. Haemolysis can increase the chance of a distorted assay, because of a difference in drug concentrations in the fluid of red cells and of plasma. If the drug is localized in red cells, haemolysis inflates the plasma concentration. If the drug fails to penetrate red cells, haemolysis reduces the plasma concentration.

Pharmacokinetic studies are the best way of studying the pharmacokinetic phenomena of absorption and elimination in their own right and, related to this, of obtaining data on such matters as bioavailability and drug interactions. They also assist detection of non-compliance in tablet-taking, although, for complex reasons associated with metabolism of oral doses during the first-pass through

[1] Address for correspondence: Dr S. H. Curry, The London Hospital Medical College, Turner Street, London E1 2AD.

the liver, urinary excretion of metabolites may be a better guide to this particular problem. However, it is in relation to effect that the subject comes into its own. In this regard there is a major problem of what to include. Most of the psychotropic drugs are converted to many metabolites. Some of these metabolites are polar and inactive. Some are rapidly removed from the body once formed and therefore not detected in plasma, in accord with the normal function of drug metabolism – to make excretion possible. Others have significant activity, for example, desipramine as a metabolite of imipramine. Investigators are faced with the need to categorize those metabolites which appear in plasma as 'active' or 'inactive' and this must usually be done with only *in vitro* work as a guide, because direct human studies with drug metabolites are rarely possible. When such studies are possible, the data are often equivocal. For example, chlorpromazine sulphoxide 'failed' in clinical studies, and a habit is developing of designating this compound as inactive. However, it has one-seventh the sedative activity of chlorpromazine and the antipsychotic effect was not really assessed in the studies concerned (Davidson *et al.* 1957; Sakalis *et al.* 1973).

When more than one apparently active compound is found in plasma, for example, imipramine and desipramine following imipramine administration, the dilemma is whether to relate effects to the two (or more) compounds separately, or to sum the various components, or to try weighting for the differential potencies of the compounds (Moody *et al.* 1967). For example, if compound A (potency one unit) is converted to compound B (potency 0·5 units) and A is found at 50 ng ml^{-1} while B is at 30 ng ml^{-1}, do we have $(1 \times 50)+(0{\cdot}5 \times 30) = 65$ ng ml^{-1} equivalents of drug? Such contortions seem excessive. Another device is the use of ratios, such as the one creeping into chlorpromazine literature (Mackay *et al.* 1974; Sakalis *et al.* 1977):

$$\frac{\text{chlorpromazine} + \text{7-hydroxychlorpromazine}}{\text{chlorpromazine sulphoxide}}.$$

This breaks all the rules, as the top line allegedly comprises active compounds, but with different potencies determined in human (chlorpromazine) and animal models (7-hydroxychlorpromazine), while the bottom line includes an allegedly inactive compound (but see earlier). Furthermore, the ratio is of two variables which are not independent, as each molecule of chlorpromazine can only be converted to one of the two metabolites (it can of course be converted to yet other metabolites). Statistically, if the concentrations of each of the compounds incorporated into such ratios in different groups of subjects are not significantly different, then any apparent significance in contrived ratios is quite fallacious. If one figure, for example chlorpromazine sulphoxide in the above ratio, is significantly different in different groups of patients, then the ratio merely confirms that this is the case, without providing any new information.

This is in fact the case with chlorpromazine. In studies of long-term patients, chlorpromazine and 7-hydroxychlorpromazine have failed to show significant differences in groups of patients categorized as responding well, indifferently, or not well. However, poor responders show elevated chlorpromazine sulphoxide levels. They also receive higher doses. So it seems that long-term patients are prescribed doses which generate common maximum plasma chlorpromazine and 7-hydroxychlorpromazine concentrations, limited by tolerability of unwanted effects, with the excess being converted to chlorpromazine sulphoxide. The clinical outcome then depends very much on non-pharmacological factors. Although there is an inverse relation between success of treatment and chlorpromazine sulphoxide concentration, there is no suggestion of the sulphoxide being psychotoxic.

Interest in the metabolites of chlorpromazine has been immense, but it now seems that only 7-hydroxychlorpromazine and demonomethylchlorpromazine are of great importance. However, there is a divergence of views. In acute patients with chlorpromazine in their plasma, in controlled studies, response occurs with negligible amounts of the metabolites present (Curry & Evans, 1976). In chronic patients, in uncontrolled studies, significant amounts of the metabolites are present (Mackay *et al.* 1974). So it seems that those metabolites which have appreciable activity (shown in animals of course, and below that of chlorpromazine itself) contribute to the action of chlorpromazine when present, but are not essential to the action of chlorpromazine.

With both chlorpromazine and tricyclic antidepressants, various other observations have been made regarding clinical outcome in relation to plasma levels. Over narrow ranges, there is no correlation to plasma levels. Over wide ranges, U-shaped relations are seen, with low concentrations inadequate, and high concentrations adverse (Åsberg *et al.* 1971; Curry, 1976). Again, it is not suggested that the drugs are psychotoxic in high concentrations. The U-shaped relation is observed using global rating scales, which take into account unwanted effects of drugs which occur when concentrations are excessive. This has been shown repeatedly with tricyclics and phenothiazines, and also with benzodiazepines and lithium. Some rules for any clinical relationship appear to be:

(1) The relation will depend heavily on the type of patients and the mode of assessment.

(2) The clinically useful range will be wide.

(3) The relation will be more obvious when individuals are studied repeatedly than when a population is sampled for a correlation.

(4) Too fine a relationship should not be expected.

This appears to be the basis for the difference of opinion among those investigating tricyclic antidepressants, a difference of opinion which has led to heated exchanges at meetings. Nobody need be making incorrect observations. Even so, rather than using clinical rating, should we be using pharmacological or biochemical measures? There is as yet no answer to this. With several examples peripheral effects, such as pulse rate and pupil size, correlate better with plasma levels than does clinical rating, but these effects do not particularly correlate with clinical rating. Also, much interest has been centred on prolactin and platelets, but not as measures of psychosis in any way (Sakalis *et al.* 1972; Loga *et al.* 1975; Boullin *et al.* 1975; Kolakowska *et al.* 1975).

So is clinical monitoring useful? When the analyst is competent, and a suitable person is available to interpret data, monitoring picks out underdosed and overdosed patients, neither of whom will always be apparent on clinical grounds alone. This can be a help in individualizing dosing regimes. Arguably, clinical monitoring should therefore always be available to the prescriber for investigation of problem cases, as Brodie's idea appears to hold true, that drug treatment in man is better controlled if pharmacokinetic variability is compensated with individually tailored dosage regimes. However, clinical monitoring costs money.

STEPHEN H. CURRY

REFERENCES

Åsberg, M., Cronholm, B., Sjöqvist, F. & Tuck, D. (1971). Relationship between plasma level and therapeutic effect of nortriptyline. *British Medical Journal* iii, 331–334.

Boullin, D. J., Woods, H. F., Grimes, R. P. J., Grahame-Smith, D. G., Wiles, D. H., Gelder, M. G. & Kolakowska, T. (1975). Increased platelet aggregation responses to 5-hydroxytryptamine in patients taking chlorpromazine. *British Journal of Clinical Pharmacology* **2**, 29–35.

Brodie, B. B. (1967). Physicochemical and biochemical aspects of pharmacology. *Journal of the American Medical Association* **202**, 600–609.

Curry, S. H. (1968). Determination of nanogram quantities of chlorpromazine and some of its metabolites in plasma using gas–liquid chromatography with an electron-capture detector. *Analytical Chemistry* **40**, 1251–1255.

Curry, S. H. (1976). Gas-chromatographic methods for the study of chlorpromazine and some of its metabolites in human plasma. *Psychopharmacology Communications* **2**, 1–15.

Curry, S. H. & Brodie, B. B. (1967). Estimation of nanogram quantities of chlorpromazine (CPZ) in plasma using gas–liquid chromatography (GLC) with an electron-capture detector. *Federation Proceedings* **26**, 761.

Curry, S. H. & Evans, S. (1976). A note on the assay of chlorpromazine *N*-oxide and its sulphoxide in plasma and urine. *Journal of Pharmacy and Pharmacology* **28**, 467–468.

Davidson, J. D., Terry, L. L. & Sjoerdsma, A. (1957). Action and metabolism of chlorpromazine sulfoxide in man. *Journal of Pharmacology and Experimental Therapeutics* **121**, 8–12.

Garattini, S., Marcucci, F., Morselli, P. L. & Mussini, E. (1973). The significance of measuring blood levels of benzodiazepines. In *Biological Effects of Drugs in Relation to their Plasma Concentrations* (ed. D. S. Davies and B. N. C. Prichard), pp. 211–225. Macmillan: London.

Hammer, W. & Brodie, B. B. (1967). Application of isotope derivative technique to assay of secondary amines. Estimation of desipramine by acetylation with H^3 acetic anhydride. *Journal of Pharmacology and Experimental Therapeutics* **157**, 503–508.

Kolakowska, T., Wiles, D. H., Gelder, M. G. & McNeilly, A. S. (1975). Correlation between plasma levels of prolactin and chlorpromazine in psychiatric patients. *Psychological Medicine* **5**, 214–216.

Loga, S., Curry, S. H. & Lader, M. H. (1975). Interactions of orphenadrine and phenobarbitone with chlorpromazine: plasma concentrations and effects in man. *British Journal of Clinical Pharmacology* **2**, 197–208.

Mackay, A. V. P., Healey, A. F. & Baker, J. (1974). The relationship of plasma chlorpromazine to its 7-hydroxy and sulphoxide metabolites in a large population of chronic schizophrenics. *British Journal of Clinical Pharmacology* **1**, 425–430.

Moody, J. P., Tait, A. C. & Todrick, A. (1967). Plasma levels of imipramine and desmethylimipramine during therapy. *British Journal of Psychiatry* **113**, 183–193.

Sakalis, G., Curry, S. H., Mould, G. P. & Lader, M. H. (1972). Physiologic and clinical effects of chlorpromazine and their relationship to plasma level. *Clinical Pharmacology and Therapeutics* **13**, 931–946.

Sakalis, G., Chan, T. L., Gershon, S. & Park, S. (1973). The possible role of metabolites in therapeutic response to chlorpromazine treatment. *Psychopharmacologia (Berlin)* **32**, 279–284.

Sakalis, G., Chan, T. L., Sathananthan, G., Schooler, N., Goldberg, S. & Gershon, S. (1977). Relationships among clinical response, extrapyramidal syndrome and plasma chlorpromazine and metabolite ratios. *Communications in Psychopharmacology* **1**, 157–166.

Schou, M. (1969). Lithium: relation between clinical effect of the drug and its absorption, distribution and excretion. In *The Present Status of Psychotropic Drugs* (ed. A. Cerletti and J. J. Bove), pp. 120–122. Excerpta Medica: Amsterdam.

Psychological Medicine, 1981, **11**, 661–667

Drug assays in neuropsychiatry[1]

INTRODUCTION AND GENERAL PRINCIPLES

The measurement and interpretation of plasma concentrations of drugs are beset by numerous problems and, up to the present time, these have militated against their routine use in neuropsychiatry. In other areas of medicine, however, drug assays have proved to be of clinical importance, and experience here has allowed the establishment of a number of principles.

Measurements of plasma steady state concentrations of anticonvulsants, for example, have led to their use in the following areas: in establishing non-compliance (especially with out-patients); for detecting abnormalities of absorption; in the differentiation of some toxic signs from those of primary brain disorder; in evaluating excessive metabolism due to liver microsomal enzyme induction from previous or concurrent treatment with other drugs, especially in non-responders; and, finally, in the evaluation of patients suspected of complex drug interactions. Measurement of plasma non-steady state concentration following single dosage has occasionally been mooted as being of predictive value in relation to therapeutic response.

Unfortunately, the situation is less clear with respect to drugs currently used in neuropsychiatry for a number of reasons.

First, less precise information is available concerning the pharmacokinetics in man, due to the high volume of distribution of lipophylic drugs and in many instances the very high degree of plasma protein binding.

Secondly, the existence of numerous metabolites, the concentrations of which vary widely and some of which are pharmacologically active, leads to a poor correlation between drug pharmacokinetics and pharmacodynamics. To this may be added the fact that many drugs used in neuropsychiatry are rapidly absorbed, leading to wide fluctuations in plasma levels, which in itself leads to difficulties in interpretation.

Thirdly, a problem exists in the laboratory concerned with the accurate measurement of the very low levels of drugs encountered and the associated metabolites.

Finally, considerable difficulties arise over precise clinical evaluation of response in patients with medium- to long-term disorders, the natural history of which is characterized by a fluctuating course and in which even precise diagnosis of a homologous group of disorders is frequently difficult.

It is perhaps not surprising, therefore, that it has proved difficult to establish therapeutic ranges; moreover, different ranges will be applicable, dependent upon whether one is interested in the management of the acute phase of illness, prophylaxis against relapse, or the identification of specific features of toxicity. By analogy with other groups of drugs, considerable individual variation, possibly genetically determined, is likely to be encountered, and different therapeutic ranges (as well as dosage) will be required for children and for the elderly. Factors such as diet and fasting which are associated with varying levels of free fatty acids in plasma will affect protein binding of drugs and where this is high, as is frequently the case with drugs used in neuropsychiatry, only small changes in binding will have large effects on the free fraction. Both pregnancy and disease states associated with alterations in plasma proteins give rise to similar problems.

Unfortunately, measurement of the free fraction of any drugs in plasma is not practicable on a routine basis at the present time for technical reasons, although trials of commercial kits are currently in progress in the United States. Estimations in saliva are also rather unsatisfactory for practical reasons and cerebrospinal fluid (c.s.f.), although ideal in many respects, is, of course, not available.

Even when these problems have been overcome, it will be appreciated that the use of serial steady

[1] Address for correspondence: Dr P. T. Lascelles, Department of Chemical Pathology, The National Hospital for Nervous Diseases, Queen Square, London WC1N 3BG.

state plasma levels of drugs is only one additional factor to be taken into account in the overall clinical management of the patient and that no account is taken in these measurements of any variations due to passage through the blood–brain barrier or of the tolerance at receptor level based on drug-induced changes of endogenous modulators.

Alternative approaches (as, for example, by analogy with measurement of prothrombin time as a monitor of anticoagulant therapy) have been suggested and, in neuropsychiatry, this has usually involved measurement of serum prolactin response to dopamine blockers or platelet monoamine oxidase (MAO) activity as a monitor of the activity of MAO inhibitors; these parameters will be considered later.

Against this background must also be set the great cost of monitoring drug therapy. Nevertheless, recent developments in both the clinical evaluation of patients and in laboratory techniques – in particular the routine application of a high performance liquid chromatography (HPLC) and radioreceptor binding – point to possible changes in the situation in the near future and warrant an evaluation at this time of the position with respect to individual groups of drugs currently used in neuropsychiatry. In this review, hypnotics and drugs used in the treatment of premenstrual tension have not been included, and no account has been given of tests for drugs of abuse, although routine rapid semiquantitative tests for a range of these by homologous enzyme immunoassay, using the EMIT (Syva) techniques, are now available.

NEUROLEPTICS

These will be considered under three headings: the phenothiazines, the thioxanthenes as illustrated by flupenthixol, and the butyrophenones as represented by haloperidol.

The phenothiazines

A vast literature exists on the measurement of blood levels of this group of drugs and the relationship of these to clinical effects. While there is some evidence that low plasma concentrations are found more frequently in non-responsive schizophrenics (Smith *et al.* 1979), and it is reported that concurrent lithium therapy may lower plasma chlorpromazine levels (Rivera-Calimlin *et al.* 1978), the value of monitoring in individual patients is very limited. As a group these drugs are lipophylic, having a large volume of distribution, and are highly bound to protein (Freedberg *et al.* 1979). Many metabolites exist, the concentrations and pharmacological activity of which vary considerably, and the absolute plasma concentrations are frequently low, being near to the limits of detection by conventional laboratory methods. Variable bio-availability as a result of hepatic metabolism and enzyme induction, and degradation within the gut wall are further complications (Dahl & Strandjord, 1977; Bergling *et al.* 1975; Smith *et al.* 1979). For details of particular drugs, the reader is referred to review articles (Cooper, 1978; May & Van Putten, 1978).

Two papers, however, warrant special attention. Creese & Snyder (1977) described a simple, sensitive radioreceptor assay (RRA) for anti-schizophrenic drugs in blood; and Tune *et al.* (1980) applied this to correlate serum neuroleptic levels with clinical state, monitored by an abbreviated version of the Present State Examination (mini-PSE). They found a significant correlation between serum neuroleptic levels and clinical response, but not between drug dosage and blood levels, or between dosage and clinical response. They argue that the failure of some reports to correlate drug levels with clinical response may be (*a*) due to the system of patient evaluation; and (*b*) because the non-receptor binding techniques might not have taken account of the activity of pharmacologically active metabolites.

Flupenthixol

Johnstone *et al.* (1980) estimated plasma levels of flupenthixol by radioimmunoassay (RIA) and RRA in acute and chronic schizophrenic patients. Both isomers were detected in blood after administration orally and by depot injection but, although a good clinical response and raised serum prolactin levels were associated with the administration of α-flupenthixol, no correlations between these and plasma levels of the drug were found. Some reduction in platelet MAO activity was also detected, but this too was unrelated directly to plasma flupenthixol levels. Concurrent administration of the anticholinergic drug, procyclidine, reduced plasma levels of flupenthixol, even when given parenterally. Trimble (personal communication), using α-flupenthixol as an antidepressant in much lower doses, also measured plasma levels and found that, although there was no direct correlation between plasma levels of the drug and improved clinical states, there was a positive correlation between drug levels and serum prolactin one month after commencing treatment and between serum prolactin and clinical improvement at two months.

Haloperidol

No convincing evidence exists for the value of measuring plasma concentrations of haloperidol as a guide to clinical response with acute or chronic disorders of any age-group, although correlates do exist between side-effects and plasma levels, especially in children (Morselli & Zarifian, 1980). According to one report, however, correlation does exist between dose and plasma levels and between plasma levels and serum prolactin, especially in higher dose regimes (Evans *et al.* 1978).

There is no evidence that in non-responders there is a lack of bio-availability of the drug (Morselli & Zarifian, 1980).

DRUGS USED IN THE TREATMENT OF DISORDERS OF MOOD

Tricyclic antidepressants

Detailed studies on the pharmacodynamics of this important group of drugs have been made since their introduction in the late 1950s. There are few differences in clinical response within the group as a whole, although amitriptyline is rather more sedative than the others. All are rapidly and completely absorbed from the gut and plasma steady states are readily achieved. Inter-patient variations occur, however, with respect to the rate of liver detoxication, possibly on a genetic basis, and are also dependent upon age, elderly patients being slow detoxicators (Nies *et al.* 1977). Demethylation converts imipramine to desimipramine and amitriptyline to nortriptyline, both of which are pharmacologically active products.

Burrows (1977) and Braithwaite (1980) have reviewed the literature with respect to the relationship between clinical response and plasma levels for individual tricyclics. Although there are some conflicting reports, there appears to be considerable evidence for the existence of a curvilinear relationship between plasma levels and clinical response, the exact reasons for which are not clear. It is certainly not simply due to the fact that non-responders are prescribed larger doses of drugs, but rather it would appear that higher levels of these drugs inhibit their own pharmacological action.

In those trials where a lack of correlation between plasma levels of tricyclic antidepressants and clinical response has been reported, possible explanations lie in the difficulties inherent in the measurement of clinical response, heterogeneity of group diagnosis, and the effects of other concurrent drug administration (Braithwaite, 1980). The relationship of blood levels to neuropsychiatric side-effects, however, is less clear. It is established that a good relationship exists between dose and plasma levels and between plasma levels and cardiotoxicity; the latter factor alone may be crucial in excluding regimes employing higher levels, especially in elderly patients (Burrows, 1977). Interactions between barbiturates and tricyclics and between neuroleptics and tricyclics which result in altered blood levels have been described; again, implications for the elderly are important (Burrows, 1977).

Most authorities would probably agree that plasma monitoring of levels of these drugs does have a place in the detection of non-compliance, the management of non-responders, and as a protection against cardiotoxicity.

It is important also to note that the tricyclic antidepressants have epileptogenic properties (Trimble, 1978; Nawiṣhy *et al.* 1980) and that, if anticonvulsants are administered concurrently, these will interact and reduce plasma levels of the tricyclics (Richens, 1976).

Maprotiline differs structurally from conventional tricyclic antidepressants only by the introduction of an ethylene bridge into the molecule, a change which is probably not sufficient to warrant its classification as a separate class of psychotropic agent. Clinical differences do exist, however, but the evidence for correlation between plasma levels and clinical response is not clear and has been reviewed by Burrows (1977) and Pinder *et al.* (1977).

Tetracyclic antidepressants

Coppen *et al.* (1976) found that plasma levels of mianserin were constant for individual patients on a standard dose, although the highest concentration was some four times the lowest in different patients. No correlation was demonstrated between plasma levels and either therapeutic response or side-effects. By contrast, Perry *et al.* (1978) did find a correlation between plasma concentration and changes in the Hamilton Rating Scale for depression.

In the largest study by Montgomery *et al.* (1978), a curvilinear relationship in plasma levels was correlated with optimum therapeutic response and a significant clinical disadvantage established with high plasma levels, particularly in endogenous depression and in patients over the age of 55 years.

Nomifensine

Nomifensine is a relatively new drug introduced for the treatment of depression. It is a non-tricyclic, non-MAO inhibitor compound which inhibits presynaptic noradrenaline re-uptake but, in addition, has dopamine agonist properties (Costall & Naylor, 1977; Brogden *et al.* 1979). Few studies have been carried out as yet on the value of monitoring plasma levels in relation to direct response but it would appear that, after the establishment of steady state kinetics, low levels are associated with sub-optimal clinical response (Nawishy *et al.* 1980). However, on the basis of acute dosage it would appear that there is a dissociation between pharmacokinetic and pharmacodynamic responses, implying either the formation of an active metabolite, or access to a deep compartment receptor, or both (Saletu & Taeuber, 1980). This is confirmed by the efficacy of once daily dosage, in spite of a half-life of 2 hours (Hanks *et al.* 1980).

Further studies of larger series are awaited but, for the present, there is no indication for routine monitoring of plasma levels.

Monoamine oxidase inhibitors

Methods exist for the direct measurement of MAO inhibitor drugs in plasma but, in practice, these are seldom used, attention being directed more towards measuring the degree of inhibition of the enzyme monoamine oxidase itself, especially in platelets (Robinson *et al.* 1978). Technical problems exist, however, in that baseline levels vary widely and different results are obtained with the use of different substrates.

Some correlation, however, does exist between high degrees of enzyme inhibition and clinical response, although there is a marked dissociation in the early stages of treatment (Robinson *et al.* 1978), suggesting that the pharmacological effect of these drugs may not be confined to this mechanism alone.

Lithium

Lithium salts have been used in the UK since 1949 but only since 1970 in the USA. They are administered for both the management and prophylaxis of manic-depressive disorders (Srinivasan & Hullin, 1980; Baldessarini, 1980). Rapid and complete absorption results in wide fluctuations in plasma levels (Crammer *et al.* 1980). Considerable variation occurs between patients but, for a given individual, the pharmacokinetics appear to be relatively constant.

The distribution of lithium in the body is wide, gradients across membranes being small (unlike sodium and potassium) and plasma protein binding is minimal. Nevertheless, penetration of the blood–brain barrier is poor and c.s.f. concentrations are only some 40 % of plasma values.

Plasma levels should be monitored regularly to assess compliance and also, in particular, as a precaution against toxicity. In this connection it is worth emphasizing the special situation of renal conservation of lithium in states of sodium depletion.

There is a lack of precise information concerning the therapeutic ranges required for the management of acute manic-depressive disorders and for prophylaxis, although it is likely that higher levels will be necessary for the former (Baldessarini, 1980).

Anxiolytics as exemplified by the benzodiazepines

Most investigators have reported a poor or absent correlation between plasma levels of benzodiazepines and clinical effect (Bellantuono *et al.* 1980; Bond *et al.* 1977), although correlations do exist between plasma levels and dose (Rutherford *et al.* 1978). Reasons for poor correlations include: difficulties in the assessment of clinical response, including those related to drug tolerance which is a particular feature of benzodiazepine therapy, and the inability to date of laboratory techniques to measure metabolites accurately. A further difficulty arises as a result of the very different pharmacokinetics of the various benzodiazepines (Bellantuono *et al.* 1980; Shader & Greenblatt, 1980).

In two surveys, however, a correlation between plasma levels and clinical response has been stressed (Curry, 1974; Dasberg *et al.* 1974); others have claimed a more limited use in relation to compliance, abuse and intoxication (Shader & Greenblatt, 1980).

Recently, an investigation has shown a good correlation between one highly specific clinical parameter capable of exact measurement by peak velocity of saccadic eye movements and serum benzodiazepine concentration in acute single dose experiments in man (Bittencourt *et al.* 1981), but the implications for this finding in the wider clinical context must remain speculative for the present. It is to be hoped, however, that this most interesting observation will pave the way for similar studies in the future.

In this connection, too, the recent development of reliable HPLC methods for the measurement of individual benzodiazepines and their metabolites (Peat *et al.* 1979) is clearly important; but perhaps of even greater significance is the development of radioreceptor binding assays for this group of drugs which are capable of measuring the total free benzodiazepine binding of pharmacologically active moieties at specific brain receptors on a regional basis, dependent upon preparation of membranes from animal tissue.

CONCLUSION

There is, at the present time, considerable interest in the monitoring of plasma levels of drugs used in neuropsychiatry and, as laboratory techniques become more sensitive and specific in the future, this is likely to increase. The range of drugs now available is too large to allow general conclusions to be drawn and each group requires to be evaluated on its own merits.

The indications for monitoring plasma levels of neuroleptics and benzodiazepines are limited at the present time but these are currently areas of intense research.

Therapeutic ranges are quoted for the antidepressants but larger trials will be needed to establish unequivocally the place for monitoring in routine patient management.

Regular measurements of lithium concentrations in plasma are essential as a precaution against toxicity.

P. T. LASCELLES

REFERENCES

Baldessarini, R. J. (1980). Drugs and the treatment of psychiatric disorders. In *The Pharmacological Basis of Therapeutics* (ed. A. Goodman Gilman, L. S. Goodman and A. Goodman), pp. 391–447. Goodman & Gilman's Sixth Edition. Macmillan: New York.

Bellantuono, C., Reggi, V., Tognoni, G. & Garattini, S. (1980). Benzodiazepines: clinical pharmacology and therapeutic use. *Drugs* **19**, 195–219.

Bergling, R., Mjorndal, T., Oreland, L., Rapp, W. & Wold, S. (1975). Plasma levels and clinical effects of thioridazine and thiothixene. *Journal of Clinical Pharmacology* **15**, 178–186.

Bittencourt, P. R. M., Wade, P., Smith, A. T. & Richens, A. (1981). The relationship between peak velocity of saccadic eye movements and serum benzodiazepine concentration. *British Journal of Clinical Pharmacology* **12**, 523–533.

Bond, A. J., Hailey, D. M. & Lader, M. H. (1977). Plasma concentrations of benzodiazepines. *British Journal of Clinical Pharmacology* **4**, 51–56.

Braithwaite, R. (1980). The role of plasma level monitoring of tricyclic antidepressant drugs as an aid to treatment. In *Drug Concentrations in Neuropsychiatry* pp. 167–197. Ciba Foundation Symposium 74 (new series). Excerpta Medica: Amsterdam.

Brogden, R. N., Heel, R. C., Speight, T. M. & Avery G. S. (1979). Nomifensine: a review of its pharmacological properties and therapeutic efficacy in depressive illness. *Drugs* **18**, 1–24.

Burrows, G. D. (1977). Plasma levels of tricyclics, clinical response and drug interactions. In *Handbook of Studies on Depression* (ed. G. D. Burrows), pp. 173–194. Excerpta Medica: Amsterdam.

Cooper, T. B. (1978). Plasma level monitoring of antipsychotic drugs. *Clinical Pharmacokinetics* **3**, 14–38.

Coppen, A., Gupta, R., Montgomery, S., Ghose, K., Bailey, J., Burns, B. & De Ridder, J. J. (1976). Mianserin hydrochloride: a novel antidepressant. *British Journal of Psychiatry* **129**, 342–345.

Costall, B. & Naylor, G. J. (1977). Further aspects of nomifensine pharmacology. *British Journal of Clinical Pharmacology* **4**, 89–99.

Crammer, J. L., Elithorn, A. C. & Lennox, R. (1980). Lithium concentrations and clinical responses. In *Drug Concentrations in Neuropsychiatry*, pp. 81–98. Ciba Foundation Symposium 74 (new series). Excerpta Medica: Amsterdam.

Creese, I. & Snyder, S. H. (1977). A simple and sensitive radioreceptor assay for antischizophrenic drugs in blood. *Nature* **270**, 180–182.

Curry, S. H. (1974). Concentration-effect relationship with major and minor tranquillizers. *Clinical Pharmacology and Therapeutics* **16**, 192–197.

Dahl, S. G. & Strandjord, R. E. (1977). Pharmacokinetics of chlorpromazine after single and chronic dosage. *Clinical Pharmacology and Therapeutics* **21** (4), 437–448.

Dasberg, H. H., van der Kleijn, E., Guelen, P. J. R. & van Praag, H. M. (1974). Plasma concentrations of diazepam and of its metabolite N-desmethyldiazepam in relation to anxiolytic effect. *Clinical Pharmacology and Therapeutics* **15** (5), 473–483.

Evans, L., Eadie, M. J., Penny, J., Cox, J., Price, J., Weston, M. J. & Tyrer, J. H. (1978). The relationship between the therapeutic effect and plasma level of high doses of haloperidol. In *Neuropsychopharmacology*, Proceedings of the 11th International Congress C.I.N.P., Vienna (ed. B. Saletu, P. Berner and L. Hollister). Pergamon: Oxford.

Freedberg, K. A., Innis, R. B., Creese, I. & Snyder, S. H. (1979). Antischizophrenic drugs: differential plasma protein binding and therapeutic activity. *Life Sciences* **24**, 2467–2474.

Hanks, G. W., Magnus, R. V., Myskova, I. & Mathur, G. (1980). Antidepressants in single daily doses: studies with nomifensine. In *The Royal Society of Medicine International Congress and Symposium*, Series Number 25, *Nomifensine* (ed. P. D. Stonier and F. A. Jenner), pp. 87–94. Grune & Stratton: London.

Johnstone, E. C., Bourne, R. C., Cotes, P. M., Crow, T. J., Ferrier, I. N., Owen, F. & Robinson, J. D. (1980). Blood levels of flupenthixol in patients with acute and chronic schizophrenia. In *Drug Concentrations in Neuropsychiatry*, pp. 99–114. Ciba Foundation Symposium 74 (new series). Excerpta Medica: Amsterdam.

May, P. R. A. & Van Putten, T. (1978). Plasma levels of chlorpromazine in schizophrenia: a critical review of the literature. *Archives of General Psychiatry* **35**, 1081–1087.

Montgomery, S., McAuley, R. & Montgomery, D. B. (1978). Relationship between mianserin plasma levels and antidepressant effect in a double-blind trial comparing a single night-time and divided daily dose regimens. *British Journal of Clinical Pharmacology* **5**, 71S–76S.

Morselli, P. L. & Zarifian, E. (1980). Clinical significance of monitoring plasma levels of psychotropic drugs. In *Drug Concentrations in Neuropsychiatry*, pp. 115–139. Ciba Foundation Symposium 74 (new series). Excerpta Medica: Amsterdam.

Nawishy, S., Trimble, M. R. & Richens, A. (1980). Antidepressants and epilepsy: the place of nomifensine. *The Royal Society of Medicine International Congress and Symposium*, Series Number 25, *Nomifensine* (ed. P. D. Stonier and F. A. Jenner), pp. 11–16. Grune & Stratton: London.

Nies, A., Robinson, D. S., Friedman, M. J., Green, R., Cooper, T. B., Ravaris, C. L. & Ives, J. O. (1977). Relationship between age and tricyclic antidepressant plasma levels. *American Journal of Psychiatry* **134** (7), 790–793.

Peat, M. A., Chem, C. & Kopjak, L. (1979). The screening and quantitation of diazepam, flurazepam, chlordiazepoxide and their metabolites in blood and plasma by electron-capture gas chromatography and high pressure liquid chromatography. *Journal of Forensic Sciences* **24**, 46–54.

Perry, G. F., Fitzsimmons, B., Shapiro, L. & Irwin, P. (1978). Clinical study of mianserin, imipramine and placebo in depression: blood level and MHPG correlations. *British Journal of Clinical Pharmacology* **5**, 35S–41S.

Pinder, R. M., Brogden, R. N., Speight, T. M. & Avery, G. S. (1977). Maprotiline: a review of its pharmacological properties and therapeutic efficacy in mental depressive states. *Drugs* **13**, 321–352.

Richens, A. (1976). Clinical pharmacology and medical treatment. In *A Textbook of Epilepsy* (ed. J. Laidlaw and A. Richens), pp. 185–247. Churchill Livingstone: Edinburgh.

Rivera-Calimlin, L., Kerzner, B. & Karch, F. E. (1978). Effect of lithium on plasma chlorpromazine levels. *Clinical Pharmacology and Therapeutics* **23**(4), 451–455.

Robinson, D. S., Nies, A., Ravaris, C. L., Ives, J. O. & Barlett, D. (1978). Clinical pharmacology of phenelzine. *Archives of General Psychiatry* **35**, 629–635.

Rutherford, D. M., Okoko, A. & Tyrer, P. J. (1978). Plasma concentrations of diazepam and desmethyldiazepam during chronic diazepam therapy. *British Journal of Clinical Pharmacology* **6**, 69–73.

Saletu, B. & Taeuber, K. (1980). Serum levels of nomifensine and pharmacodynamics assessed by the computer-pharmaco-EEG. *The Royal Society of Medicine International Congress and Symposium*, Series Number 25, *Nomifensine* (ed. P. D. Stonier and F. A. Jenner), pp. 31–38. Grune & Stratton: London.

Shader, R. I. & Greenblatt, D. J. (1980). Benzodiazepines: some aspects of their clinical pharmacology. In *Drug Concentrations in Neuropsychiatry*, pp. 141–155. Ciba Foundation Symposium 74 (new series). Excerpta Medica: Amsterdam.

Smith, R. C., Crayton, J., Dekirmenjian, H., Klass, D. & Davis, J. M. (1979). Blood levels of neuroleptic drugs in nonresponding chronic schizophrenic patients. *Archives of General Psychiatry* **36**, 579–584.

Srinivasan, D. P. & Hullin, R. P. (1980). Current concepts of lithium therapy. *British Journal of Hospital Medicine* **24**(5), 466–475.

Trimble, M. (1978). Non-monoamine oxidase inhibitor antidepressants and epilepsy: a review. *Epilepsia* **19**, 241–250.

Tune, L. E., Creese, I., DePaulo, J. R., Slavney, P. R., Coyle, J. T. & Snyder, S. H. (1980). Clinical state and serum neuroleptic levels measured by radioreceptor assay in schizophrenia. *American Journal of Psychiatry* **137**(2), 187–190.

Psychological Medicine, 1982, **12**, 689–693

The benzodiazepines: recent trends[1]

The benzodiazepines have now been available to the clinician for over 20 years, since the introduction of chlordiazepoxide (Librium) in 1960. The broad and unique spectrum of activity of these compounds as anxiolytics, hypnotics/sedatives, anticonvulsants and muscle relaxants, together with their low toxicity and an essential absence from peripheral side-effects, has resulted in compounds of this class becoming the most frequently prescribed of all psychotropic drugs. Although it is difficult to obtain an accurate estimate of their usage in England, in Canada 1 in 10 of the population receives a prescription for these drugs each year, while over 30% of hospitalized patients is given one or other of these agents (Ban *et al.* 1981).

USE OR OVER-USE

The indications are that the benzodiazepines are suffering a significant though small decline in their popularity, but their continued widespread use has resulted in some disquiet concerning their over-use. A number of cases of dependence on these compounds has been reported, though with respect to their widespread usage the percentage of such difficulties is extremely small and rarely becomes apparent without long-term administration of the compounds. However, with regard to their anxiolytic activity recent evidence from Davis *et al.* (1981) in Oxford would contra-indicate such prescription habits. It is well known that animals subjected to certain stressful situations are able to adapt to their new environment over a period of time. The Oxford group has found that the benzodiazepines are able to inhibit this adaptation response, and the results of experiments so far indicate that such inhibition can occur in situations normally experienced by man (J. A. Gray, personal communication). This would imply that, while short-term usage of the benzodiazepines to overcome some acute anxiety problem is acceptable, continued ingestion of the compounds would reduce the ability to cope with stressful situations.

THE PROLIFERATION OF COMPOUNDS

There is little evidence that the pharmacological profile of any single compound among the many now available to the clinician is significantly different from any other: i.e. all produce sedation/anxiolysis in approximately the same proportions. It is, however, possible to use an appropriate drug to accentuate a particular effect by relying on the differing pharmacokinetic profiles of the compounds; for example, the choice of one of short biological half-life for night time sedation and a compound with a longer biological half-life if the drug effects are to be protracted, as in the treatment of anxiety. The fact that all of the compounds currently available display the varying aspects of their pharmacological profile to a similar extent has provided a considerable impetus for research into the mechanisms of action of these drugs, in the hope that compounds might be found with a more restricted spectrum of activity.

THE BENZIODIAZEPINE RECEPTOR: EARLY DAYS

The observations made independently in 1977 by Squires & Braestrup in Copenhagen and Möhler & Okada in Basle, that the mammalian brain possesses specific receptors for the benzodiazepines,

[1] Address for correspondence: Dr I. L. Martin, MRC Neurochemical Pharmacology Unit, Medical Research Council Centre, Medical School, Hills Road, Cambridge CB2 2QH.

produced a remarkable explosion of research interest in these compounds. These initial experiments showed, with the use of radioactively labelled diazepam, that binding sites existed on cell membranes in the mammalian CNS which recognized the benzodiazepines specifically and with high affinity. Many further experiments have since been carried out which suggest that these 'binding-sites' are part of the receptor complex through which the benzodiazepines exert their effects.

Initially, it was thought that the benzodiazepine receptors consisted of a single homogeneous population, and the inference was therefore that all of the pharmacologial actions of these drugs were mediated via this single receptor. However, work by Squires *et al.* (1979) indicated that the triazolopyridazine CL 218872 (see Fig. 1) was able to displace diazepam from its binding sites in

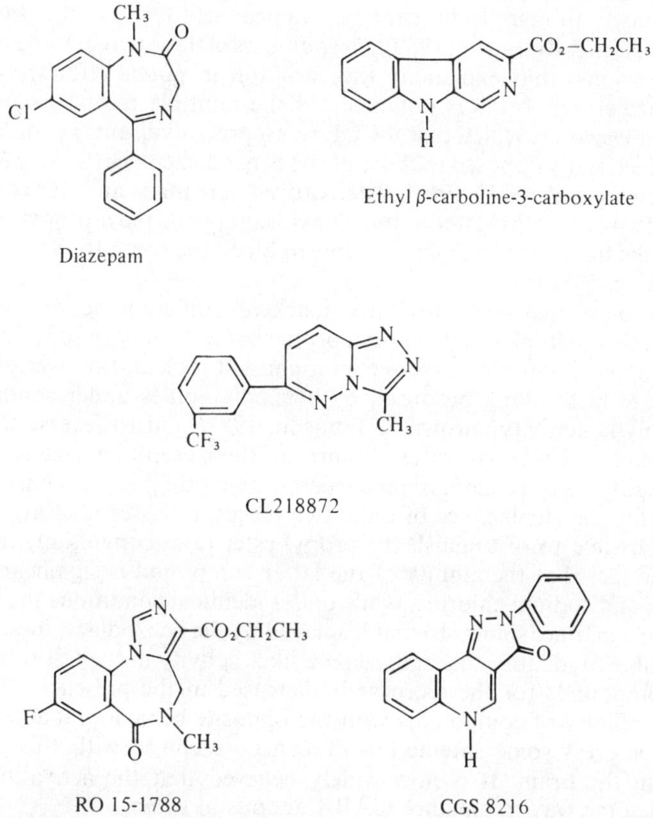

FIG. 1.

a manner which indicated that two binding sites existed: sites which could be differentiated by this compound but not by diazepam. The further claim (not since confirmed) that this compound produced anxiolytic and anti-convulsant effects but little sedation aroused intense interest, the hypothesis being that one of the receptor subtypes was responsible for the sedative effects of the benzodiazepines, while the other mediated the anxiolytic and anti-convulsant actions. Further support was added to the multiple site hypothesis by studies on the thermal inactivation of benzodiazepine receptors, the stability of which could not be adequately explained by the assumption that only a single homogeneous population of receptors existed (Squires *et al.* 1979).

THE BENZODIAZEPINE RECEPTOR: ONE OR TWO?

In searching for the endogenous ligand for the benzodiazepine receptor Braestrup *et al.* (1980) obtained a compound ethyl β-carboline-3-carboxylate (β-CCE) from human urine (see Fig. 1). Although it is now clear that this compound was an experimental artefact, β-CCE nevertheless has an extremely high affinity for the benzodiazepine receptor and has proved to be an extremely valuable experimental tool.

This compound was found to be potent in displacing radiolabelled diazepam from CNS membranes, but its potency varied depending on which brain region had been used to prepare the membranes. It was suggested that the explanation of this phenomenon was that two subtypes of benzodiazepine existed, a Bz_1 type with a high affinity for β-CCE (1 nM) and a Bz_2 type with a lower affinity (about 12 nM), though both subtypes appeared to show the same affinity for the benzodiazepines (Nielsen & Braestrup, 1980). The numbers of these two subtypes varied independently in different brain regions, thus explaining the variation in potency for the displacement of the diazepam. Thus further support was obtained for the multiple receptor hypothesis. Subsequent behavioural work, however, revealed that β-CCE was a proconvulsant: i.e. the compound appeared to have actions diametrically opposed to those of the benzodiazepines (Oakley & Jones, 1980; Tenen & Hirsch, 1980; Cowan *et al.* 1981). Further derivatives were made and subsequent work with these compounds has shown the methyl ester to be a convulsant, while the *n*-propyl ester exhibits no overt actions alone but, like the benzodiazepines, is able to block the convulsions produced by the methyl ester (Jones & Oakley, 1981).

While the β-carboline-3-carboxylates have markedly different actions with regard to anti-convulsant activity, their complete behavioural profile has not yet been fully investigated, due to the extremely short biological half-life of these compounds. It is clear, however, that β-CCE is able to suppress the increase in drinking produced by benzodiazepines under conditions thought to be predictive of anxiolytic acitivity (Brown & Johnson, 1982) and to reverse the sedative effects of flurazepam (Cowan *et al.* 1981). However, all three of these esters are able to differentiate between the two proposed subtypes of benzodiazepine receptor in binding experiments with the same degree of preference, making the significance of these two receptor classes unclear.

It is, however, possible to distinguish the propyl ester (anti-convulsant) from the methyl ester (convulsant) by the fact that the affinity of the latter compound is significantly decreased by the presence of GABA and sodium chloride, while under identical conditions the affinity of the propyl ester is increased, in a manner similar to that displayed by the benzodiazepines. (Doble *et al.* 1982*b*). It is therefore possible to identify 'benzodiazepine-like' activity in the test tube by the fact that the affinity of such compounds for the receptor is increased in the presence of GABA and sodium chloride, while the affinity of compounds with the opposite behavioural actions is decreased. The effects of GABA suggest some interaction of benzodiazepines with this important inhibitory neurotransmitter in the brain. It is now widely believed that the activation of benzodiazepine receptors serves in some way to enhance GABA actions in brain.

While there is now considerable support for the hypothesis of multiple subtypes of the benzodiazepine receptor, other biochemical evidence suggests that the observations may be explained by different states, or conformations of the same receptor (Doble *et al.* 1982*a*). The significance of the existence of multiple subtypes of the receptor, in any case, remains unclear, although it continues to provide a considerable impetus to the research effort.

BENZODIAZEPINE ANTAGONISTS

Changes in the basic structure of the benzodiazepine molecule by the group at Hoffman la Roche have led to the development of antagonists to the actions of these compounds (Hunkeler *et al.* 1981). Ro 15-1788 (see Fig. 1) is one such example, having a high affinity for the benzodiazepine receptor. It is assumed that its remarkable ability to reverse specifically the actions of the benzodiazepines is due to its interaction at the receptor itself. However, the compound is also able to reverse effectively the actions of β-CCE, and this antagonism of two diametrically opposed actions has led to considerable speculation as to the nature of the interaction of these compounds with the benzodiazepine receptor (Nutt *et al.* 1982). While Ro 15-1788 is structurally related to the benzodiazepines, the compound CGS 8216 (see Fig. 1), from Ciba-Geigy, shows little such resemblance, though it exhibits a very high affinity for the receptor. Little further information is available about this compound so far, except that it is reported to antagonize the actions of the benzodiazepines by a direct interaction at the benzodiazepine receptor itself (Czernik *et al.* 1981).

ENDOGENOUS LIGANDS FOR THE BENZODIAZEPINE RECEPTOR

As the discovery of opiate receptor sites in the brain led, in turn, to the discovery of endogenous opioids (the enkephalins), so it was hoped that it might be possible to identify endogenous benzodiazepine-like compounds in the brain. This area of research, however, has proved to be a graveyard of dashed hopes (Martin, 1980), and arguments have been put forward concerning the necessity to envisage such a compound (see Möhler, 1981). The most recent reports concern a polypeptide found in the small intestine and bile duct which is able to displace competitively the benzodiazepines from their binding sites (Woolf & Nixon, 1981). This compound, named nepenthin, has now been purified to apparent homogeneity and appears to have a molecular weight of ~ 16000, though the stability of its displacing activity after treatment with proteases suggests that a lower molecular weight fragment retains activity. Little is yet known about the compound, though anti-bodies prepared to the purified material have been used in double antibody labelling experiments on rat brain slices, the result of which suggest that an immunologically similar material is present in some cells of deep cortical regions of the forebrain.

SUMMARY AND CONCLUSIONS

The discovery of non-benzodiazepinoid compounds which are able to displace effectively the benzodiazepines from their receptors, together with the apparent existence of multiple types of this receptor, have resulted in new hopes that the different behavioural actions of these drugs can be effectively separated. Indeed, chemical modifications of the molecule have resulted in the preparation of effective antagonists and to compounds with a greater anxiolytic/sedative ratio than those currently available to the clinician. However, although we have a great deal of information concerning the neurochemical actions of these compounds, a detailed understanding of the structure–activity relationships in this series can only be attempted with similarly detailed clinical/behavioural evidence concerning the profile of action of the individual compounds. Such a task is, of course, a daunting one but, unless we are to continue to rely on serendipity to provide us with compounds which exhibit more restricted profiles of action, this information must be obtained. Therefore it is perhaps in this field of endeavour where greater efforts and support must be sought in the future.

I. L. MARTIN

REFERENCES

Ban, T. A., Brown, W. T., Da Silva, T., Gagnon, M. A., Lamont, H. E., Leeman, H. E., Lowy, F. W., Ruedy, J. & Sellers, E. M. (1981). Therapeutic monograph on anxiolytic–sedative drugs. *Canadian Pharmaceutical Journal* **114**, 301–308.

Braestrup, C., Nielsen, M. & Olsen, C. E. (1980). Urinary and brain β-carboline-3-carboxylates as potent inhibitors of brain benzodiazepine receptors. *Proceedings of the National Academy of Sciences* (*USA*) **77**, 2288–2292.

Brown, C. L. & Johnson, A. M. (1982). Ethyl β-carboline-3-carboxylate reverses the effects of benzodiazepines in a test for detecting anxiolytic activity. *British Journal of Pharmacology* **75**, 43P.

Cowan, P. J., Green, A. R., Nutt, D. J. & Martin, I. L. (1981). Ethyl β-carboline carboxylate lowers seizure threshold and antagonises flurazepam induced sedation in rats. *Nature* **290**, 54–55.

Czernik, A. J., Petrack, B., Tsai, C., Granat, R. F., Rinehart, R. K., Kalinsky, H. J., Lovell, R. A. & Cash, W. D. (1981). High affinity occupancy of benzodiazepine receptors by the novel antagonist CGS-8216. *Pharmacologist* **23**, 160.

Davis, N. M., Brookes, S., Gray, J. A. & Rawlins, J. N. P. (1981).

Chlorodiazepoxide and resistance to punishment. *Quarterly Journal of Experimental Psychology* **33B**, 227–239.
Doble, A., Iversen, L. L. & Martin, I. L. (1982*a*). The benzodiazepine binding site: one receptor or two. *British Journal of Pharmacology* **75**, 42P.
Doble, A., Martin, I. L. & Richards, D. A. (1982*b*). GABA modulation predicts biological activity of ligands for the benzodiazepine receptor. *British Journal of Pharmacology* **76**, 238*P*.
Hunkeler, W., Möhler, H., Pieri, L., Polc, P., Bonetti, E. P., Cumin, R., Schaffner, R. & Haefely, W. (1981). Selective antagonists of benzodiazepines. *Nature* **290**, 514–516.
Jones, B. J. & Oakley, N. R. (1981). The convulsant properties of methyl β-carboline-3-carboxylate in the mouse. *British Journal of Pharmacology* **74**, 884P.
Martin, I. L. (1980). Endogenous ligands for benzodiazepine receptors. *Trends in Neurosciences* **3**, 299–301.
Möhler, H. (1981). Benzodiazepine receptors: are there endogenous ligands in the brain? *Trends in Pharmacological Sciences* **1**, 116–119.
Möhler, H. & Okada, T. (1977). Benzodiazepine receptor: demonstration in the central nervous system. *Science* **198**, 849–851.
Nielsen, M. & Braestrup, C. (1980). Ethyl β-carboline-3-carboxylate shows differential benzodiazepine receptor interaction. *Nature* **286**, 606–607.
Nutt, D. J., Cowan, P. J. & Little, H. J. (1982). Unusual interactions of benzodiazepine receptor antagonists. *Nature* **295**, 436–438.
Oakley, N. R. & Jones, B. J. (1980). The proconvulsant and diazepam reversing effects of ethyl β-carboline-3-carboxylate. *European Journal of Pharmacology* **68**, 381–382.
Squires, R. F. & Braestrup, C. (1977). Benzodiazepine receptors in rat brain. *Nature* **266**, 732–734.
Squires, R. F., Benson, D. I., Braestrup, C., Coupet, J., Klepner, C. A., Myers, V. & Beer, B. (1979). Some properties of brain specific benzodiazepine receptors: new evidence for multiple receptors. *Pharmacology, Biochemistry and Behaviour* **10**, 825–830.
Tenen, S. S. & Hirsch, J. D. (1980). Antagonism of diazepam activity by β-carboline-3-carboxylic acid ethyl ester. *Nature* **288**, 609–610.
Woolf, J. H. & Nixon, J. C. (1981). Endogenous effector of the benzodiazepine binding site: purification and characterisation. *Biochemistry* **20**, 4263–4269.

PSYCHOLOGY

Psychological Medicine, 1975, **5**, 219–221

Psychological theories and behaviour therapy

There can be no doubt about the fact that behaviour therapy has won a firm place in psychiatry and clinical psychology. In a dozen years or so, the number of articles on the subject has risen meteorically from almost nothing to the point where, in 1972, it exceeded the total contribution of psychoanalysis (Hoon and Lindsley, 1974). Special commissions set up to pronounce on its value, such as that of the American Psychiatric Association, have reported very favourably (1973). What is more, the number of well-planned, well-conducted clinical and experimental studies comparing the results of behaviour therapy with those of no treatment, placebo treatment, and various forms of psychotherapeutic treatment is increasing, and demonstrates beyond cavil the efficacy of these new techniques of desensitization, flooding, modeling, reinforcement, aversive conditioning, and so on. Critics have almost ceased to argue that the methods do not work, or that they 'merely' cure symptoms; the failure of relapses and symptom substitutions to occur has by now been recognized through a variety of follow-up studies. Instead, critics are concentrating their fire on the fundamental proposition that behaviour therapy is an applied science, and that its methods derive from modern learning theory (Eysenck, 1959). They now claim that there is no unified theory of learning on which behaviour therapy is based; that the principles of treatment are not rigorously deduced from such (non-existent) theory: and that quite generally theoretical considerations do not play much part in the work of the clinician (Breger and McGaugh, 1965; Locke, 1971; London, 1972). What in fact is the relation between psychological theory and behaviour therapy?

A rational appraisal of the situation must take into account two sets of facts. The first relates to the present situation in psychology, and particularly in learning theory. It is certainly true that there is no unified learning theory, and that many alternative formulations are being put forward. It is certainly true that the principles of treatment are not 'rigorously' deduced from learning theory, but that instead well-established laboratory phenomena suggest modes of application which are tried out by clinicians, elaborated when successful, and abandoned or altered and improved when unsuccessful. When successful variants are discovered—for example, desensitization or 'flooding'—clinicians seldom worry overmuch about the theoretical background of these successful methods, but use them on a hand-to-mouth basis, as valuable tools in their therapeutic armamentarium. Thus it would at first glance seem as if the critics were right; psychological theory does not play as much part in the genesis of behaviour therapy methods as had originally been claimed.

The second set of facts, however, suggests that this would be an erroneous interpretation, because it views behaviour therapy from an impossibly idealistic angle, such that no applied science, even in the fields of physics and chemistry, would pass muster. The situation which obtains in psychology is precisely analogous to that obtaining in other sciences; there also unified theories are sadly lacking, 'rigorous' applications of firmly established principles turn out to be less rigorous than imagined, and practitioners often do not worry very much about the ultimate truth of the principles on which the methods they use are based. The famous case of the discovery of the planet Neptune, for instance, is often quoted as an inspiring example of rigorous deduction from unified theory leading to great discovery. When Herschel discovered Uranus, the slight deviations of this planet's path from prediction suggested that another planet might be present which affected the motions of Uranus; LeVerrier in France and Adams in England calculated the position of this hypothetical planet, and when astronomers in Berlin and London directed their telescopes to the precise spot indicated, there was Neptune. So much for the textbook story. Reality, alas, is somewhat different. The discovery of Neptune was possible only because an approximate estimate of its distance from the sun was available through Bode's Law, a rough-and-ready empirical rule showing a regularly increasing distance from planet to planet as we go from the sun outwards; this 'law' cannot be deduced from Newton's equations, and is just an accidental property of our planetary system which would probably not obtain in other such systems. In addition, Bode's Law does not apply to Neptune; astronomers were very lucky that they looked for the planet when it was roughly at the distance predicted; six months earlier or later it would have been very far from the predicted spot, and would not have been found! Thus deduction, even in this classical case, was far from rigorous; it was based on an empirical rule which has no basis in theory; and successful prediction depended to a considerable extent on sheer luck. This is a more realistic point from which to view scientific prediction!

Nor does the notion of a 'unified theory' fare any better in this example. Newton's theory of gravitation postulates action at a distance, which was in fact disowned by Newton himself; Faraday and Maxwell later substituted a field theory, which was applied to gravitational problems by Einstein. Now, however, we are back at square one; 'action-at-a-distance electrodynamics' has been introduced, and Narlikar has shown that ADE fits in with Einstein's general theory of relativity and gives predictions which are indistinguishable from conventional field theory. There are many other examples of alternative theories with the same experimental consequences, but a very different conceptual basis: Newtonian and Lagrangian mechanics, for instance, and the Schroedinger and Heisenberg interpretations of quantum mechanics. The same may be true of cognitive and conditioning-type theories of learning; the fact that alternative interpretations exist does not excommunicate learning theory from science! It simply indicates that learning theory is similar, in this as in other respects, to what is common in the hard sciences.

Consider an example of the application of psychological theory to treatment. We can regard enuresis nocturna as a failure of conditioning to occur: the enlargement of the bladder, the conditioning stimulus (CS), does not produce the conditioned response (CR), of waking up and going to the toilet. We can mediate this conditioning process by means of the well-known bell-and-blanket method; this leads us to make three predictions. (1) Repeated application of the method should lead to the formation of the missing conditioned link, and the patient should learn to wake up in time and urinate in the toilet. This has been shown to be true over and over again. (2) The conditioned response, through failure of reinforcement to occur once it has become established, should extinguish again; we should have many relapses. This too has been demonstrated. (3) Extinction is known to be much less marked after partial reinforcement than after 100% reinforcement; we would predict that if the bell-and-blanket device was activated only on some of the trials, but not on others, relapses should occur much less frequently. This too has been demonstrated (Finley *et al.*, 1973). Can it really be denied that the discovery of the appropriate method owed much to well-known principles of learning theory? Much the same can be said for another successful method (overlearning) for reducing relapse (Young and Morgan, 1972).

But is it not true that contradictory results are often reported, both from laboratory work and from clinical experience? 'Flooding' methods—that is, extinction through response prevention—should work theoretically in eliminating phobic fears and obsessive-compulsive symptoms; some studies have shown the method to be very successful, others have shown it to make the patient worse. Is this not a grievous failure of theory to direct therapeutic work? The answer is that theory suggests the importance of a temporal parameter in making predictions. Short-term exposure to the CS (the phobic object, or the prevention of the obsessive-compulsive motor component) without reinforcement enhances the fear–anxiety component; long-term exposure reduces it. This has been found to be true both in animal (laboratory) experiments, and with clinical experiments on neurotic patients. The theory works perfectly well when it is properly applied; it seems to fail when important and relevant parameters are not taken sufficiently into account.

Criticisms of observed clinical facts as being contrary to theory are often based on a partial view of systematic theory. Thus it has often been observed that aversive conditioning of alcoholism, for instance, seems to imply 'backward conditioning'; in other words, the unconditioned stimulus (UCS) (nausea produced by drugs) precedes the CS (drinking alcoholic beverages). Backward conditioning, so it is said, is known not to work; it seems to follow that the clinical facts contradict the theoretical formulation. But this is not true; the rule that backward conditioning does not work applies only when certain parameters of the experiment follow a given pattern. There is no backward conditioning when the CS is weak and the UCS strong; this is the typical pattern in American work. But when both CS and UCS are strong (as in the work of Asratyan in the USSR) or weak (as in the work of Dostalek in Czechoslovakia) backward conditioning has been demonstrated to be quite strong. Now the aversive conditioning situation closely resembles Asratyan's type of strong–strong association, and, consequently, backward conditioning would properly be predicted; it is only the failure to consider the parametric details of the theory which leads to erroneous prediction.

It will be apparent now what our answer is to the oft-repeated criticism that the theory underlying behaviour therapy is in a chaotic and incoherent state. The charge is true, but it would be equally true of most scientific theories. Ever since I began taking an interest in subatomic physics 40 years ago theories in that field have been in an incoherent state; yet the field has prospered and has had its unarguable applied successes. The same could be said of cryogenics, where one expert pointed out that it consumed theories at the rate of one every six months. We are not quite as lavish with our theories—perhaps we ought to be. Scientific theories are not Simon-pure, ethereal constructs of eternal beauty, Platonic ideas paraded at the mouth of the cave; they are tools of greater or lesser usefulness, to be discarded when they do not serve their function any longer, and replaced by better ones. As J. J. Thomson said, 'A theory in science is a policy rather than a creed'. Such theories as we have in psychology are far from perfect, but they have shown considerable usefulness. More than anything, perhaps, they serve to denote a policy; it is this policy that sets off behaviour therapy from its predecessors. That policy is to rely on laboratory experiments and general laws deriving from these; to deal with facts rather than with speculation; and to pay particular attention to the outcome problem—do patients actually get measurably better when I apply this, that, or the other general law? The imperfect state of the underlying theory will make certain that it never becomes a creed!

H. J. EYSENCK

REFERENCES

American Psychiatric Association Task Force on Behavior Therapy (1973). *Behavior Therapy in Psychiatry*. Task Force Report 5. American Psychiatric Association: Washington.

Breger L., and McGaugh, J. L. (1965). Critique and reformulation of 'learning-theory' approaches to psychotherapy and neurosis. *Psychological Bulletin*, **63**, 338–358.

Eysenck, H. J. (1959). Learning theory and behaviour therapy. *Journal of Mental Science*, **105**, 61–75.

Finley, W. W., Besserman, R. L., Bennett, L. F., Clapp, R. K., and Finley, P. M. (1973). The effect of continuous, intermittent, and 'placebo' reinforcement on the effectiveness of the conditioning treatment for enuresis nocturna. *Behaviour Research and Therapy*, **11**, 289–297.

Hoon, P. W., and Lindsley, O. R. (1974). A comparison of behavior and traditional therapy publication activity. *American Psychologist*, **29**, 694–697.

Locke, E. A. (1971). Is 'behavior therapy' behavioristic? *Psychological Bulletin*, **76**, 318–327.

London, P. (1972). The end of ideology in behavior modification. *American Psychologist*, **27**, 913–920.

Young, G. C., and Morgan, R. T. T. (1972). Overlearning in the conditioning treatment of enuresis. *Behaviour Research and Therapy*, **10**, 147–151.

Psychological Medicine, 1979, **9**, 605–609

Anxiety and the brain: not by neurochemistry alone[1]

There has recently been a great flurry of excitement over the discovery of receptors in the central nervous system that specifically bind benzodiazepines (Squires & Braestrup, 1977; Möhler & Okada, 1977). This might be the long-awaited clue that will direct us to the brain systems on which the anti-anxiety drugs act, and which therefore presumably mediate anxiety. Clue it certainly is; but one which will need cautious interpretation alongside the evidence gathered by other means of studying the neuropsychology of anxiety. Taken in isolation it could yet turn out to be a sign-post which points clearly, but in the wrong direction; indeed, there are already indications that this may be so.

Benzodiazepine receptors have been found all over the brain, with a particularly heavy concentration in the neocortex (Braestrup & Squires, 1977; Williamson *et al.* 1978). I shall argue later that, if one is to do justice to the complexities of anxiety, it is essential to recognize that it has cognitive as well as emotional aspects. Even so, the neocortex does not look right as the primary site of action of an anti-anxiety drug. Experiments with animals suggest that the limbic system would be a better candidate for the seat of emotional experience and the mediator of emotional behaviour. While there is a reasonably dense concentration of benzodiazepine receptors in various parts of the limbic system, there is also a high concentration in the cerebellum (Braestrup & Squires, 1977; Williams *et al.* 1978); yet the latter structure is mainly concerned with motor behaviour. Worse still, there is quite a high concentration of benzodiazepine receptors in the spinal cord (Möhler & Okada, 1977; Robertson *et al.* 1978); and while this might have comforted an earlier generation of animal psychologists (e.g. Mowrer, 1947), who sought a purely peripheral account of fear, it is unlikely to find favour today as a site for anxiety in human beings.

The ubiquity of benzodiazepine receptors in the nervous system is perhaps linked to their association with γ-amino butyric acid (GABA), the equally wide-spread inhibitory neurotransmitter. There has been evidence for some time that the benzodiazepines facilitate the action of GABA-ergic systems (Costa & Greengard, 1975; Macdonald & Barker, 1978). The elegant biochemical experiments of Costa's group at NIMH (Guidotti *et al.* 1978) now suggest that benzodiazepine receptors are closely associated with (but not identical to) GABA receptors. This group has proposed that the endogenous ligand which normally occupies the benzodiazepine receptor is an inhibitor of GABA's binding to its own receptor (Guidotti *et al.* 1978). The action of the benzodiazepines *in vivo* is then seen to consist in the displacement of this endogenous inhibitor of GABA binding, with a consequent facilitation of GABA-ergic activity. The logic of this argument turns GABA itself into a kind of endogenous anti-anxiety agent. There is some support for this view in the recent experiments of Soubrié *et al.* (1978), who have found that picrotoxin, which can block the inhibitory action of GABA, alters the behaviour of the rat in a number of ways which are consistent with an increase in anxiety. But the key prediction that follows from the argument – namely, that drugs which promote the activity of GABA should possess anti-anxiety action – has so far not been confirmed, in spite of efforts to demonstrate such an action using amino-oxyacetic acid, which increases the level of GABA in the brain (Cook & Sepinwall, 1975). There is, as yet, no good explanation for these inconsistent findings with picrotoxin and amino-oxyacetic acid; however, the exact neurochemical effects produced by both these drugs are still obscure.

The solution to these problems might lie in the realization that the benzodiazepines are more than simply anti-anxiety drugs: they are also, among other things, centrally acting muscle-relaxants and anti-convulsants (Randall & Kappell, 1973; Schallek *et al.* 1972; Browne & Perry, 1973). The benzodiazepine receptors in the spinal cord might be related to either or both of these effects. As to

[1] Address for correspondence: Dr J. A. Gray, Department of Experimental Psychology, South Parks Road, Oxford OX1 3UD.

the receptors in the brain, there is at least as good a case for linking them to the anti-convulsant properties of the benzodiazepines as to their anti-anxiety action. There is a considerable amount of evidence which suggests a relation between lowered GABA-ergic activity and convulsions (Meldrum, 1975); thus facilitation of GABA-ergic function is exactly what one would expect of an anti-convulsant drug. Furthermore, a recent report provides direct evidence of a relationship between benzodiazepine receptors and seizures: the experimental induction of seizures by electro-convulsive shock or by pentylenetetrazol was followed by a substantial and rapid increase in benzodiazepine binding in the brain (Paul & Skolnick, 1978).

It is important to keep these other relationships of the benzodiazepines and their receptors in mind when interpreting evidence which, on the face of it, fits well with the anti-anxiety activity of these drugs. For example, our group in Oxford has recently collaborated with Professor P. B. Bradley's group in Birmingham in an investigation of benzodiazepine binding in the brains of rats from the Maudsley reactive and nonreactive strains, which have been selectively bred for, respectively, high and low fearfulness (Broadhurst, 1975). It was found that the Nonreactives had a higher density of benzodiazepine receptors throughout the brain (and the spinal cord) than the Reactives (Robertson *et al.* 1978), a finding which it is tempting to relate to the strain difference in fearfulness. However, the Nonreactive rats are also more susceptible to seizures than the Reactives (Gray, 1964), and this is an equally plausible behavioural correlate of the strain difference in benzodiazepine binding.

It might be thought that the fact that the benzodiazepines have other behavioural effects besides their ability to reduce anxiety renders nugatory the strategy of deducing the brain systems that mediate anxiety from an investigation of the brain systems on which the benzodiazepines act. But there are ways round this problem.

First, the benzodiazepines are not the only anti-anxiety drugs. Alcohol has always been ingested in large quantities for this purpose, and the barbiturates and meprobamate were extensively prescribed for it before the benzodiazepines swept them from favour. A review of the behavioural effects in animals of the barbiturates, alcohol and the benzodiazepines shows that, with minor exceptions, these three classes of drug affect behaviour in tasks relevant to anxiety (a phrase which is explained below) in an almost identical manner (Gray, 1977). The benzodiazepine receptor does not bind these other anti-anxiety drugs (Squires & Braestrup, 1977; Möhler & Okada, 1977); had it done so, it would have been a more plausible sign-post to the brain systems which mediate anxiety. Since it does not, there must be a final common pathway for the anti-anxiety drugs which lies beyond the benzodiazepine receptor. We can use the existence of different classes of anti-anxiety drug as a means to triangulate this final common pathway: it is where the actions of these classes of drug *intersect* that we should seek the brain systems which mediate anxiety.

Secondly, the benzodiazepines and other anti-anxiety drugs produce behavioural changes in animals which have been well described, of which we have a good theoretical understanding (derived from learning theory: Gray, 1975), and which are plausible as the changes one would expect to be produced by anti-anxiety agents (Gray, 1977, 1978). An economical and reasonably accurate description of these changes is that the anti-anxiety drugs block the behavioural effects of stimuli which warn of impending punishment, of stimuli which warn of frustrative non-reward (as defined by Amsel, 1962), and of novel stimuli (Gray, 1977). From this, one might deduce that anxiety consists in the state which is elicited by these three classes of stimuli (Gray, 1978). This definition of anxiety is based entirely on animal experiments. Yet it does not do badly as a description of clinical anxiety in man, especially with a little re-phrasing: anxiety is a state elicited by the threat of pain, loss or failure and by unfamiliar circumstances. Furthermore, the behavioural effects produced in experimental animals by these three classes of 'adequate stimuli for anxiety' (as one might boldly call them) are also plausible as analogues of the behavioural signs of human anxiety. They consist in the inhibition of ongoing behaviour (especially rewarded behaviour), an increased level of arousal, and increased attention to environmental cues, especially novel ones (Gray, 1975, 1977, 1978).

The existence in animals of these theoretical and experimental parallels to human anxiety gives one an invaluable double-check on the validity of any proposed identification of a particular brain structure as part of a system mediating anxiety. For it follows that intervention in the normal functioning of this structure should produce predictable effects on behaviour. If the intervention is such as to impair its normal functioning (e.g. a lesion), we should observe a reduction in anxiety (i.e. a reduction in the behavioural effects of the adequate stimuli for anxiety), as when we administer an anti-anxiety drug. Conversely, if the intervention is such as to increase its normal functioning (e.g. electrical stimulation), we should observe an increase in anxiety. Notice that one is not always in such a fortunate position in attempting to deduce relevant brain structures from drug action. For example, one of the greatest handicaps faced by workers interested in the neural basis of schizophrenia is that, while much is known about the neurochemical effects of anti-psychotic drugs, there is no behaviour in experimental animals to which these effects can be related and which is at the same time a plausible analogue of psychotic behaviour in man.

Arguments and experiments along these lines have been used to identify the septo-hippocampal system and its noradrenergic and serotonergic afferents as candidates for structures which mediate anxiety (Gray, 1970, 1978; Gray *et al.* 1978; Stein *et al.* 1973). This is not the place to repeat the evidence which supports these inferences. Rather, I should like briefly to relate this hypothesis to certain other views of the functions of the same structures.

The first of these alternative views has been expressed by Crow (1973) in this country and Stein (1968) in the United States. It is that the dorsal ascending noradrenergic bundle, which originates in the locus coeruleus in the brain stem and innervates much of the forebrain, including the septal area and the hippocampus (Ungerstedt, 1971), is the neural substrate of reward (Stein) or reinforcement (Crow). This suggestion is, of course, diametrically opposed to the hypothesis (Gray *et al.* 1975) that the dorsal noradrenergic bundle mediates responses to stimuli which warn of frustrative *non*-reward (a component of anxiety, as defined above). The reward hypothesis of the function of the dorsal noradrenergic bundle is largely based on the results of experiments on electrical self-stimulation of the brain (Rolls, 1975). Like the non-reward hypothesis, it too has been said by some of its proponents to have significance for psychiatry, though now it is schizophrenia (Stein & Wise, 1972) rather than anxiety which occupies the centre of the stage. But recent experiments which have examined responses to natural reward (e.g. food), as distinct from electrical stimulation of the brain, in animals with virtually total destruction of the dorsal noradrenergic bundle have clearly disproved the reward hypothesis, while offering good support for the non-reward hypothesis. These animals learn and perform the rewarded response without difficulty, but show retarded extinction (Mason & Iversen, 1975) and loss of the normal 'partial reinforcement effects' produced when non-rewarded trials are randomly intermixed with rewarded trials (Owen *et al.* 1979).

The second alternative view which I wish to consider is harder to summarize succinctly. It is not a single hypothesis, but rather a distillation of a variety of different views of the functions of the septo-hippocampal system, as expressed at a recent CIBA symposium on this topic (Elliott & Whelan, 1978). These views differed in detail from one another in very many ways. But they all had in common the assumption that the septo-hippocampal system is concerned with *cognitive* rather than emotional functions. This might seem to imply that the hypothesis proposed here, that the septo-hippocampal system mediates anxiety, is excessively idiosyncratic. But this inference would be based on a false dichotomy between thought and emotion. Anxiety is as distinctive a state cognitively as it is emotionally: it shows itself as clearly in obsessional ruminations as in poundings of the heart, in indecision as much as in sweating of the palms.

After much discussion, the participants at the CIBA symposium were able to find common ground in their differing proposals as to the functions of the septo-hippocampal system. This lay in the proposal that this system functions as a match–mismatch comparator (A. H. Black, in Elliott & Whelan, 1978, p. 418). This proposal is congenial to the theory of anxiety outlined here. For this theory may be stated as follows: the septo-hippocampal system has the task of monitoring ongoing activities, comparing achieved with desired goals, registering discrepancies (punishment, non-reward, failure) and threats of discrepancies, bringing ongoing activities to a halt when such registrations occur, and searching for better alternative courses of action. On this analysis, the clinical symptom which is most characteristic of anxiety is obsessional checking, not the simple phobia (which has more traditionally fallen easy prey to accounts based on learning theory). In sum, as the Soviet physiologist, Simonov, put it, the septo-hippocampal system is 'an organ of hesitation and doubt'. We all need such an organ; it is when it becomes pathologically over-active (usually in predisposed individuals: Eysenck, 1967; Gray, 1973) that one sees the clinical phenomena of anxiety.

An important question remains: what synaptic and neural events intervene between the binding of the benzodiazepines to their receptor and the action which (*ex hypothesi*) they exert on the septo-hippocampal system? To this question there is, as yet, no answer. The ubiquity of benzodiazepine binding in the brain makes it difficult to see how a precisely localized site of action can be attributed to these drugs. The ubiquity of GABA poses an analogous problem. But the demonstration of increased anxiety after picrotoxin administration (Soubrié *et al.* 1978), and the evidence that the barbiturates (like the benzodiazepines) facilitate the action of GABA (Ransom & Barker, 1976; Barker & Ransom, 1978), both reinforce the likelihood that this neurotransmitter is intimately concerned with the regulation of anxiety. Fuxe *et al.* (1975) have suggested that GABA-ergic afferents to the locus coeruleus play a critical role in this regulation. Alternative possibilities lie in the GABA-ergic terminals in the lateral septal area (McLennan & Miller, 1974, 1976) or in the hippocampus (Storm-Mathisen, 1978). Resolution of this problem will provide a lively challenge to research in the next few years.

J. A. GRAY

My thanks are due to Drs Jane Mellanby and Ian Martin for helpful comments on the manuscript.

REFERENCES

Amsel, A. (1962). Frustrative nonreward in partial reinforcement and discrimination learning: some recent history and a theoretical extension. *Psychological Review* **69**, 306–328.

Barker, J. L. & Ransom, B. R. (1978). Pentobarbitone pharmacology of mammalian central neurones grown in tissue culture. *Journal of Physiology* **280**, 355–372.

Braestrup, G. & Squires, R. F. (1977). Specific benzodiazepine receptors in rat brain characterized by high-affinity [^{3}H]-diazepam binding. *Proceedings of the National Academy of Sciences, USA* **74**, 3805–3809.

Broadhurst, P. L. (1975). The Maudsley reactive and non-reactive strains of rats: a survey. *Behavior Genetics* **5**, 299–319.

Browne, T. R. & Perry, J. K. (1973). Benzodiazepines in the treatment of epilepsy, *Epilepsia* **14**, 277–310.

Cook, L. & Sepinwall, J. (1975). Behavioral analysis of the effects and mechanisms of action of benzodiazepines. In *Mechanism of Action of Benzodiazepines* (ed. E. Costa and P. Greengard), pp. 1–28. Raven Press: New York.

Costa, E. & Greengard, P. (eds.) (1975). *Mechanism of Action of Benzodiazepines*. Raven Press: New York.

Crow, T. J. (1973). Catecholamine-containing neurones and electrical self-stimulation. 2. A theoretical interpretation and some psychiatric implications. *Psychological Medicine* **3**, 66–73.

Elliott, K. & Whelan, J. (eds.) (1978). *Functions of the Septo-Hippocampal System*. CIBA Foundation Symposium no. 58 (new series). Elsevier: Amsterdam.

Eysenck, H. J. (1967). *The Biological Basis of Personality*. C. C. Thomas: Springfield, Ill.

Fuxe, K., Agnati, L. F., Bolme, P., Hökfelt, T., Lidbrink, P., Ljungdahl, A., Perez de la Mora, M. & Ögren, S.-O. (1975). The possible involvement of GABA mechanisms in the action of benzodiazepines on central catecholamine neurons. In *Mechanism of Action of Benzodiazepines* (ed. E. Costa and P. Greengard), pp. 45–61. Raven Press: New York.

Gray, J. A. (1964). The relation between stimulus intensity and response strength in the context of Pavlovian personality theory. Unpublished Ph.D. thesis: University of London.

Gray, J. A. (1970). Sodium amobarbital, the hippocampal theta rhythm and the partial reinforcement extinction effect. *Psychological Review* **77**, 465–480.

Gray, J. A. (1973). Causal theories of personality and how to test them. In *Multivariate Analysis and Psychological Theory* (ed. J. R. Royce), pp. 409–463. Academic Press: London.

Gray, J. A. (1975). *Elements of a Two-Process Theory of Learning*. Academic Press: London.

Gray, J. A. (1977). Drug effects on fear and frustration: possible limbic site of action of minor tranquillizers. In *Handbook of Psychopharmacology* (ed. L. L. Iversen, S. D. Iversen and S. H. Snyder), pp. 433–529. Plenum: New York.

Gray, J. A. (1978). The 1977 Myers Lecture: The neuropsychology of anxiety. *British Journal of Psychology* **69**, 417–434.

Gray, J. A., McNaughton, N., James, D. T. D. & Kelly, P. H. (1975). Effect of minor tranquillisers on hippocampal theta rhythm mimicked by depletion of forebrain noradrenaline. *Nature* **258**, 424–425.

Gray, J. A., Feldon, J., Rawlins, J. N. P., Owen, S. & McNaughton, N. (1978). The role of the septo-hippocampal system and its noradrenergic afferents in behavioural responses to nonreward. In *Functions of the Septo-Hippocampal System* (ed. K. Elliott and J. Whelan), pp. 275–300. CIBA Foundation Symposium no. 58 (new series). Elsevier: Amsterdam.

Guidotti, A., Toffano, G. & Costa, E. (1978). An endogenous protein modulates the affinity of GABA and benzodiazepine receptors in rat brain. *Nature* **275**, 553–555.

Macdonald, R. L. & Barker, J. L. (1978). Benzodiazepines specifically modulate GABA-mediated postsynaptic inhibition in cultured mammalian neurones. *Nature* **271**, 563–564.

Mason, S. T. & Iversen, S. D. (1975). Learning in the absence of forebrain noradrenaline. *Nature* **258**, 422–424.

McLennan, H. & Miller, J. J. (1974). The hippocampal control of neuronal discharges in the septum of the rat. *Journal of Physiology* **237**, 607–624.

McLennan, H. & Miller, J. J. (1976). Frequency-related inhibitory mechanisms controlling rhythmical activity in the septal area. *Journal of Physiology* **254**, 827–841.

Meldrum, B. S. (1975). Epilepsy and γ-aminobutyric acid-mediated inhibition. *International Review of Neurobiology* **17**, 1–36.

Möhler, H. & Okada, T. (1977). Benzodiazeipne receptor: demonstration in the central nervous system. *Science* **198**, 849–851.

Mowrer, O. H. (1947). On the dual nature of learning: a re-interpretation of 'conditioning' and 'problem-solving'. *Harvard Educational Review* **17**, 102–148.

Owen, S., Boarder, M. R., Feldon, J., Gray, J. A. & Fillenz, M. (1979). Role of forebrain noradrenaline in reward and nonreward. *Proceedings of the 4th International Catecholamine Symposium*, California, September 1978 (ed. E. Usdin) (in the press).

Paul, S. M. & Skolnick, P. (1978). Rapid changes in brain benzodiazepine receptors after experimental seizures. *Science* **202**, 892–894.

Randall, L. O. & Kappell, B. (1973). Pharmacological activity of some benzodiazepines and their metabolites. In *The Benzodiazepines* (ed. S. Garattini, E. Mussini and L. O. Randall), pp. 27–51. Raven Press: New York.

Ransom, B. R. & Barker, J. L. (1976). Pentobarbital selectively enhances GABA-mediated post-synaptic inhibition in tissue cultured mouse spinal neurons. *Brain Research* **114**, 530–535.

Robertson, H. A., Martin, I. L. & Candy, J. M. (1978). Differences in benzodiazepine receptor binding in Maudsley reactive and Maudsley non-reactive rats. *European Journal of Pharmacology* **50**, 455–457.

Rolls, E. T. (1975). *The Brain and Reward*. Pergamon: Oxford.

Schallek, W., Schlosser, W. & Randall, L. O. (1972). Recent developments in the pharmacology of the benzodiazepines. *Advances in Pharmacology and Chemotherapy* **10**, 119–181.

Soubrié, P., Thiébot, M. H. & Simon, P. (1978). Enhanced suppressive effects of aversive events induced in rats by picrotoxin: evidence for a GABA control on behavioral inhibition. *Abstracts of the 11th Congress of the Collegium Internationale Neurophychopharmacologicum*, p. 426.

Squires, C. & Braestrup, R. F. (1977). Benzodiazepine receptors in rat brain. *Nature* **266**, 732–734.

Stein, L. (1968). Chemistry of reward and punishment. In *Psychopharmacology: A Review of Progress* 1957–1967 (ed. D. H. Efron), pp. 105–123. US Government Printing Office: Washington, D.C.

Stein, L. & Wise, D. C. (1972). Possible etiology of schizophrenia: progressive damage to the noradrenergic reward system by endogenous 6-hydroxydopamine. In *Neurotransmitters* (ed. I. J. Kopin). *Research Publications of the Association for Nervous and Mental Disease* **50**, 298–311.

Stein, L., Wise, C. D. & Berger, B. D. (1973). Anti-anxiety action of benzodiazepines: decrease in activity of serotonin neurons in the punishment system. In *The Benzodiazepines* (ed. S. Garattini E. Mussini and L. O. Randall), pp. 299–326. Raven Press: New York.

Storm-Mathisen, J. (1978). Localization of putative transmitters in the hippocampal formation (with a note on the connections to septum and hypothalamus). In *Functions of the Septo-Hippocampal System* (ed. K. Elliott and J. Whelan), pp. 49–79. CIBA Foundation Symposium no. 58 (new series). Elsevier: Amsterdam.

Ungerstedt, U. (1971). Stereotaxic mapping of the monoamine pathways in the rat brain. *Acta Physiologica Scandinavica* **82**, Suppl. 367, 1–48.

Williamson, M. J., Paul, S. M. & Skolnick, P. (1978). Labelling of benzodiazepine receptors *in vivo*. *Nature* **275**, 551–553.

Psychological Medicine, 1981, **11**, 449–453

Artificial intelligence[1]

Artificial intelligence (AI) is a fundamentally interdisciplinary subject, combining ideas from psychology, computer science, linguistics, mathematics and even philosophy (see, for example, Sloman, 1978). It is also a very young field. One consequence of its youth and interdisciplinary nature is that until fairly recently one of its most distinctive characteristics was its state of confusion. In the last few years, however, AI has begun to take on a much more coherent form. Reasons for this include the identification of key issues and fundamental areas and the development of approaches possessing considerable generality. I shall, very briefly, outline some of these below, but before doing so I shall explain why I believe AI to have a very important role to play in psychiatric research (indeed, also in psychological and sociological research and in the behavioural sciences generally).

The study of AI has two primary motivations. The first is to build computers (or, more correctly, to write programs) which behave in an intelligent way; and the second is to investigate the nature of human intelligence. Clearly, although these aims are related, they are not identical. In particular, we may note that while being an adequately close model of human brain function is a sufficient attribute for a program to demonstrate intelligent behaviour, it is not a necessary one. One can make an analogy with flying: while the study of flying animals (birds) can lead to ideas about flying (the use of wings), this is not a necessary approach (use rockets instead). Nevertheless, it is obvious that a mutual enrichment must follow from the interaction between AI and the human based mental sciences. Certainly, AI and cognitive psychology exhibit parallel theoretical developments and the hard formalism imposed by the rigorous theory formulation necessitated by the AI methodology has aided the testing of psychiatric (Colby, 1975) and sociological (Abelson, 1973) hypotheses. At present, both human-based models (for example, in natural language processing – see below) and abstract mathematical approaches (for example, in pattern recognition, Duda & Hart, 1973) have been successful. Some, however (for example, Hayes-Roth, 1978), believe that ultimately the best approach to AI may not be via the non-human information processing paradigms but via closer modelling of human memory and cognition. And, conversely, it may also be the case that the best approach to the study of human mentation is via the new field of AI. The point is that it is all very well formulating psychological and psychiatric theories verbally but, when using natural language (even technical jargon), it is difficult to recognize when a theory is complete; oversights are all too easily made, gaps too readily left. This is a point which is generally recognized to be true and it is for precisely this reason that the behavioural sciences attempt to follow the natural sciences in using 'classical' mathematics as a more rigorous descriptive language. However, it is an unfortunate fact that, with a few notable exceptions, there has been a marked lack of success in this application. It is my belief that a different approach – a different mathematics – is needed, and that AI provides just this approach (see also Boden, 1977). When formulating a theory as a program, which is exactly what AI does, the oversights are spotted, the gaps made apparent, and the oversimplifications made explicit. And a theory so formulated can be rigorously tested and appropriately refined. Weizenbaum (1976) puts it thus:

> The very eloquence that natural language permits sometimes illuminates our words and seems (falsely, to be sure) to illuminate our undeserving logic just as brightly. An interpreter of programming language texts, a computer, is immune to the seductive influence of mere eloquence.

It is, however, equally important to emphasize the qualitative distinction between the AI approach and the 'classical' mathematical or statistical approach. The former permits rigorous formulation

[1] Address for correspondence: Dr D. J. Hand, Biometrics Unit, Institute of Psychiatry, De Crespigny Park, Denmark Hill, London SE5 8AF.

and testing of hypotheses concerning the underlying psychological motivations (etc.), and not merely superficial ('mechanical', 'trivial') and easily observed variables.

In the remainder of this editorial I shall mention a few of the areas of research within AI which have been recognized as of fundamental importance, and also indicate a few of the many applications for which programs have been implemented. Thus, in view of the significant implications (social, philosophical, and so on), I shall not constrain myself merely to those formulations which are explicit models of human information processing. I have also attempted to refer mainly to key articles or review papers.

The single most important issue is probably that of knowledge representation: that is, the issue of how to describe or encode knowledge or information. (Here the parallel with certain areas of psychology is obvious.) A particular kind of behaviour may be almost impossible to model in one type of representation but trivial in another. Having said this, however, there are obvious advantages to be gained from general representations, representations which can be applied usefully in a large number of areas. One such is the concept of the 'frame'. This was first developed at the Massachusetts Institute of Technology (MIT) in the context of vision but has also been applied extremely effectively in the domain of natural language processing. A key paper is one by Minsky (1975), who states:

> A *frame* is a data-structure for representing a stereotyped situation like being in a certain kind of living room or going to a child's birthday party. Attached to each frame are several kinds of information. Some of this information is about how to use the frame. Some is about what one can expect to happen next. Some is about what to do if these expectations are not confirmed.

As the focus of attention moves from one situation to another, so different frames are implemented. More correctly, different frames are *instantiated* (Bobrow & Brown, 1975; Kuipers, 1975): detailed information from the new situation is slotted into the chosen frame, replacing default values by values obtained from the currently experienced environment, be it verbal, visual, or in some abstract universe. Since the extra information may itself be in the form of frames, quite complex structures can be built up. The frame concept has led to the development of special high-level frame representation programming languages (see, for example, Bobrow & Winograd, 1977; Hayes, 1980). Related ideas include those of the script (Schank & Abelson, 1977; Lehnert, 1980) and the plan (Abelson, 1975; Schank & Abelson, 1975).

Given that a particular type of behaviour may appear simple or difficult to model, according to the representation chosen to realize it, the fact that it is not always obvious which of several competing representations is the best has led to some controversy. A good example of this is the fundamental choice between the opposing epistemologies of representing knowledge as procedures (i.e. program segments) or as declarations (i.e. as facts in a database): as Winograd (1975) puts it, choosing between 'knowing how' and 'knowing that'. The declarative approach, by separating the 'that' from the 'how' and concentrating on the former, leads to independence of distinct facts and hence to generalizability, modularity, and comprehensibility. Conversely, the procedural approach yields the capability for very rich interaction. While it is true that the two representations are trivially isomorphic at some level, the question is: what are the advantages to be gained by adopting one or the other (or a compromise) viewpoint? Frequently (always, some would say), either can be chosen for a particular domain and it is not clear which is the more efficient. Examples of the proceduralists' standpoint are given by Hewitt *et al.* (1973) and Winograd (1972), and of the declarativists' view by McCarthy & Hayes (1969). A thoughtful outline of the difference is provided by Winograd (1975) and an amusing 'imaginary, yet somehow representative conversation' from the procedural–declarativist feud appears at the end of Winston (1977).

Another related and important example of a fundamental choice in representation is that between conventional computer programs which operate 'on expected data in known formats using a prespecified and inflexible control structure' and *pattern-directed* systems in which parts of the program are activated whenever certain patterns or structures occur in the data (Waterman &

Hayes-Roth, 1978*b*). Pattern-directed inference systems and *production systems* are being used more and more often in practical applications and I shall list some below.

Representation is one issue which has been identified as being of fundamental importance. Another is that of *search*. In the case of vision or natural language processing, for example, incoming information has to gain access to and interact with the appropriate part of the model, so that some efficient way has to be used to locate this part. Or consider the game of chess. In principle, one could list all possible games and choose the best move from a particular position by studying this list. In practice, this is inconceivable for even the fastest computer imaginable, so some simplified search method has to be found for identifying a good move in a reasonable amount of time. Once again, both abstract mathematics and the emulation of hypothesized human abilities have led to methods (Nilsson, 1971; Newell & Simon, 1972; Knuth & Moore, 1975). An interesting discovery of search theory, which seems at first counterintuitive, is the advantage to be gained by additional complexity. Waltz (1975), for example, shows how the introduction of the apparently additional complication of shadows into scenes makes it easier rather than harder to interpret the scene (the introduction imposes extra constraints on the number of possible interpretations).

It will be evident from the preceding brief sampling of some important issues that certain areas of study crop up again and again. Particular examples are the topics of natural language processing and vision. It is perhaps hardly surprising that natural language understanding has attracted a lot of interest since it can be argued that the same issues are involved in this limited domain as are involved in more general problems of intelligence, and it is also obvious that language understanding systems have direct practical application. Once again, many different approaches have been studied and a vast literature has accumulated. Examples of two different approaches are those of Winograd (1972) and Weizenbaum (1965). The former uses an internal representation which enables it to recognize the identity of paraphrases, to understand anaphora, and generally 'to infer the meaning of questions and commands that would otherwise remain opaque' (Boden, 1977) about its own (limited) universe. Weizenbaum's program uses pattern-matching processes and applies simple transformations to input sentences (so it can 'recognize' but not 'understand'). While the pattern-matching approach is not powerful enough to demonstrate the subtleties of parsing and comprehension exhibited by the knowledge-based approach, it does have the advantage that, whenever the input sentence contains a recognizable pattern, a response of some kind is given. Important recent developments include attempts to integrate the two approaches (for example, Schank, 1972, 1973; Wilks, 1972, 1976). It may be noted that in testing theories of language it is possible to adopt different viewpoints: Lehnert (1978) takes question-answering as the main aim, while Davey (1978) concentrates on discourse production. Examples of frame-based text processing are given by Cullingford (1977) and Rosenberg (1980). Further, different grammatical theories can be used (Winograd, 1972, for example, uses Halliday's (1970) 'systemic' grammar rather than Chomsky's syntactic theory).

Like language, vision is an area of immediate practical relevance (we have all heard how the latest generation of industrial robots have TV camera eyes to guide their work). Mathematical approaches (for example, Roberts, 1965) have been used, as also have more psychological based theories. Winston (1975) provides an excellent introduction. One thing which has become evident as understanding has grown is that much computation occurs in natural vision systems. This is only made feasible by massive computational parallelism – which is again being emulated in artificial systems (such as the CLIP4).

Natural language and vision are limited domains which have obvious relevance both to theoretical understanding and to practical applications. Another limited domain, but one which does not have any obvious practical relevance, is the development of games-playing programs. In fact, many of the fundamental ideas of AI have been developed in the game arena – and I can do no better than quote Clarke (1977):

> Many of us would maintain that chess, with its simple representation yet deep structure and richly developed culture, may even be the best system in which to study these problems (that is, AI) in their purest and most readily quantifiable form.

Recently, a new branch of AI has become important, namely, the *expert system* (Waterman & Hayes-Roth, 1978*a*; Michie, 1979, 1980). These are systems which hold representations of a particular limited domain and can respond intelligently and easily to questions and suggestions. They can thus act as consultants. I shall illustrate with a few medical examples, though such systems have been implemented in many different fields. MYCIN (Shortliffe, 1976) identifies bacteria in blood and urine samples and prescribes appropriate antibiotic treatments; INTERNIST (Pople *et al.* 1977) yields diagnoses in internal medicine (within their limited domains MYCIN and INTERNIST perform better than clinical consultants); PUFF (Kunz, 1978) diagnoses pulmonary function disorder; VM (Fagan, 1978) gives advice on the mechanical ventilation of patients in intensive care. An interesting spin-off of expert systems (perhaps one to be expected in the light of the comments above) is that the formalization of the domains as computer programs has led to improved understanding and clearer explanations of the subject matter. Michie (1980) calls this *knowledge refining*.

It is implicit in the above that such systems can improve their knowledge base by interacting with a human tutor. It is not so obvious that artificial systems can generate original material. Lenat (1976), however, has developed a system that searches for potentially interesting mathematical theorems (as distinct from other systems, which prove theorems). Boden (1977) also makes some telling points about creativity in AI. Research in other areas within AI has resulted in programs which can do geometric analogy tests as well as humans, perform symbolic integration better than humans, beat the world backgammon champion (Berliner, 1980), and make moves which even world champion chess players initially supposed to be poor until they had thought about it overnight.

We commented above that AI is a young discipline – and as with any young organism it is growing very rapidly. (There are already several journals devoted solely to AI research.) The reason for its youth is simply that effective experimentation in AI is entirely dependent on electronic computers, and these are a relatively recent development. It is even more recently that the importance of *user-friendliness* has been recognized. The expert systems discussed above do not give cursory diagnoses based on statistical analyses of databases: they arrive at their conclusions by interacting (usually in some subset of natural language) with the user. If asked why they have made an assertion they can answer – in as much detail as the user requires (see also Fox *et al.* 1980). One's thoughts inevitably turn to psychiatric interviews and diagnosis. To some, the very idea is immoral (Weizenbaum, 1976). But others (Colby, 1967) point out that if computers are helpful and if staffing problems mean there are too few psychiatrists, then we really have no choice. One must also remember the evidence that people prefer computer interviews when delicate or anxiety-causing topics are being discussed (Walton *et al.* 1973; Lucas *et al.* 1977).

These points are, however, quite distinct from that which I made at the beginning. Namely, that when we view AI as modelling man it follows a basically humanist approach, but one which nevertheless permits formal hypothesis formulation and testing.

D. J. HAND

REFERENCES

Abelson, R. P. (1973). The structure of belief systems. In *Computer Models of Thought and Language* (ed. R. C. Schank and K. M. Colby), pp. 287–340. W. H. Freeman: San Francisco.

Abelson, R. P. (1975). Concepts for representing mundane reality in plans. In *Representation and Understanding* (ed. D. G. Bobrow and A. Collins), pp. 273–309. Academic Press: New York.

Berliner, H. (1980). Computer backgammon. *Scientific American* **242**, 54–62.

Bobrow, D. G. & Winograd, T. (1977). An overview of KRL. *Cognitive Science* **1**, 3–46.

Bobrow, R. J. & Brown, J. S. (1975). Systematic understanding: synthesis, analysis, and contingent knowledge in specialised understanding systems. In *Representation and Understanding* (ed. D. G. Bobrow and A. Collins), pp. 103–130. Academic Press: New York.

Boden, M. (1977). *Artificial Intelligence and Natural Man.* Harvester Press: Brighton.

Clarke, M. R. B. (ed.) (1977). *Advances in Computer Class – I.* Edinburgh University Press. Edinburgh.

Colby, K. M. (1967). Computer simulation of change in personal belief systems. *Behavioural Science* **12**, 253.

Colby, K. M. (1975). *Artificial Paranoia.* Pergamon: New York.

Cullingford, R. C. (1977). Script application: computer understanding of newspaper stories. Research Report no. 116, Dept. of Computer Science. Yale University: New Haven, Ct.

Davey, A. (1978). *Discourse Production.* Edinburgh University Press: Edinburgh.

Duda, R. & Hart, P. (1973). *Pattern Classification and Scene Analysis.* Wiley: New York.

Fagan, L. M. (1978). Ventilator management. A program to provide on-line consultative advice in the intensive care unit. Memo no. 78-16. Stanford University Department of Computer Science: Stanford, Ca.

Fox, J., Barber, D. & Bardhan, K. D. (1980). Alternatives to Bayes? A quantitation comparison with rule-based diagnostic inference. *Methods of Information in Medicine* **19**, 210–215.

Halliday, M. A. K. (1970). Functional diversity in language as seen from a consideration of modality and mood in English. *Foundations of Language* **6**, 322–361.

Hayes, P. J. (1980). The logic of frames. In *Frame Conceptions and Text Understanding* (ed. D. Metzing), pp. 46–61. De Gruyter: Berlin.

Hayes-Roth, F. (1978). Implications of human pattern processing for the design of artificial knowledge systems. In *Pattern Directed Inference Systems* (ed. D. A. Waterman and F. Hayes-Roth), pp. 333–346. Academic Press: New York.

Hewitt, C., Bishop, P. & Steiger, R. (1973). A universal modular ACTOR formalism for artificial intelligence. In *Proceedings of the Third International Joint Conference on Artificial Intelligence*, pp. 235–245. Stanford, Ca.

Knuth, D. E. & Moore, R. W. (1975). An analysis of alpha–beta pruning. *Artificial Intelligence* **6**, 293–326.

Kuipers, B. J. (1975). A frame for frames: representing knowledge for recognition. In *Representation and Understanding* (ed. D. G. Bobrow and A. Collins), pp. 151–184. Academic Press: New York.

Kunz, J. (1978). A physiological rule-based system for interpreting pulmonary function test results. Memo HPP no. 78-19. Stanford University Department of Computer Science: Stanford, Ca.

Lehnert, W. G. (1978). *The Process of Question Answering*. Laurence Erlbaum: Hillsdale, N.J.

Lehnert, W. G. (1980). The role of scripts in understanding. In *Frame Conceptions and Text Understanding* (ed. D. Metzing), pp. 79–95. De Gruyter: Berlin.

Lenat, D. (1976). AM. an artificial intelligence approach to discovery in mathematics as heuristic search. Memo AIM no. 286. Stanford University AI Lab.: Stanford, Ca.

Lucas, R. W., Mullin, P. J., Luna, C. B. X. & McInroy, D. C. (1977). Psychiatrist and a computer as interrogators of patients with alcohol-related illnesses: a comparison. *British Journal of Psychiatry* **131**, 160–167.

McCarthy, J. & Hayes, P. (1969). Some philosophic problems from the standpoint of AI. In *Machine Intelligence* vol. 4 (ed. B. Meltzer and D. Michie), pp. 463–502. Edinburgh University Press: Edinburgh.

Michie, D. (1979). *Expert Systems in the Micro-electronic Age*. Edinburgh University Press: Edinburgh.

Michie, D. (1980). Expert systems. *The Computer Journal* **23** 369–376.

Minsky, M. (1975). A framework for representing knowledge. In *The Psychology of Computer Vision* (ed. P. H. Winston), pp. 211–277. McGraw-Hill: New York.

Newell, A. & Simon, H. A. (1972). *Human Problem Solving*. Prentice-Hall: Englewood Cliffs, N.J.

Nilsson, N. J. (1971). *Problem Solving Methods in Artificial Intelligence*. McGraw-Hill: New York.

Pople, H. E., Myers, J. D. & Miller, R. A. (1977). DIALOG: a model of diagnostic logic for internal medicine. In *Proceedings of the Fifth International Joint Conference on Artificial Intelligence*. Pittsburgh, USA.

Roberts, L. G. (1965). Machine perception of three-dimensional solids. In *Optical and Electro-optical Information Processing* (ed. J. T. Tippett, D. A. Berkowitz, L. C. Clapp, C. Clapp, C. J. Koester and A. Vanderburgh), pp. 159–198. MIT Press: Cambridge, Mass.

Rosenberg, St T. (1980). Frame-based text processing. In *Frame Conceptions and Text Understanding* (ed. D. Metzing), pp. 96–119. De Gruyter: Berlin.

Schank, R. C. (1972). Conceptual dependency: a theory of natural language understanding. *Cognitive Psychology* **3**, 552–631.

Schank, R. C. (1973). Identification of conceptualisation underlying natural language. In *Computer Models of Thought and Language* (ed. R. C. Schank and K. M. Colby), pp. 187–248. W. H. Freeman: San Francisco.

Schank, R. C. & Abelson, R. P. (1975). Scripts, plans and knowledge. In *Proceedings of the Fourth International Joint Conference on Artificial Intelligence*, pp. 151–157. Tbilisi, USSR.

Schank, R. C. & Abelson, R. P. (1977). *Scripts, Plans, Goals and Understanding*. Laurence Erlbaum: Hillsdale, N.J.

Shortliffe, E. H. (1976). *Computer-based Medical Consultations: MYCIN*. Elsevier/North Holland: New York.

Sloman, A. (1978). *The Computer Revolution in Philosophy*. Harvester Press: Brighton.

Walton, H. J., Kiss, G. R. & Farvis, K. M. (1973). A computer program for the on-line exploration of attitude structures of psychiatric patients. MRC Speech and Communication Research Unit: Edinburgh.

Waltz, D. (1975). Understanding line drawings of scenes with shadows. *The Psychology of Computer Vision* (ed. P. H. Winston), pp. 19–92. McGraw-Hill: New York.

Waterman, D. A. & Hayes-Roth, F. (eds.) (1978*a*). *Pattern Directed Inference Systems*. Academic Press: New York.

Waterman, D. A. & Hayes-Roth, F. (1978*b*). An overview of pattern-directed inference systems. In *Pattern Directed Interference Systems* (ed. D. A. Waterman and F. Hayes-Roth), pp. 3–22. Academic Press: New York.

Weizenbaum, J. (1965). ELIZA – a computer program for the study of natural language communication between man and machine. *Communications of the ACM* **9**, 36–45.

Weizenbaum, J. (1976). *Computer Power and Human Reason*. W. H. Freeman: San Francisco.

Wilks, Y. A. (1972). *Grammar, Meaning, and the Machine Analysis of Language*. Routledge and Kegan Paul: London.

Wilks, Y. A. (1976). *Natural Language Understanding Systems Within the AI Paradigm*. Edinburgh University AI Dept: Edinburgh.

Winograd, T. (1972). *Understanding Natural Language*. Academic Press: New York.

Winograd, T. (1975). Frame representation and the declarative/procedural controversy. In *Representation and Understanding* (ed. D. G. Bobrow and A. Collins), pp. 185–210. Academic Press: New York.

Winston, P. H. (1975). *The Psychology of Computer Vision*. McGraw-Hill: New York.

Winston, P. H. (1977). *Artificial Intelligence*. Addison-Wesley: London.

Psychological Medicine, 1981, **11**, 219–227

Cerebral laterality and psychopathology: fact and fiction[1]

The plethora of reports on lateralization and psychopathology is part of the *Zeitgeist* that spawned 'neuroscience', and in psychology the concern with brain behaviour relations. The underpinning of abnormal behaviour with a disturbance in lateralization has long been a source of speculation (Zangwill, 1960) and more recently gained impetus from the association of schizophreniform psychoses with left-sided temporal lobe dysfunction and affective psychoses with a corresponding right hemisphere disturbance (Flor-Henry, 1969, 1974). After a decade of intensive research what can be concluded?

For those who acknowledge *terra firma* when morphological deficits are proven, Luchins *et al.* (1979) found with computer tomography that normally occurring lateral asymmetries in the width of frontal and occipital lobes were reversed more often in schizophrenia than in controls. The coincidence between the two asymmetries was not given, but frontal asymmetries were reversed in 13 % of controls and 33 % of patients, with 9 % and 25 % the corresponding percentages for occipital reversals. If reversals of function follow, they may confound comparisons between patients and controls so that in schizophrenia, and to a lesser extent in controls, group distributions of laterality scores will show asymmetries in both directions.

This serves to introduce the complex methodological problems that laterality research faces. One may construe a lateralized disorder in patients not only if the normal asymmetry is absent, or reversed, but also in the presence of the normal asymmetry, provided that performance is reduced below the level of controls. It is essential, therefore, to equate the patient and comparison groups for task difficulty. Nevertheless, quite apart from the results of Luchins *et al.*, it is not entirely satisfactory that all three possible outcomes may be considered evidence of a lateralized deficit to a single hemisphere.

Fortunately, not all approaches are prone to this qualification. If a deficit is defined in terms of the nature of the psychological processing measured, instead of laterality, a conclusion may run that verbal processing compared with spatial processing was deficient, in which case the question 'to which hemisphere do verbal functions belong?' is of secondary importance. With this strategy an experiment should include tasks specific to each hemisphere which in themselves are of equal difficulty. When such requirements are met they also circumvent a major criticism that bedevils psychological studies: namely, the intrusion of factors such as motivation, test anxiety, institutionalism, etc.; such issues will usually affect both hemispheres, and the nature of a lateralized deficit is likely to be neurophysiological. Furthermore, as a global hemispheric deficit is not an issue in current theories, a matter sometimes overlooked, the tests specific to each hemisphere should possess a neuro-anatomical equivalence. This requirement is more easily met when measuring the earlier stages of processing or in tasks processed by either hemisphere. The transmission of information between the hemispheres may also be examined by comparing material transmitted directly to the specialized hemisphere with that directed via the non-specialized one.

Returning to the review of evidence, an association between abnormal lateralization and schizophrenia has been found in the handedness of twins, one or both of whom have psychosis (Boklage, 1977; Luchins *et al.* 1980). Concordance for schizophrenia was 93 % when both twins were dextral, but merely 23 % when one was sinistral. Left-handed cases also showed milder forms of the disorder. Surveys of handedness in psychotic populations are contradictory, with evidence of more sinistrality (Dvirskii, 1976; Gur, 1977; Lishman & McMeekan, 1976; Flor-Henry, 1979*a*), and dextrality (Taylor *et al.* 1980), or no difference from controls (Oddy & Lobstein, 1972; Wahl, 1976). Neverthe-

[1] Address for correspondence: Dr John H. Gruzelier, Department of Psychiatry, Charing Cross Hospital Medical School, Fulham Palace Road, London W6 8RF.

less, given that when distributions of handedness in psychotic patients differ from control distributions the differences are marginal, data from this source are of peripheral interest in elucidating the mechanisms of dysfunction. Left and mixed handedness have also been associated with non-psychotic psychopathology (Bakan, 1973; Fitzhugh, 1973; Orme, 1970; Zangwill, 1960).

Attempts to lateralize dysfunction with neuropsychological tests have had limited success. While some have found evidence of a disturbance to the speech dominant hemisphere in schizophrenia, or the opposite hemisphere in mania and depression (Klonoff *et al.* 1970; Gruzelier & Hammond, 1976; Flor-Henry & Yeudall, 1979; Abrams & Taylor, 1979), this is a far from universal finding (Malek, 1978). Undoubtedly problems of sampling, inappropriate comparison groups, difficulty in controlling drugs, Parkinsonian side-effects and fatiguability of patients when faced with large batteries of tests contribute to the confusion. Also, such tests were designed to measure brain damage and there is little evidence that brain damage in a gross form, even when detected (e.g. Johnstone *et al.* 1978), is necessary for the primary schizophrenic disturbance.

In their attempts to measure more discrete processes experimental psychologists have devoted most attention to the schizophrenic psychoses. In the case of visual processing there are eight studies using a tachistoscope, a device which enables stimuli to be transmitted to one hemisphere before the other. In the first (Beaumont & Dimond, 1973) a deficiency was revealed in the integration of information between the hemispheres as well as a left hemisphere deficit. Others have revealed a deficiency when information is projected directly to the left hemisphere, rather than indirectly via the transcallosal pathway. Gur (1978) found for both paranoid and non-paranoid patients that accuracy in recalling letters was poorer when projected over the direct pathway. This contrasted with adequate performance on a right hemisphere task irrespective of input channel. Connolly *et al.* (1979) found similar results insofar as schizophrenic and hypomanic patients took *longer* to process verbal material when presented directly to the left hemisphere – accuracy was not affected. While the same phenomenon was not reproduced by Eaton (1979), who examined patients both on and off drugs, her mean results suggest that the effect may have existed on drugs but not before. As the patients of Gur and Connolly *et al.* were medicated, the possibility of a drug explanation should be investigated. Eaton found a left hemisphere advantage in processing verbal material in both schizophrenic patients and controls; but the performance of schizophrenic patients was poorer, indicating a verbal deficit, particularly as both groups showed a similar ability on tasks involving the right hemisphere. Hillsberg (1979) also found in schizophrenics poorer left than right hemisphere processing in deciding whether pairs of arrows pointed in the same or opposite directions. There was no interhemispheric transfer deficit. In a study of symptomatic schizophrenic out-patients, maintained on drugs, male patients failed to show the normal advantage in processing verbal material in the left hemisphere (Colbourn & Lishman, 1979).

Unlike the above studies which found no evidence of right hemisphere deficits in detecting spatial information, Pic'l *et al.* (1979) report a verbal deficit in schizophrenia coupled with a spatial deficit in non-paranoid patients. The latter was attributed to a problem in integrating information between the hemispheres because normals and paranoid patients counted dots in a serial fashion, thereby requiring analytic processes of the left hemisphere integrated with spatial abilities of the right hemisphere. Non-paranoids utilized the right hemisphere only. An alternative explanation might be that non-paranoid patients were restricted to right hemisphere processing because the analytic ability of their left hemisphere was deficient. The authors explained away the verbal deficit found in both types of schizophrenia because it correlated with years spent at school. However, in the case of paranoids, this explanation is unconvincing – their education was no different from that of controls. Furthermore, paranoids showed a deficit on a similarities test, which is indicative of a left hemisphere deficit (McFie, 1975) and one previously found in chronic schizophrenia (Gruzelier & Hammond, 1976). Turning to the non-paranoid group, even if a deficit does correlate with years of schooling this does not exclude the possibility that the left hemisphere disability predisposes a vulnerability to schizophrenia and limits educational progress. A similar deficiency in children with a schizophrenic parent (Gruzelier *et al.* 1979) supports this supposition. Thus a left-sided deficit could account for their results.

This is not to exclude the possibility of a dysfunctional right hemisphere in schizophrenia. Gur (1979) required paranoid and non-paranoid patients with unrestricted vision to detect the difference between pairs of pictures placed side by side or seen successively. While all groups were less accurate with successive presentation, and schizophrenic patients were poorer overall, patients of both categories were *slower* when pictures were presented side by side. This was likened to the results of an unpublished study of neurological patients with right hemisphere brain damage which, on the face of it, would appear to support a right hemisphere deficit in schizophrenia. Instead, this was interpreted as evidence of an over-reliance on a dysfunctional left hemisphere. Perhaps in the service of parsimony a right hemisphere explanation should be preferred or be an alternative.

Returning to the divided field tachistoscope studies, Clooney & Murray (1977) required patients to identify an array of letters as the same or different. While no lateral asymmetries in processing were found in schizophrenic patients or controls, patients were slower overall than controls, and paranoid patients were progressively slower as the size of the array increased. This anomaly in paranoids was interpreted as arising from their dependence on serial (left hemisphere) rather than parallel (right hemisphere) processing.

When we turn to studies of auditory function, the plot thickens further, though the auditory symptoms that accompany psychosis, auditory functions of the temporal lobe, and psychotic-like states that accompany temporal lobe dysfunction (Davison & Bagley, 1969) led us to suppose a more coherent outcome. The functional neuroanatomy of the auditory system is such that each ear projects to both hemispheres but the contralateral pathways are dominant. Ipsilateral input may be suppressed by requiring the immediate recall of competing input presented to both ears simultaneously. This was verified in patients with sections of the transcallosal pathway (Sparks & Geschwind, 1968). Recall of verbal material from the right ear was normal, whereas from the left ear it was substantially reduced. Presumably right ear input was processed by the contralateral pathway and left ear input depended on the transcallosal pathway from the right to left hemisphere. Using a closely similar procedure, three studies (Lerner *et al.* 1977; Lishman *et al.* 1978; Gruzelier & Hammond, 1979, 1980) have shown a *larger* lateral asymmetry in favour of the right ear in many schizophrenic patients compared with controls. Two of the studies found that this characterized paranoid schizophrenia (Gruzelier & Hammond, 1979, 1980; Lerner *et al.* 1977, as reanalysed by Nachshon, 1980). This might imply a deficit in transferring information between the hemispheres but, by controlling attentional bias to either side, the asymmetry could be explained as an over-reliance on direct right ear input to the left hemisphere rather than as a defective transcallosal pathway (Gruzelier & Hammond, 1979); levels of performance did not differ between patients and controls. The dependence on left hemisphere processing in paranoid schizophrenia is consistent with evidence in the visual modality (Clooney & Murray, 1977; Pic'l *et al.* 1979).

Green and colleagues (Green *et al.* 1979; Green & Kotenko, 1980) report a larger than normal right ear preference in the speech comprehension of schizophrenic patients. The level of performance with which the lateral difference was correlated was below that of controls. These results are open to a number of interpretations: for example, a left hemisphere verbal deficit coupled with an attentional bias to the right ear, or an attentional bias coupled with a lack of motivation which lowered performance. However, poorer comprehension when speech was heard binaurally rather than monaurally suggests a problem in integrating information between the hemispheres, as does evidence of longer reaction times to binaural than to monaural stimuli in schizophrenic patients (Gruzelier & Hammond, 1979). The locus of dysfunction might be lateralized or reside in interhemispheric pathways. Dichotic listening studies have shown a left hemisphere inhibitory deficit through the inability of schizophrenic patients to withhold recall of words in the right ear in favour of the left ear when right ear words were twenty decibels louder than left ear words (Bull, 1972; Gruzelier & Hammond, 1980). Performance of a corresponding condition which required suppression of left ear words was no worse than controls. By examining serial position effects the latter authors conclude that there were a number of left hemisphere deficits of higher order processing, which involved semantic encoding, retrieval and response organization. These could include the reception of information transmitted from the right hemisphere.

Other studies, while showing the normal right ear advantage in processing language-related tasks, found a poorer level of performance in schizophrenic patients than controls, consistent with a left hemisphere deficit in patients (Bruder & Yozawitz, 1979; Caudrey & Kirk, 1979). In fact, Caudrey & Kirk showed in schizophrenia impairments in a left hemisphere task coexisting with normal performance on a right hemisphere task, whereas in depression there was the reverse asymmetry. In two other studies the expected right ear preference was absent in schizophrenia. This was shown by Colbourn & Lishman (1979) in a subgroup of male patients, and by Wexler & Heninger (1979) who examined patients repeatedly before and during treatment and found the normal asymmetry reinstated with improvement of symptoms on drugs. The magnitude of the asymmetries was within normal limits.

A systematic reversal of asymmetries in auditory processing with the withdrawal and later reinstatement of drug was reported by Hammond & Gruzelier (1978). The effect was related to dose level. Phenothiazines appeared to increase the arousability of the left hemisphere relative to the right, an effect which may facilitate or impair performance depending on existing arousal levels and intensity of input (Gruzelier, 1979*a*). Alterations of lateralized differences on drug have also been found in the electroencephalogram (Goldstein *et al.* 1965; Serafetinides, 1972, 1973), palmar electrodermal activity (Gruzelier & Yorkston, 1978), visual processing (Eaton, 1979) and reaction times (Gruzelier & Hammond, 1979).

Studies of the tactile modality have provided the main evidence of Dimond and his colleagues for a disorder of interhemispheric communication in schizophrenia (Green, 1978; Dimond, 1979; Dimond *et al.* 1979; Carr, 1980). Other workers (Kugler & Henley, 1979; Weller & Kugler, 1979), as reviewed elsewhere (Gruzelier, 1979*a*), have not found conclusive support for the theory, though they have obtained evidence of left hemisphere dysfunction. In a more recent report of 24 middle-aged, institutionalized schizophrenic patients a third were found to exhibit errors in naming objects with eyes closed, particularly when placed in the left hand, a condition which required callosal transmission to the language processors of the left hemisphere (Dimond *et al.* 1979). However, on one of the four test occasions no errors were made in either hand. The study would appear to substantiate the impression that the callosal deficit when manifested in schizophrenia is an elusive one and often coexists with left hemisphere dysfunction. The problem may be spasmodic and has been attributed to one of impaired transmission (Beaumont & Dimond, 1973), a noisy channel (Butler, 1979; Dimond *et al.* 1979), a loss of contralateral inhibition (Gruzelier, 1978; Wexler & Heninger, 1979) and a dominance of transcallosal influences (Tress *et al.* 1979).

A variety of psychophysiological indices have provided evidence of an abnormal balance of activity between the hemispheres in psychosis. Under controlled conditions the majority of studies show that schizophrenic patients direct their eyes rightwards more often than patients with affective disorders or controls (Gur, 1978; Schweitzer *et al.* 1978; Myslobodsky *et al.* 1979; Schweitzer, 1979). This was attributed to an over-activation of the left hemisphere. However, Sandel & Alcorn (1980) found more leftward movements in non-paranoid schizophrenia, as well as in depression and alcoholism, with movements in both directions in manic-depression, schizo-affective disorders and psychopathy. No normal controls were tested. Measures of activation with electro-encephalographic techniques obtained in the resting state or during cognitive activity have produced complex results implicating both hemispheres in psychosis and providing evidence of activation inappropriate to the nature of the task (Flor-Henry *et al.* 1979; Perris & Monakhov, 1979; Goldstein, 1979; Shaw *et al.* 1979; Weller & Montague, 1979; and see Gruzelier, 1979*a* for a review). These studies, together with those which average discrete changes to trains of identical stimuli (Buchsbaum *et al.* 1979; Shagass *et al.* 1979; Tress *et al.* 1979), suggest that topographic analysis may prove rewarding in differentiating between psychiatric groups (e.g. Shagass *et al.* 1980). Greater clarity may also arise in correlating symptoms rather than diagnostic categories with EEG topography and coherence between recording sites within and between the hemispheres (Perris & Monakhov, 1979). The recording of phasic changes in experimental tasks will assist in localizing and defining processing deficits.

An abnormal balance in hemispheric influences has also been shown in the electrical conductivity of the skin recorded from palmar surfaces. Schizophrenic patients, particularly chronic ones, tend to have larger orienting and non-specific responses on the right hand, with the opposite asymmetry shown in some depressives (Fisher & Cleveland, 1959; Gruzelier, 1973, 1979*b*; Gruzelier & Hammond, 1977; Gruzelier & Venables, 1974; Myslobodsky & Horesh, 1978; Uherik, 1975). On the whole normal subjects have symmetrical responses or small deviations in either direction. The limbic influence on these asymmetries is reinforced by recent evidence suggesting that it is predominantly an emotional component that determines the direction of the electrodermal asymmetry. By relating them to syndromes from the Present State Examination (Wing *et al.* 1974) and ratings on the Brief Psychiatric Rating Scale (Overall & Gorham, 1962) it was found that hypomania, depressive delusions and pressure of speech were among the characteristics of admissions for schizophrenia with larger left-sided responses, whereas blunted affect, emotional withdrawal, slowness, catatonia, motor retardation and conceptual disorganization characterized the schizophrenic patients with larger right-sided responses (Gruzelier *et al.* 1981).

Regarding the affective disorders and lateralization, essentially there have been two rival notions. One is that mania and depression are a result of right hemisphere dysfunction, and are thereby distinguished from schizophrenia. The second is that emotional polarity differs between the hemispheres, with positive emotions and mania on the left side and negative emotions and depression on the right side. Certainly there is a growing body of experimental data with normal subjects indicating that mood is controlled by the right hemisphere (see Gainotti, 1979). Furthermore, in patients, schizophrenia and affective disorders have been distinguished by lateral differences in facets of auditory processing, neuropsychological tests, and measures of muscle activity, electrodermal responses, conjugate eye movements and EEG, most of which implicate the right hemisphere in affective disorders (Abrams & Taylor, 1979; Caudrey & Kirk, 1979; Flor-Henry & Yeudall, 1979; Flor-Henry *et al.* 1979; Gruzelier & Venables, 1974; Myslobodsky & Horesh, 1978; Bruder & Yozawitz, 1979). Equally there is support for an association of euphoria and depression, and corresponding psychopathology, with the left and right hemispheres respectively (see Gainotti, 1979). This has led Flor-Henry (1979*a*, *b*) to conceive a complex model of how mood is organized by both hemispheres, with transcallosal influences posited to explain hemispheric differences in the polarity of mood and with distinctions made between the syndromes of mania and depression, on the one hand, and normal reactions of euphoria and depression, on the other. While some of the evidence is compelling, it is also true that there is evidence of the opposite relation: namely, euphoric reactions deriving from the right hemisphere and depressive reactions from the left hemisphere. Evidence with normals indicates reciprocal influences between the hemispheres in the control of arousal and habituation (Gruzelier *et al.* 1980) and offers a means whereby each hemisphere has the potential to evoke euphoria or depression, depending on the state of imbalance between excitatory and inhibitory subsystems with contralateral projections. Divergent findings on the lateralization of the emotions may be reconciled through elucidating mechanisms of this type.

Psychopathy and various neurotic disorders have also been associated with a disturbance of lateralization (Zangwill, 1960). Yeudall & Fromm-Auch (1979) amassed evidence largely from neuropsychological tests of a dominant hemisphere deficit in various groups of children and adults with behaviour disturbances. Hare (1979) was unable to support this in a tachistoscope study with psychopaths. The lateralization of some neurotic disorders, such as conversion hysteria and psychogenic pain to the left side of the body, has been explained as a mode of expression for the non-verbal, right hemisphere (Galin, 1974; Fleminger *et al.* 1980). However, not all reports indicate a preponderance of left-sided symptoms.

The simple notions that have generated much of the research reviewed above have now given way to more complex models (e.g. Flor-Henry, 1979*a*, *b*). Schizophrenia is unlikely to be a disorder of strictly one hemisphere or a disconnection syndrome in the conventional sense (cf. Geschwind, 1965). This review of evidence suggests a new working model as follows. In schizophrenia the moment to moment allocation of capacity between the hemispheres is often at odds with hemispheric specialization. In paranoid schizophrenia and schizo-affective cases with hypomania there is an over-reliance on the left or speech dominant hemisphere. In non-paranoid schizophrenia and schizo-affective cases with depression reliance is on the right hemisphere. Such a distinction between paranoid and non-paranoid schizophrenia, invoked because of the differences revealed in many reports above, may need qualifying and be replaced by partially overlapping syndromes, perhaps incorporating an arousal/motility dimension (cf. Gruzelier & Hammond, 1979, 1980). Primary delusions, as well as flat incongruous affect and catatonic features, all correlated with left hemisphere lesions in the survey by Davison & Bagley (1969) of schizophrenic-like psychoses associated with organic disorders. Therefore it is likely that the primary disturbance in schizophrenia is in the left hemisphere and affects the right hemisphere through transcallosal influences. It would be parisimonous, though too good to be true, if the affective disorders involved corresponding right hemisphere dysfunction with mania showing a dependence on the left hemisphere and depression a dependence on the right hemisphere.

It has been suggested (Weller & Montague, 1979; Venables, 1980) that in schizophrenia the disturbance develops in the right hemisphere and spreads to the left with chronicity. There is scant evidence in support of this and it should be noted that the evidence called upon of Itil *et al.* (1974), whereby there was an accentuation of EEG abnormalities in the right hemisphere in children with a schizophrenic parent, coexisted with evidence of verbal deficits and in some children superior spatial–perceptual ability (Gruzelier *et al.* 1979).

From this review it is clear that, while the neuropsychology of psychopathological states is in its infancy, it is a new and promising line of enquiry which provides some integration of hitherto numerous and unrelated reports of patient–control differences. Apart from its scientific interest, it may have clinical applications. Evidence of objective, biological differences between patients will assist with diagnosis. The likelihood of hemispheric asymmetries in neurotransmitter systems (Glick *et al.* 1977; Oke *et al.* 1978), and the evidence of alterations in lateralized processes on neuroleptics, may elucidate the therapeutic actions of drugs in psychiatric practice. Whatever the outcome, the fact of the matter is that the study of the abnormal brain has already led to insights about the workings of the normal brain.

JOHN H. GRUZELIER

REFERENCES

Abrams, R. & Taylor, M. A. (1979). Laboratory studies in the validation of psychiatric diagnoses. In *Hemisphere Asymmetries of Function in Psychopathology* (ed. J. H. Gruzelier and P. Flor-Henry), pp. 363–372. Elsevier/North Holland Biomedical Press: Amsterdam.

Bakan, P. (1973). Left-handedness and alcoholism. *Perceptual and Motor Skills* **36**, 514.

Beaumont, J. G. & Dimond, S. J. (1973). Brain disconnection and schizophrenia. *British Journal of Psychiatry* **123**, 661–662.

Boklage, C. E. (1977). Schizophrenia, brain asymmetry development and twinning: cellular relationship with etiological and possibly prognostic implication. *Biological Psychiatry* **12**, 17–35.

Bruder, G. E. & Yozawitz, A. (1979). Central auditory processing and lateralization in psychiatric patients. In *Hemisphere Asymmetries of Function in Psychopathology* (ed. J. H. Gruzelier and P. Flor-Henry), pp. 561–580. Elsevier/North Holland Biomedical Press: Amsterdam.

Buchsbaum, M. S., Carpenter, W. T., Fedio, P., Goodwin, F. K., Murphy, D. L. & Post, R. M. (1979). Hemispheric differences in evoked potential enhancement by selective attention to hemiretinally presented stimuli in schizophrenic, affective and post-temporal lobectomy patients. In *Hemisphere Asymmetries of Function in Psychopathology* (ed. J. H. Gruzelier and P. Flor-Henry), pp. 317–328. Elsevier/North Holland Biomedical Press: Amsterdam.

Bull, H. C. (1972). Speech perception and short-term memory in schizophrenia. Unpublished doctoral dissertation: University of London.

Butler, S. (1979). Interhemispheric relations in schizophrenia. In *Hemisphere Asymmetries of Function in Psychopathology* (ed. J. H. Gruzelier and P. Flor-Henry), pp. 47–63. Elsevier/North Holland Biomedical Press: Amsterdam.

Carr, S. A. (1980). Interhemispheric transfer of stereognostic information in chronic schizophrenics. *British Journal of Psychiatry* **136**, 53–58.

Caudrey, D. J. & Kirk, K. (1979). The perception of speech in schizophrenia and affective disorders. In *Hemisphere Asymmetries of Function in Psychopathology* (ed. J. H. Gruzelier and P. Flor-Henry), pp. 581–601. Elsevier/North Holland Biomedical Press: Amsterdam.

Clooney, J. L. & Murray, D. J. (1977). Same–different judgments in paranoid and non-paranoid patients: a laterality study. *Journal of Abnormal Psychology* **86**, 655–658.

Colbourn, C. J. & Lishman, W. A. (1979). Lateralisation of function and psychotic illness: a left hemisphere deficit? In *Hemisphere Asymmetries of Function in Psychopathology* (ed. J. H. Gruzelier and P. Flor-Henry), pp. 539–560. Elsevier/North Holland Biomedical Press: Amsterdam.

Connolly, J. F., Gruzelier, J. H., Kleinman, K. M. & Hirsch, S. R. (1979). Lateralised abnormalities in schizophrenic, depressive and non-psychotic patients in hemispheric specific tachistoscopic tasks. In *Hemisphere Asymmetries of Function in Psychopathology* (ed. J. H. Gruzelier and P. Flor-Henry), pp. 647–672. Elsevier/North Holland Biomedical Press: Amsterdam.

Davison, K. & Bagley, C. R. (1969). Schizophrenia-like psychoses associated with organic disorders of the central nervous system: a review of the literature. In *Current Problems in Neuropsychiatry* (ed. R. N. Herrington), pp. 113–184. Royal Medico-Psychological Association, Headley Bros.: Ashford, Kent.

Dimond, S. J. (1979). Disconnection and psychopathology. In *Hemisphere Asymmetries of Function in Psychopathology* (ed. J. H. Gruzelier and P. Flor-Henry), pp. 35–46. Elsevier/North Holland Biomedical Press: Amsterdam.

Dimond, S. J., Scammell, R. E., Pryce, J. Q., Huss, D. & Gray, C. (1979). Callosal transfer and left-hand anomia in schizophrenia. *Biological Psychiatry* **14**, 735–739.

Dvirskii, A. E. (1976). Functional asymmetry of the cerebral hemispheres in clinical types of schizophrenia. *Neuroscience and Behavioral Physiology (Washington)* **7**, 236–239.

Eaton, E. M. (1979). Hemisphere-related visual information processing in acute schizophrenia before and after neuroleptic treatment. In *Hemisphere Asymmetries of Function in Psychopathlogy* (ed. J. H. Gruzelier and P. Flor-Henry), pp. 511–526. Elsevier/North Holland Biomedical Press: Amsterdam.

Fisher, S. & Cleveland, S. E. (1959). Right–left body reactivity problems in disorganised states. *Journal of Nervous and Mental Disease* **128**, 396–400.

Fitzhugh, K. B. (1973). Some neuropsychological features of delinquent subjects. *Perceptual and Motor Skills* **36**, 494.

Fleminger, J. J., McClure, G. M. & Dalton, R. (1980). Lateral response to suggestion in relation to handedness and the side of psychogenic symptoms. *British Journal of Psychiatry* **136**, 562–566.

Flor-Henry, P. (1969). Psychoses and temporal lobe epilepsy: a controlled investigation. *Epilepsia* **10**, 363–395.

Flor-Henry, P. (1974). Psychosis, neurosis and epilepsy. *British Journal of Psychiatry* **124**, 144–150.

Flor-Henry, P. (1979*a*). Laterality, shifts of cerebral dominance, sinistrality and psychosis. In *Hemisphere Asymmetries of Function in Psychopathology* (ed. J. H. Gruzelier and P. Flor-Henry), pp. 3–20. Elsevier/North Holland Biomedical Press: Amsterdam.

Flor-Henry, P. (1979*b*). On certain aspects of the localisation of the cerebral systems regulating and determining emotions. *Biological Psychiatry* **14**, 677–697.

Flor-Henry, P. & Yeudall, L. T. (1979). Neuropsychological investigation of schizophrenia and manic-depressive psychoses. In *Hemisphere Asymmetries of Function in Psychopathology* (ed. J. H. Gruzelier and P. Flor-Henry), pp. 341–362. Elsevier/North Holland Biomedical Press: Amsterdam.

Flor-Henry, P., Koles, Z. J., Howarth, B. G. & Burton, L. (1979). Neurophysiological studies of schizophrenia, mania and depression. In *Hemisphere Asymmetries of Function in Psychopathology* (ed. J. H. Gruzelier and P. Flor-Henry), pp. 189–222. Elsevier/North Holland Biomedical Press: Amsterdam.

Gainotti, G. (1979). The relationships between emotions and cerebral dominance: a review of clinical and experimental evidence. In *Hemisphere Asymmetries of Function in Psychopathology* (ed. J. H. Gruzelier and P. Flor-Henry), pp. 21–34. Elsevier/North Holland Biomedical Press: Amsterdam.

Galin, D. (1974). Implications for psychiatry of left and right cerebral specialisations. A neuropsychological context for unconscious processes. *Archives of General Psychiatry* **31**, 572–583.

Geschwind, N. (1965). Disconnection syndromes in animals and man. *Brain* **88**, 237–294.

Glick, S. D., Jerussi, T. P. & Zimmersberg, B. (1977). Behavioural and neuropharmacological correlates of nigrostriatal asymmetry in rats. In *Lateralisation in the Nervous System* (ed. S. Harnad, R. W. Doty, L. Goldstein, J. Jaynes and S. Krauthamer), pp. 213–250. Academic Press: London.

Goldstein, L. (1979). Some relationships between quantified hemispheric EEG and behavioural states in man. In *Hemisphere Asymmetries of Function in Psychopathology* (ed. J. H. Gruzelier and P. Flor-Henry), pp. 237–254. Elsevier/North Holland Biomedical Press: Amsterdam.

Goldstein, L., Sugerman, A. A., Stolberg, H., Murphee, H. B. & Pfeiffer, C. C. (1965). Electro-cerebral activity in schizophrenics and non-psychotic subjects: quantitative EEG amplitude analyses. *Electroencephalography and Clinical Neurophysiology* **19**, 350–361.

Green, P. (1978). Defective interhemispheric transfer in schizophrenia. *Journal of Abnormal Psychology* **87**, 472–480.

Green, P. & Kotenko, V. (1980). Superior speech comprehension in schizophrenics under monaural *versus* binaural listening conditions. *Journal of Abnormal Psychology* **89**, 399–408.

Green, P., Glass, A. & O'Callaghan, M. A. J. (1979). Some implications of abnormal hemisphere interaction in schizophrenia. In *Hemisphere Asymmetries of Function in Psychopathology* (ed. J. H. Gruzelier and P. Flor-Henry), pp. 431–448. Elsevier/North Holland Biomedical Press: Amsterdam.

Gruzelier, J. H. (1973). Bilateral asymmetry of skin conductance orienting activity and levels in schizophrenia. *Journal of Biological Psychology* **1**, 21–41.

Gruzelier, J. H. (1978). Bimodal states of arousal and lateralised dysfunction in schizophrenia: the effect of chlorpromazine. In *The Nature of Schizophrenia: New Approaches to Research and Treatment* (ed. L. Wynne, R. Cromwell and S. Matthysse), pp. 167–187. Wiley: New York.

Gruzelier, J. H. (1979*a*). Synthesis and critical review of the evidence for hemisphere asymmetries of function in psychopathology. In *Hemisphere Asymmetries of Function in Psychopathology* (ed. J. H. Gruzelier and P. Flor-Henry), pp. 647–672. Elsevier/North Holland Biomedical Press: Amsterdam.

Gruzelier, J. H. (1979*b*). Lateral asymmetries in electrodermal activity and psychosis. In *Hemisphere Asymmetries of Function in Psychopathology* (ed. J. H. Gruzelier and P. Flor-Henry), pp. 149–168. Elsevier/North Holland Biomedical Press: Amsterdam.

Gruzelier, J. H. & Hammond, N. V. (1976). Schizophrenia: a dominant hemisphere temporal-limbic disorder? *Research Communications in Psychology, Psychiatry and Behaviour* **1**, 33–72.

Gruzelier, J. H. & Hammond, N. V. (1977). The effect of chlorpromazine upon bilateral asymmetries of bioelectric skin reactivity in schizophrenia. *Studia Psychologica* **19**, 40–50.

Gruzelier, J. H. & Hammond, N. V. (1979). Lateralised auditory processing in medicated and unmedicated schizophrenic patients. In *Hemisphere Asymmetries of Function in Psychopathology* (ed. J. H. Gruzelier and P. Flor-Henry), pp. 603–638. Elsevier/North Holland Biomedical Press: Amsterdam.

Gruzelier, J. H. & Hammond, N. V. (1980). Lateralised deficits and drug influences on the dichotic listening of schizophrenic patients. *Biological Psychiatry* **15**, 759–779.

Gruzelier, J. H. & Venables, P. H. (1974). Two-flash threshold sensitivity and β in normal subjects and schizophrenics. *Quarterly Journal of Experimental Psychology* **26**, 594–604.

Gruzelier, J. H. & Yorkston, N. J. (1978). Propranolol and schizophrenia: objective evidence of efficacy. In *Biological Basis of Schizophrenia* (ed. W. and G. Hemmings), pp. 127–146. MTP Press: Lancaster.

Gruzelier, J. H., Mednick, S. A. & Schulsinger, F. (1979). Lateralised impairments in the WISC profiles of children at genetic risk for psychopathology. In *Hemisphere Asymmetries of Function in Psychopathology* (ed. J. H. Gruzelier and P. Flor-Henry), pp. 105–110. Elsevier/North Holland Biomedical Press: Amsterdam.

Gruzelier, J. H., Eves, F. F. & Connolly, J. F. (1980). Reciprocal hemispheric influences on response habituation in the electrodermal system. Paper presented to conference on Lateral Asymmetries and Cerebral Function, Leicester, September 1980. (Submitted for publication.)

Gruzelier, J. H., Connolly, J. C. & Hirsch, S. R. (1981). Altered brain functional organisation in psychosis: brain

behaviour relationships. In *Clinical Neurophysiological Aspects of Psychopathological Conditions.* Karger: Basle (in the press).
Gur, R. E. (1977). Motoric laterality imbalance in schizophrenia: a possible concomitant of left hemisphere dysfunction. *Archives of General Psychiatry* **34**, 33–37.
Gur, R. E. (1978). Left hemisphere dysfunction and left hemisphere overactivation in schizophrenia. *Journal of Abnormal Psychology* **87**, 226–238.
Gur, R. E. (1979). Cognitive concomitants of hemispheric dysfunction in schizophrenia. *Archives of General Psychiatry* **36**, 269–274.
Hammond, N. V. & Gruzelier, J. H. (1978). Laterality, attention and rate effects in the auditory temporal discrimination of chronic schizophrenics: the effect of chlorpromazine. *Quarterly Journal of Experimental Psychology* **30**, 91–103.
Hare, R. D. (1979). Psychopathy and laterality of cerebral function. *Journal of Abnormal Psychology* **28**, 605–610.
Hillsberg, B. (1979). A comparison of visual discrimination performance of the dominant and nondominant hemispheres in schizophrenia. In *Hemisphere Asymmetries of Function in Psychopathology* (ed. J. H. Gruzelier and P. Flor-Henry), pp. 527–538. Elsevier/North Holland Biomedical Press: Amsterdam.
Itil, T. M., Hsu, W., Saletu, B. & Mednick, S. A. (1974). Computer EEG and auditory evoked potential investigations in children at high risk for schizophrenia. *American Journal of Psychiatry* **131**, 892–900.
Johnstone, E. C., Crow, T. J., Frith, C. D., Stevens, M., Kreel, L. & Husband, J. (1978). The dementia of dementia praecox. *Acta psychiatrica scandinavica* **57**, 305–324.
Klonoff, H., Fibiger, C. G. & Hutton, G. H. (1970). Neuropsychological problems in chronic schizophrenia. *Journal of Nervous and Mental Disease* **150**, 291–300.
Kugler, B. T. & Henley, S. H. A. (1979). Laterality effects in the tactile modality in schizophrenia. In *Hemisphere Asymmetries of Function in Psychopathology* (ed. J. H. Gruzelier and P. Flor-Henry), pp. 475–489. Elsevier/North Holland Biomedical Press: Amsterdam.
Lerner, J., Nachshon, I. & Carmon, A. (1977). Responses of paranoid and non-paranoid schizophrenics in a dichotic listening task. *Journal of Nervous and Mental Disease* **164**, 247–252.
Lishman, W. A. & McMeekan, E. R. L. (1976). Hand preference in psychiatric patients. *British Journal of Psychiatry* **129**, 158–166.
Lishman, W. A., Toone, B. K., Colbourn, C. J., McMeekan, E. R. L. & Mance, R. M. (1978). Dichotic listening in psychotic patients. *British Journal of Psychiatry* **132**, 333–341.
Luchins, D. J., Weinberger, D. R. & Wyatt, R. J. (1979). Schizophrenia: evidence of a subgroup with reversed cerebral asymmetry. *Archives of General Psychiatry* **36**, 1309–1311.
Luchins, D., Pollin, W. & Wyatt, R. J. (1980). Laterality in monozygotic schizophrenic twins: an alternative hypothesis. *Biological Psychiatry* **15**, 87–94.
Malek, J. (1978). Neuropsychological assessment of schizophrenia *versus* brain damage: a review. *Journal of Nervous and Mental Disease* **166**, 507–516.
McFie, J. (1975). *The Assessment of Organic Impairment.* Academic Press: London.
Myslobodsky, M. S. & Horesh, N. (1978). Bilateral electrodermal activity in depressive patients. *Biological Psychiatry* **6**, 111–120.
Myslobodsky, M., Mintz, M. & Tomer, R. (1979). Asymmetric reactivity of the brain and components of hemispheric imbalance. In *Hemisphere Asymmetries of Function in Psychopathology* (ed. J. H. Gruzelier and P. Flor-Henry), pp. 125–148. Elsevier/North Holland Biomedical Press: Amsterdam.
Nachshon, G. (1980). Hemispheric dysfunctions in schizophrenia. *Journal of Nervous and Mental Disease* **168**, 241–242.
Oddy, H. C. & Lobstein, T. J. (1972). Hand and eye dominance in schizophrenia. *British Journal of Psychiatry* **120**, 331–332.
Oke, A., Keller, R., Mefford, I. & Adams, R. (1978). Lateralisation of norepinephrine in human thalamus. *Science* **200**, 1411–1433.
Orme, J. E. (1970). Left-handedness, ability and emotional instability. *British Journal of Social and Clinical Psychology* **9**, 87–88.
Overall, J. E. & Gorham, D. R. (1962). The Brief Psychiatric Rating Scale. *Psychological Reports* **10**, 799–812.
Perris, C. & Monakhov, K. (1979). Depressive symptomatology and systemic structural analysis of the EEG. In *Hemisphere Asymmetries of Function in Psychopathology* (ed. J. H. Gruzelier and P. Flor-Henry), pp. 223–236. Elsevier/North Holland Biomedical Press: Amsterdam.
Pic'l, A. K., Magaro, P. A. & Wade, E. A. (1979). Hemispheric functioning in paranoid and nonparanoid schizophrenia. *Biological Psychiatry* **14**, 891–903.
Sandel, A. & Alcorn, J. D. (1980). Individual hemisphericity and maladaptive behaviors. *Journal of Abnormal Psychology* **89**, 514–517.
Schweitzer, L. (1979). Differences of cerebral lateralisation among schizophrenic and depressed patients. *Biological Psychiatry* **14**, 721–733.
Schweitzer, L., Becker, E. & Walsh, H. (1978). Abnormalities of cerebral lateralisation in schizophrenic patients. *Archives of General Psychiatry* **35**, 982–985.
Serafetinides, E. A. (1972). Laterality and voltage in the EEG of psychiatric patients. *Diseases of the Nervous System* **33**, 422.
Serafetinides, E. A. (1973). Voltage laterality in the EEG of psychiatric patients. *Diseases of the Nervous System* **34**, 190–191.
Shagass, C., Roemer, R. A., Straumanis, J. J. & Amadeo, M. (1979). Evoked potential evidence of lateralized hemispheric dysfunction in the psychoses. In *Hemisphere Asymmetries of Function in Psychopathology* (ed. J. H. Gruzelier and P. Flor-Henry), pp. 293–316. Elsevier/North Holland Biomedical Press: Amsterdam.
Shagass, C., Roemer, R. A., Straumanis, J. F. & Amadeo, M. (1980). Topography of sensory evoked potentials in depressive disorders. *Biological Psychiatry* **15**, 183–207.
Shaw, J. C., Brooks, S., Colter, N. & O'Connor, K. P. (1979). A comparison of schizophrenic and neurotic patients using EEG power and coherence spectra. In *Hemisphere Asymmetries of Function in Psychopathology* (ed. J. H. Gruzelier and P. Flor-Henry), pp. 257–284. Elsevier/North Holland Biomedical Press: Amsterdam.
Sparks, R. & Geschwind, N. (1968). Dichotic listening in man after section of neocortical commissures. *Cortex* **4**, 3–16.
Taylor, P. J., Dalton, R. & Fleminger, J. J. (1980). Handedness in schizophrenia. *British Journal of Psychiatry* **136**, 375–383.
Tress, K. H., Kugler, B. T. & Caudrey, D. J. (1979). Interhemispheric integration in schizophrenia. In *Hemisphere Asymmetries of Function in Psychopathology* (ed. J. H. Gruzelier and P. Flor-Henry), pp. 449–462. Elsevier/North Holland Biomedical Press: Amsterdam.
Uherik, A. (1975). Interpretations of bilateral asymmetry of bioelectrical skin reactivity in schizophrenics. *Studia Psychologica* **17**, 51–59.
Venables, P. H. (1980). Primary dysfunction and cortical lateralisation in schizophrenia. In *Functional States of the Brain: Their Determinants* (ed. M. Kkou-Lehmann), pp. 243–264. Elsevier/North Holland Biomedical Press: Amsterdam.

Wahl, O. F. (1976). Handedness in schizophrenia. *Perceptual and Motor Skills* **42**, 944–946.

Weller, M. & Kugler, B. T. (1979). Tactile discrimination in schizophrenic and affective psychoses. In *Hemisphere Asymmetries of Function in Psychopathology* (ed. J. H. Gruzelier and P. Flor-Henry), pp. 463–474. Elsevier/North Holland Biomedical Press: Amsterdam.

Weller, M. & Montague, J. D. (1979). Electroencephalographic coherence in schizophrenia: a preliminary study. In *Hemisphere Asymmetries of Function in Psychopathology* (ed. J. H. Gruzelier and P. Flor-Henry), pp. 285–292. Elsevier/North Holland Biomedical Press: Amsterdam.

Wexler, B. F. & Heninger, G. R. (1979). Alterations in cerebral laterality in acute psychotic illness. *Archives of General Psychiatry* **36**, 278–284.

Wing, J. K., Cooper, J. E. & Sartorius, N. (1974). *The Measurement and Classification of Psychiatric Symptoms*. Cambridge University Press: Cambridge.

Yeudall, L. T. & Fromm-Auch, D. (1979). Neuropsychological impairments in various psychopathological populations. In *Hemisphere Asymmetries of Function in Psychopathology* (ed. J. H. Gruzelier and P. Flor-Henry), pp. 401–428. Elsevier/North Holland Biomedical Press: Amsterdam.

Zangwill, O. L. (1960). *Cerebral Dominance and its Relation to Psychological Function*. Oliver and Boyd: Edinburgh.

Psychological Medicine, 1982, **12**, 225–230

Interhemispheric integration in man[1]

Twenty years ago a group of distinguished scientists – physiologists, neurologists, anatomists, psychologists and linguists – met at the Johns Hopkins School of Medicine to discuss the functional relationships between the two cerebral hemispheres. Their discussion centred around the simple question 'Why have we two brains?', and details of the proceedings of this conference are contained in a monograph entitled *Interhemispheric Relations and Cerebral Dominance* (Mountcastle, 1962). In summing up these proceedings, it was pointed out that the lack of any clear understanding of the ways in which brain commisures act to provide a transfer of information between the two cerebral hemispheres forms a major gap in the field of neuroscience.

Ten years later, in 1971, another group of eminent research workers gathered for the third study programme in the neurosciences at Colorado (Schmitt & Worden, 1974). At this meeting Teuber (1974) presented a paper entitled 'Why two brains?', in which he stressed the limitations of existing knowledge concerning the fundamental question of 'How commisures act in providing information transfer between the hemispheres and in constraining, or modulating, the activities of the parallel halves of the brain in such a way that a functional asymmetry arises and is maintained'.

Today the question of how interaction between the two hemispheres is obtained still remains unanswered.

This gap in our knowledge might be at least partly explained by the almost exclusive interest, over recent years, in establishing differential specialization of the right and left hemispheres in the normal brain (see Dimond, 1972; Kinsbourne, 1978; Bradshaw & Nettleton, 1981). To a great extent this is a consequence of techniques becoming available which permit a behavioural analysis of the two halves of the intact brain. Previously, the only way to obtain information about the dual functional asymmetry of the human brain had been by experimental investigations carried out on patients with unilateral brain lesions (see Hécaen, 1962; Zangwill, 1963). The studies of normal individuals were designed in an attempt, not only to determine those crucial aspects of cognitive function which distinguish right and left hemispheres, but also to demonstrate differences that exist between different groups of individuals – for example, between men and women (see Buffery & Gray, 1972; Harshman & Remington, 1975), children and adults (see Harnard *et al.* 1977; Dimond & Blizard, 1977), right and left handers (see Hécaen & Ajuriaguerra, 1964; Corballis & Beale, 1976). These studies have taught us a great deal and, as a result, the concept of left cerebral dominance has been abandoned, to be replaced by one of complementary specialization. For some time the roles of the left and the right cerebral hemispheres were described in terms of a verbal/non-verbal dichotomy, with the left hemisphere dominant for language functions and the right for visuo-spatial abilities. This view, however, has now been challenged, and the roles of the hemispheres have been interpreted on an entirely different basis (see Bradshaw & Nettleton, 1981). For instance, the left hemisphere is no longer described as possessing a specialized mechanism for the processing of speech; rather, its function is explained as having a unique specialization for the organization of temporal order sequencing and segmentation. Although the question of what, precisely, are the special functions of the two hemispheres remains open, the fact of a dual functional asymmetry of the two halves of the brain is now generally accepted.

At present, however, it is felt that too much time has been devoted to separating the functions of the respective cerebral hemispheres and too little to analysing how they interact. And it might, at this point, be instructive to bear in mind that between the 'two brains' there is one of the most

[1] This paper is based on a talk given at the Institute of Psychiatry, on 13 February 1980. Address for correspondence: Dr Maria Wyke, Department of Psychology, Institute of Psychiatry, De Crespigny Park, Denmark Hill, London SE5 8AF.

extensive bands of fibres in the nervous system: the corpus callosum, which must serve some other purpose than simply carrying a one-way traffic of information, or as has been stated in the past 'to aid the transmission of epileptic seizures from one side of the body to the other', or, just to perform a simple mechanical role 'to keep the hemispheres from sagging' (see Sperry, 1962). It is now time to turn our attention to establishing how the two distinct and dissimilar brains interact in order to bring about the organized and integrated behaviour of normal individuals.

Others have already drawn attention to the need to solve this problem, among them Broadbent (1974) who, in the same study programme of neurosciences in 1972, argued convincingly for the need to see the cerebral hemispheres as 'performing different parts of an integrated performance, rather than completely separate and parallel functions'.

This paper presents behavioural evidence in support of the notion that the functional specialization of the two hemispheres does not necessarily imply a parallel function or total independence, but that their functions do, in fact, interact. Much of this evidence for interaction between the two cerebral hemispheres has been derived from the very same techniques used to study cerebral specialization, and a brief description of these techniques will follow. They have involved comparing differences in performance between the right and left side of the visual field, by analysing responses to stimuli presented to the left and right ear, and also assessing the performance of voluntary movements with the right and left arms.

The anatomical and physiological arrangement of the visual system – with stimuli presented to the left visual field being processed by the right hemisphere and vice versa – provides us with the opportunity to study effectively the different modes of action of the two hemispheres. The possible interference of eye movements can be eliminated by making the presentation brief – in milliseconds. The accuracy and speed with which these presentations are reported has been taken as evidence of cerebral specialization. For example, when printed words are presented to the left and right of the fixation points and the subject reports more accurately those shown in the right field, this has been taken to imply that the left hemisphere is superior, or dominant, in the processing of verbal material. Similarly, evidence of hemispheric specialization in the auditory modality has been obtained by using the dichotic listening technique. This involves the simultaneous presentation of different messages to the two ears. Greater cortical responses to stimulation of the contralateral ear than to stimulation of the ipsilateral ear reveal the asymmetry of function, and this effect is accentuated when stimulation is simultaneous and competitive (Rosenzweig, 1951). For example, when a different set of words is simultaneously presented to each ear and there is greater accuracy of identification in the right ear, this is taken as evidence that the left hemisphere is dominant in the perception of verbal material (see Milner, 1971; Hécaen & Albert, 1978).

The neural organization of the motor system is somewhat similar to that of the auditory system. The left hemisphere controls mainly the somatosensory and motor functions of the right limbs, while the right hemisphere controls the functions of the left arm and leg. Separation is not complete, as there is ample physiological and anatomical evidence for the existence of an ipsilateral control of sensory–motor function (Terzulo & Adey, 1960; Patton *et al.* 1962; Goff *et al.* 1962).

Evidence for cerebral specialization can be, and frequently is, taken too literally – that is, it is taken to imply that the two halves of the normal brain perform separate and parallel functions. There is, however, substantial evidence of interaction which may suggest that integration of the activity of the two hemispheres is, in fact, the normal and customary mode of function of the intact brain. The term 'interaction' is used here to mean 'mutual and reciprocal' influence between the two halves of the brain. This definition goes well beyond that which describes a simple one-way traffic of information and attributes a role to the cerebral commissures which is much more than merely informing one hemisphere of the activities of the other. Rather, the commissures' function is that of exerting reciprocal influence between the two hemispheres. There are a number of ways in which we can demonstrate the presence of such interaction. For instance, by showing the existence of *cooperative activity* between the hemispheres – that is to say, an increased proficiency at performing a task when the two hemispheres are involved; and by demonstrating *interference* – that is, when one hemisphere interferes with, or hinders, the activity of the other. It could also be demonstrated by showing *transfer of learning* – for example, when activity learned by one hemisphere is transferred to the other; by showing *inhibition* – that is, when one hemisphere inhibits or takes control of the latent activity of the other; and by showing *suppression* – that is, when one hemisphere suppresses the outgoing activity of the other.

Evidence for interhemispheric interaction comes from various behavioural studies. The first example of cooperative activity comes from a study made by Dimond & Beaumont (1972). They presented, tachistoscopically, simple non-verbal stimuli to a group of normal subjects. The stimulus material consisted of pairs of semicircles with various symmetrical designs. The subjects were shown two of these designs in succession and were simply required to identify whether the first and second designs were the same. There were three different modes of presentation of the stimuli to the right visual field, to the left visual field, and to both fields.

There were two different means of response: vocal and manual, the latter requiring the subject to depress two micro switches, one held in each hand. On the basis of existing information it might be assumed that, since this was a non-verbal task, the right hemisphere would be superior in processing this type of information. This would mean that the responses to stimuli presented to the left visual field alone would be significantly faster. In fact, this was not the case. The fastest responses actually occurred when the stimuli were presented to both visual fields: that is, when the two hemispheres were involved in the decision. Dimond & Beaumont interpreted their findings as showing that when the perceptual load was divided between the two hemispheres, efficiency was accentuated.

Another experimental study demonstrating cooperative interaction comes from Basso *et al.* (1977). They based their study on the well known perceptual experience of brightness contrast (see Forgus, 1966). It has been shown that if a shade of grey is surrounded by a white background it appears darker than if it is surrounded by a black background. Basso *et al.* used cards with areas of grey half surrounded by a white background and the other half by a black background. Their subjects were asked to fixate their eyes on the middle of the card in such a way that half the card (for instance, the grey area with white background) was processed by one hemisphere while the other half (in this case the grey with the black background) was simultaneously processed by the other hemisphere. The subjects were then asked to match the grey that they perceived with one on a multiple choice display. This experimental condition, with a different perception of the greyness reaching each hemisphere, provided a perceptual ambiguity. Decision regarding the greyness of the area would, according to existing information, be determined by the right hemisphere which is dominant for the perception of non-verbal material. Thus it was predicted that the subjects would opt for the grey which matched that presented in their left visual field. The results, however, showed that the subjects' responses were an averaging of the information available to each hemisphere. In other words, the grey selected was neither of the two stimuli processed by the respective hemispheres, but rather the decision was based on the information derived from both. Thus it clearly demonstrated a case of mutual cooperation between the two halves of the brain.

As has been mentioned above, if the activity of one hemisphere is seen to interfere with the activity of the other this may be taken as evidence of inter-hemispheric interaction, as the two following studies show precisely. The first comes from Broadbent & Gregory (1965) and Broadbent (1974). These authors argued that, if the two cerebral hemispheres were indeed two parallel channels of communication, then it ought to be possible for a normal subject to perform two different activities simultaneously: one which is known to be subserved by the left hemisphere, the other by the right. To test this notion they studied the reaction time to the stimulation of the finger tip of the left hand. The stimulation occurred every five seconds and the subjects were required to depress a key with the finger stimulated. At the same time they were receiving, every five seconds, a spoken letter of the alphabet. These letters were normally different, but within each minute one letter occurred twice. The subjects were required to report verbally, each minute, which letter appeared most frequently. Thus the subject was simultaneously performing a manual reaction to touch and a spoken reaction based upon memory of speech stimuli – with the right hemisphere controlling the somatosensory and motor performances of the left hand and the left hemisphere, dominant for the language function, subserving the verbal task. This experimental situation would allow the two halves of the brain to work simultaneously in an independent and parallel fashion. Broadbent & Gregory, however, found that when the two stimuli coincided the subject had both a diminished memory for the spoken letters and a significantly slower reaction time to the finger stimulation. The implication of these results is that, since the two hemispheres interfere with each other's action, they cannot be working independently or in parallel; rather, they must be interacting.

It could be argued, however, that the tasks which Broadbent & Gregory required their subjects to perform were too complex, and that the interference arose because their subjects had to divide their attention. But this argument cannot be maintained if interference can be demonstrated when the subject is performing simple, identical, repetitive tasks. Wyke (1969) studied the ability of subjects to perform simple tapping movements with the two hands. The subject's task was simply to tap on a board with a stylus in an up-and-down movement. All the subjects were tested using the right and left hands independently and also using both hands simultaneously. Tapping with the right hand (all the subjects were right-handed) was invariably faster than tapping with the left hand, but when both hands were tapping simultaneously the speed dropped to a level which was significantly lower than for the left hand alone. So, even when they are performing simple repetitive tasks, the arms cannot be regarded as independent moving parts controlled, in parallel, by the two cerebral hemispheres. There is interference, even at this level.

The point concerning the transfer of learning between the two hemispheres is demonstrated by looking at an example of negative transfer. Heap & Wyke (1972) studied the learning of a unimanual motor skill in normal subjects. They used a target pursuit rotor apparatus, consisting of an illuminated target which moves in a circular manner around the glass top of the apparatus, and asked their subjects to follow the target with the probe using one hand. Accuracy of performance was assessed by measuring the total length of time that the subject managed to keep the probe in contact with the target.

Subjects attempted 10 trials of fifteen seconds, each using one hand followed immediately by the same number of trials using the other hand. Subjects were sub-divided into two groups: those who started the test with the right arm and followed with the left, and those who carried out the task in reverse sequence. Results showed that the efficiency of the right arm at performing the task significantly decreased when it was used second in the testing sequence. A decrease in performance was also recorded when the left arm was used second in the sequence, but here the difference was not statistically significant. So it can be said that decreased efficiency of performance with the right arm was a case of negative transfer of learning, although it is of interest that this negative transfer of learning only occurs when the left hand is trained first. The findings, however, reinforce the view that the arms are not independent units controlled in a simple manner by the contralateral hemisphere.

Finally, the information obtained on the two areas of hemispheric interactions mentioned above – the control, by one hemisphere, of the latent activity of the other and the suppression, by one hemisphere, of the outgoing activities of the other – has been derived from the clinical field. Several workers (see von Békésy, 1967) have provided evidence for inhibitory control of one hemisphere over the other. One instance refers to the inhibition of speech function. It has been argued that the right hemisphere possesses a limited ability for verbal expression (Gazzaniga & Hillyard, 1971). This ability, however, is restricted by the left hemisphere's predominance in the control of the neuro-muscular mechanisms involved in speech (Butler & Norrsell, 1968; Levy *et al.* 1971). Release of the inhibition of speech mechanisms by the left hemisphere has been demonstrated in the case of some aphasic patients. Kinsbourne (1971) studied three right-handed patients who had suffered left hemisphere strokes which caused aphasia. All three subjects had some residual speech functions. Injection of sodium amylobarbitone into the right carotid circulation caused a complete arrest of speech, while this was not the case when the injection was on the left. These observations were interpreted by claiming that whatever speech these patients retained was subserved by the right and not by the left hemisphere. This implies that only when the left hemisphere relinquishes control of the neuro-muscular mechanisms can the right hemisphere 'speak'. In other words, the right hemisphere is capable of speech production and can, in fact, subserve oral language when, as a result of brain damage, the left hemisphere surrenders control of the peripheral apparatus of speech production.

Analysis of voluntary movements can also demonstrate a similar suppression of outgoing activity. It is well known that in young children voluntary movements of one limb, and especially the hand, are frequently accompanied by contralateral movements (Fog & Fog, 1963; Abercrombie *et al.* 1964). The natural tendency is for these movements to disappear after the first decade (Fog & Fog, 1963). Their suppression, however, is not total as it has been demonstrated, by means of electromyography, that during voluntary movements of one arm there is contraction of the symmetrical muscles on the opposite side (Cernacek, 1961; Hopf *et al.* 1974). Occasionally, diseases can damage these suppression mechanisms (see Schott & Wyke, 1977, 1981) and give rise to abnormal synkinesias. There are also rare cases in which the mechanism fails to develop altogether, producing abnormal obligatory movements in otherwise normal subjects (Schott & Wyke, 1977). The conclusion we can draw from the suppression of this contralateral motor activity is that there is a constant interaction between the two cerebral hemispheres.

At present, the mechanisms of interaction between the two hemispheres are poorly understood. Moreover, theoretical models which might explain the different aspects of this interaction are lacking. A great deal of research remains to be done. We may at least hope that, in the future, the same zeal which has been applied to separating the activities of the two cerebral hemispheres can be applied to unifying them.

MARIA WYKE

REFERENCES

Abercrombie, M. L., Lindon, R. L. & Tyson, M. C. (1964). Associated movements in normal and physically handicapped children. *Developmental Medicine and Child Neurology* **6**, 573–580.

Basso, A., Bisiach, E. & Capitani, E. (1977). Decision in ambiguity: hemispheric dominance or interaction? *Cortex* **13**, 96–99.

Békésy, G. von (1967). *Sensory Inhibition*. Princeton University Press: Princeton, N.J.

Bradshaw, J. L. & Nettleton, N. C. (1981). The nature of hemisphere specialization in man. *Behavioural and Brain Sciences* **4**, 51–91.

Broadbent, D. E. (1974). Division of function and integration of behaviour. In *The Neurosciences Third Study Program* (ed. F. O. Schmitt and F. G. Worden), pp. 31–41. MIT Press: Cambridge, Mass.

Broadbent, D. E. & Gregory, M. (1965). On the interaction of S–R compatibility with other variables affecting reaction time. *British Journal of Psychology* **56**, 61–67.

Buffery, A. W. H. & Gray, J. A. (1972). Sex differences in the development of perceptual and linguistic skills. In *Gender Differences: Their Ontogeny and Significance* (ed. C. Ounsted and D. C. Taylor), pp. 123–157. Churchill: London.

Butler, S. R. & Norrsell, U. (1968). Vocalisation possibly initiated by the minor hemisphere. *Nature* **220**, 793–794.

Cernacek, J. (1961). Contralateral motor irradiation – cerebral dominance. *Archives of Neurology and Psychiatry* **4**, 165–172.

Corballis, M. C. & Beale, I. L. (1976). *The Psychology of Left and Right*. Lawrence Erlbaum: Hillsdale, N.J.

Dimond, S. J. (1972). *The Double-Brain*. Churchill Livingstone: London & Edinburgh.

Dimond, S. & Beaumont, G. (1972). Processing in perceptual integration between and within the cerebral hemispheres. *British Journal of Psychology* **63**, 509–514.

Dimond, S. J. & Blizard, D. A. (1977). *Evolution and Lateralisation of the Brain*. New York Academy of Sciences: New York.

Fog, E. & Fog. M. (1963). Cerebral inhibition examined by associated movements. In *Minimal Cerebral Dysfunction* (ed. R. MacKeith and M. Bax), pp. 52–57. Little Club Clinics in Developmental Medicine, No. 10. Heinemann: London.

Forgus, R. H. (1966). *Perception*. McGraw-Hill: New York.

Gazzaniga, M. S. & Hillyard, S. A. (1971). Language and speech capacity of the right hemisphere. *Neuropsychologia* **9**, 273–280.

Goff, W. R., Rosner, B. S. & Allison, T. (1962). Distribution of cerebral somatosensory evoked responses in normal man. *Electroencephalography and Clinical Neurophysiology* **14**, 697–713.

Harnard, S., Doty, R. W., Goldstein, L., Jaynes, J. & Krauthamer, G. (eds.) (1977). *Lateralization in the Nervous System*. Academic Press: New York.

Harshman, R. A. & Remington, R. (1975). Sex, language and the brain: 2. Adult sex differences in lateralization. Mimeographed.

Heap, M. & Wyke, M. (1972). Learning of a unimanual skill in patients with brain lesions. *Cortex* **8**, 1–18.

Hécaen, H. (1962). Clinical symptomatology in right and left hemisphere lesions. In *Interhemispheric Relations and Cerebral Dominance* (ed. V. B. Mountcastle), pp. 215–243. Johns Hopkins University Press: Baltimore.

Hécaen, H. & Ajuriaguerra, J. de (1964). *Left-handedness, Manual Superiority and Cerebral Dominance*. Grune & Stratton: New York.

Hécaen, H. & Albert, M. L. (1978). *Human Neuropsychology*. Wiley: New York.

Hopf, H. C., Schlegel, H. J. & Lowitzsch, K. (1974). Irradiation of voluntary activity to the contralateral site in movements of normal subjects and patients with central motor disturbances. *European Neurology* **12**, 142–147.

Kinsbourne, M. (1971). The minor cerebral hemisphere. *Archives of Neurology* **25**, 302–306.

Kinsbourne, M. (ed.) (1978). *Asymmetrical Function of the Brain*. Cambridge University Press: Cambridge.

Levy, J., Nebes, R. D. & Sperry, R. W. (1971). Expressive language in the surgically separated minor hemisphere. *Cortex* **7**, 49–58.

Milner, B. (1971). Interhemispheric differences and psychological process. *British Medical Bulletin* **27**, 272–277.

Mountcastle, V. B. (ed.) (1962). *Interhemispheric Relations and Cerebral Dominance*. Johns Hopkins University Press: Baltimore.

Patton, H. D., Towe, A. L. & Kennedy, T. T. (1962). Activation of pyramidal tract neurons by ipsilateral cutaneous stimuli. *Journal of Neurophysiology* **25**, 501–514.

Rosenzweig, M. R. (1951). Representation of the two ears at the auditory cortex. *American Journal of Physiology* **67**, 147–158.
Schmitt, F. O. & Worden, F. G. (eds.) (1974). *The Neurosciences Third Study Program.* MIT Press: Cambridge, Mass.
Schott, G. D. & Wyke, M. A. (1977). Obligatory bimanual associated movements. *Journal of the Neurological Sciences* **33**, 301–312.
Schott, G. D. & Wyke, M. A. (1981). Congenital mirror movements. *Journal of Neurology, Neurosurgery and Psychiatry* **44**, 586–599.
Sperry, R. W. (1962). Some general aspects of interhemispheric integration. In *Interhemispheric Relations and Cerebral Dominance* (ed. V. B. Mountcastle), pp. 5–19. Johns Hopkins University Press: Baltimore.
Terzulo, C. A. & Adey, W. R. (1960). Sensorimotor activities. In *Handbook of Physiology, Section I* (*Neurophysiology*), vol. 2 (ed. J. Field, H. W. Magoun and V. Z. Hall), pp. 797–835. American Physiological Society: Washington, D.C.
Teuber, H. L. (1974). Why two brains? In *The Neurosciences Third Study Program* (ed. F. O. Schmitt and F. G. Worden), pp. 71–74. MIT Press: Cambridge, Mass.
Wyke, M. (1969). Influence of direction in the rapidity of bilateral arm movements. *Neuropsychologia* **7**, 189–194.
Zangwill, O. L. (1963). The cerebral localisation of psychological function. *The Advancement of Science* **XX**, 1963–64.

Psychological Medicine, 1982, **12**, 7–11

Psychological aspects of employment and unemployment[1]

The central role of employment in society and in individual lives is increasingly being addressed by specialists from several disciplines. For the psychologist and psychiatrist concerned to understand and assist everyday functioning, issues of personal effectiveness and relationships in occupational settings clearly warrant careful examination; and for the epidemiologist and sociologist investigating environmental stressors, life events and vulnerability factors, a range of important work-related themes have emerged. Issues of contemporary concern may be considered under two general headings. I shall first examine some features and processes of paid employment, before moving on to illustrate the links between these and psychological aspects of being unemployed. The latter are of particular concern at present, when the number of people in Britain registered as unemployed and seeking work has almost doubled in a single year.

THE PSYCHOLOGICAL MEANINGS OF PAID EMPLOYMENT

Six benefits of having a job may be identified: the provision of money, activity, variety, temporal structure, social contacts, and a status and identity within society's institutions and networks.

The major importance of the first of these, financial gain, has sometimes been underemphasized by psychological and medical writers, yet a job is clearly essential for most people as their principal source of income and as a means to consequential gains of many kinds. Secondly, employment provides outlets for physical and mental energy, and offers rewards through the development and exercise of personal skills. One basis of mental health may be considered to be the establishment and attainment of realistic goals, and it is partly through work that these may be achieved.

Thirdly, a job provides variety by taking one out of unchanging domestic surroundings and permitting access to facilities and tasks which are not otherwise available. Paid employment serves, fourthly, to divide time into segments, each with its own built-in structure and goals. To move between employment responsibilities and routines and the greater freedom and ease associated with leisure activities provides a contrast which can enhance the value of both. Fifthly, the majority of jobs require social interactions, giving access to a range of shared experiences and supports, as well as providing opportunities for social comparisons which are important for stability and change in self-concept. Finally, employment also provides a personal identity and status within social institutions. The employed person occupies a role, with associated rights and obligations which are not possessed by those out of work; in a sense the latter are not full members of society as it is currently organized.

However, we should also note the psychological costs of being employed. In the first place, many jobs are unquestionably tedious and unattractive. Research has recently focused upon the 'intrinsic' features of tasks such as their variety, autonomy, identity and feedback of results, often observing a marked absence of these characteristics in contemporary employment settings. Strong associations have been recorded between the extent to which they are present and employees' job satisfaction, work motivation, job involvement, commitment, alienation, and measures of mental health and individual or work group effectiveness (e.g. Kornhauser, 1965; Hackman & Lawler, 1971; Coburn, 1978; Wall, 1978). As a result there has been much interest in 'job redesign', suggesting that work tasks may be reorganized to increase their intrinsically valued components and thus yield psychological benefits as well as greater productivity (e.g. Den Hertog, 1976; Hackman & Oldham, 1980). Controlled experiments in this area are difficult, and too many studies which introduce operational

[1] Address for correspondence: Professor Peter Warr, MRC/SSRC Social and Applied Psychology Unit, Department of Psychology, The University, Sheffield S10 2TN.

changes (rather than merely recording correlations at one point in time) are scientifically flawed. However, there is growing evidence that the redesign of jobs can enhance mental health generally, as well as increase specific satisfactions with work (e.g. Wall, 1980). Several authors have stressed that it is lack of personal control of one's work activities which is most strongly predictive of low psychological well-being, especially in circumstances of high task demands (e.g. Karasek, 1979).

Other negative features of employment which have recently been examined include overload, conflict, role ambiguity, excessive responsibility for people, environmental turbulence and uncertainty, bad working conditions, and troubled interpersonal relationships (e.g. Kasl, 1978; Fletcher & Payne, 1980). These negative aspects of having a job have provoked an extensive literature on 'occupational stress', in which a large number of job-related correlates of strain reactions have been suggested. However, this literature needs to be approached with care. Without doubt some jobs are stressful and some job-holders are often under strain, but there are few jobs which cause continuing psychological strain for all people who undertake them.

In their search for stressors and strain reactions, many authors cite merely the correlations between reported job characteristics and reported psychological problems. Apart from the methodological limitation that these studies examine only self-reports, it is important to note that authors rarely cite average values of the variables examined. On those infrequent occasions when mean occupational stressor or employee strain scores are published, they are typically quite low.

Estimated prevalence of course depends upon where the threshold is set, but several sources of evidence suggest that about 5 % of employees are at any one time under work-related strain severe enough to warrant help. Some are likely to be seriously impaired, and over a period (a year, for example) the absolute number of cases becomes substantial. Among those cases will be many who have succumbed to repeated failure in attempts to cope with chronic job pressures. In that respect it is important to view occupational stressors in conjunction with non-occupational difficulties. (Conversely, the medical practitioner exploring non-occupational stressors should also investigate employment difficulties.) It is when problems accumulate from both domains that strain reactions are most probable.

THE PSYCHOLOGICAL IMPACT OF UNEMPLOYMENT

Research over many decades has indicated that the large majority of people say they would continue to work even if they could afford not to, so that it would appear that the psychological benefits of employment outweigh the costs. On this basis those who become unemployed may be expected to suffer.

Their suffering would be due to withdrawal of the positive features described earlier: money, activity, variety, temporal structure, social contacts, and a status and identity within society's institutions. Furthermore, we might expect the negative effects of unemployment to combine together, so that (for example) lack of money, social contact and self-confidence would aggravate each other to yield a cumulatively large deterioration and a reduced ability to find fresh work. This process might be accentuated by the generally dispiriting consequences of prolonged uncertainty, anxiety and self-doubt.

Such effects of unemployment are indeed reported from studies of two general kinds. A wealth of case study material has been gathered, illustrating in detailed narrative form the psychological deterioration which accompanies a period of unemployment (e.g. Jahoda *et al.* 1933; Bakke, 1940; Marsden & Duff, 1975; Sinfield, 1981; Swinburne, 1981). Parallel studies from a more quantitative base have used inventories of depression, anxiety, life satisfaction, minor psychiatric morbidity, self-esteem, and positive and negative affect, and have consistently revealed substantial decrements for the unemployed (e.g. Warr, 1978; Dooley & Catalano, 1980; Hepworth, 1980; Stafford *et al.* 1980). For example, research from the Social and Applied Psychology Unit in Sheffield has found unemployed teenagers to be at least twice as likely as those with jobs to suffer from minor psychiatric disorder (e.g. Warr, 1981).

However, although in general terms the psychological correlates of unemployment are established as strongly negative, there are many important specific questions waiting to be answered. Several of these concern possible moderating variables: what other features influence the strength of the association between employment status (having or not having a job) and psychological health? A number of these will be considered next.

Length of unemployment is an obvious candidate for study: do unemployed people become progressively more impaired with time out of a job, or do processes of adjustment reverse an initial decline? Sadly, we have no detailed information here. Several sequences of response stages have been suggested (e.g. Eisenberg & Lazarsfeld, 1938; Hill, 1978; Schlossberg & Leibowitz, 1980), but these differ considerably between themselves and are not based adequately upon longitudinal data. This area is particularly difficult, since direction and speed of development are dependent upon many factors, such as job-seeking success, financial resources or social supports. One variable of interest is age: for example, it may be that unemployed people in their 50s come to adjust to the idea of 'early retirement', whereas younger people with dependent children find continuing unemployment increasingly painful. Differential hypotheses of this kind have not yet been tested.

It should be emphasized that there is a disturbing lack of psychological research into longer-term unemployment (more than 12 months is one definition). Long-term unemployed people differ from those out of work for shorter periods in a number of respects, for example being older, less healthy and having fewer qualifications and skills (Colledge & Bartholomew, 1980). Generalizations to this group from present psychological data are unlikely to be fully justified. By the same token, we lack adequate information about possible long-term irreversible effects of unemployment; research has not looked for these in any systematic way, concentrating more upon measures of current psychological state during periods of unemployment up to a few months.

One variable which has been shown clearly to moderate the impact of short-term unemployment is 'work involvement', the degree to which having paid employment is salient within a person's system of values. It is firmly established that the negative psychological effects of unemployment are greater for those people with high work involvement (Warr, 1978; Stafford *et al.* 1980). In a general motivational sense this is not surprising, but it has several important practical implications. For example, the strength of influence of this variable means that in examining psychological correlates of unemployment we should attempt to assess average work involvement levels in each sample; without that information, comparisons between studies in terms of the degree and mechanisms of impairment are extremely difficult.

A second practical implication of the importance of work involvement is seen in therapy and counselling interventions. Much counselling of unemployed people aims to assist them to cope with present problems through sustained job-seeking motivation and better self-presentation, in effect through the maintenance or enhancement of work involvement. Yet research findings make clear that this very process will increase distress if the person fails to find a job. Solutions to this counselling dilemma will presumably hinge upon a separation between several different bases of self-esteem, some employment-related but others having no occupational content.

Work involvement is also important in considering possible sex differences in the impact of unemployment. The literature on women's employment and mental health is generally excessively simple-minded (notable exceptions being the projects by Brown & Harris (1978) and Bebbington *et al.* (1981)), but the literature may be interpreted to suggest that for women who see themselves as being in the labour market, employment and unemployment are as influential in determining mental health as they are for men. Women who currently see themselves as out of the labour market (many mothers of young children, for instance) appear, in general, to show no differences in mental health associated with employment status, although having a job may be psychologically important for particular disadvantaged groups. Unfortunately, very little research in this area has examined personal work involvement, and these generalizations require further testing (cf. Warr & Parry, 1981).

To the possible moderating variables of length of unemployment, age, work involvement and sex may be added those of occupational status, financial position, family unemployment, social support networks, local levels of unemployment, hobbies and personal interests. Almost no research has included these in examinations of the psychological consequences of being out of work. Other desirable research developments would extend the range of dependent variables which are examined. Up to now there has been an emphasis upon measures of well-being and of job-seeking activities. This has been appropriate and valuable, but hints that unemployed people may become less able to retain and retrieve information, to concentrate for long periods, or to make difficult decisions have not yet been followed by empirical enquiry. These cognitive aspects of personal functioning deserve early attention.

Also important is the possibility that in comparison with certain psychologically harmful jobs (of the kinds mentioned earlier) unemployment might in some cases be beneficial. It is likely that the next decade will see substantial changes in traditional work patterns, so that we shall have to build upon the positive features of being out of work as well as to search for alternative sources of those benefits which jobs themselves provide. Financial rewards from an employment relationship are not easily replaced in full, but the other five psychological benefits from work summarized above could increasingly be generated by new forms of social institution. What these will be is at present unclear, but one possible step towards their specification may be to examine to what degree and through what mechanisms shorter work-weeks or forms of work-sharing can increase psychological health, especially for those in undesirable jobs.

Most studies from a more traditional perspective have been of a cross-sectional kind, comparing outcome measures for unemployed and employed samples. These leave open the question of causality: perhaps the cross-sectional findings are a result of self-selection, such that people with lower psychological health are likely to become or remain unemployed, whereas their counterparts with higher scores are liable to retain or find work. This is another issue in urgent need of empirical investigation, although the small amount of evidence available argues against the self-selection interpretation. For example, we have recorded a significant increase in minor psychiatric morbidity among a small group of employed people when they subsequently become unemployed, and the opposite effect for another small sample moving from unemployment to employment (e.g. Warr, 1981). Incidentally, we have observed that, in terms of psychological well-being, government schemes to provide short-term training and work experience for young adults are as effective as genuine employment. (There are of course differences of other kinds, in terms of occupational role, duration, payment levels and so on.)

Finally, some comments should be made about aggregate time-series studies. Investigations reviewed above have all been at the level of the individual person, but there is an important tradition of research which examines relationships between national or local economic conditions and aggregate medical data, for example in terms of suicide rates or hospital admissions. Several recent studies of this kind have been based upon econometric prediction methods, crucial to which is the identification of an appropriate time lag between an economic change and the outcome measure.

The work of Brenner (1973, 1980) has been influential in this field. For example, one study found a strong relationship between changes in the manufacturing employment index and admissions to New York State public mental hospitals between 1914 and 1967, after an appropriate temporal lag had been introduced. Such research has important implications for the planning and provision of services, and it deserves extension. However, the findings reported so far in respect of psychiatric indices are not without problems. For example, the investigators' omission of data from private mental hospitals and state general hospitals has been criticized, and variations between years and discrepancies between subgroups have been noted to weaken the general argument. There are also problems associated with the capacity of hospitals (a natural constraint on admissions), and the matching of community areas for economic and medical indices. The model assumes a cyclical pattern of relationships, such that improvements as well as decrements in economic conditions both yield higher morbidity, and there has been controversy about that possibility. Another issue of contention is the validity of assessing hospitalization rather than community prevalence. These themes have been discussed by Catalano & Dooley (1977), Dooley & Catalano (1980), Marshall & Funch (1979, 1980), Ratcliff (1980) and others. It seems appropriate to accept that, despite the problems, some relationships of the kind described do exist in North American data, but that further exploration is required. The important point here is that uncertainty about the validity or otherwise of aggregate time-series data does not prevent a conclusion at the individual level; as described above, it is clear that unemployment is in general associated with individual psychological distress.

PETER WARR

REFERENCES

Bakke, E. W. (1940). *Citizens without Work*. Yale University Press: New Haven.

Bebbington, P., Hurry, J., Tennant, C., Sturt, E. & Wing, J. K. (1981). Epidemiology of mental disorders in Camberwell. *Psychological Medicine* **11**, 561–579.

Brenner, M. H. (1973). *Mental Illness and the Economy*. Harvard University Press: Cambridge, Mass.

Brenner, M. H. (1980). Industrialization and economic growth: estimates of their effects on the health of populations. In *Assessing the Contributions of the Social Sciences to Health* (ed. M. H. Brenner, A. Mooney and T. J. Nagy), pp. 65–115. American Academy for the Advancement of Science: Washington, D.C.

Brown, G. W. & Harris, T. (1978). *Social Origins of Depression: A Study of Psychiatric Disorder in Women*. Tavistock: London.

Catalano, R. & Dooley, C. D. (1977). Economic predictors of depressed mood and stressful life events in a metropolitan community. *Journal of Health and Social Behavior* **18**, 292–307.

Coburn, D. (1978). Work and general psychological and physical well-being. *International Journal of Health Services* **8**, 415–435.

Colledge, M. & Bartholomew, R. (1980). The long-term unemployed: some new evidence. *Employment Gazette* **88**, 9–12.

Den Hertog, F. J. (1976). Work structuring. In *Personal Goals and Work Design* (ed. P. B. Warr), pp. 43–65. Wiley: London.

Dooley, D. & Catalano, R. (1980). Economic change as a cause of behavioral disorder. *Psychological Bulletin* **87**, 450–468.

Eisenberg, P. & Lazarsfeld, P. F. (1938). The psychological effects of unemployment. *Psychological Bulletin* **35**, 358–390.

Fletcher, B. C. & Payne, R. L. (1980). Stress at work: a review and theoretical framework, parts 1 and 2. *Personnel Review* **9**(1), 19–29; **9**(2), 5–8.

Hackman, J. R. & Lawler, E. E. (1971). Employee reactions to job characteristics. *Journal of Applied Psychology* **55**, 259–286.

Hackman, J. R. & Oldham, G. R. (1980). *Job Redesign*. Addison-Wesley: Reading, Mass.

Hepworth, S. J. (1980). Moderating factors of the psychological impact of unemployment. *Journal of Occupational Psychology* **53**, 139–145.

Hill, J. M. M. (1978). The psychological impact of unemployment. *New Society* **43**, no. 798, 118–120.

Jahoda, M., Lazarsfeld, P. F. & Zeisel, H. (1933). *Marienthal: The Sociography of an Unemployed Community* (English edition). Aldine-Atherton: Chicago, 1971.

Karasek, R. A. (1979). Job demands, job decision latitude, and mental strain: implications for job redesign. *Administrative Science Quarterly* **24**, 285–308.

Kasl, S. V. (1978). Epidemiological contributions to the study of work stress. In *Stress at Work* (ed. C. L. Cooper and R. L. Payne), pp. 3–48. Wiley: London.

Kornhauser, A. W. (1965). *Mental Health of the Industrial Worker*. Wiley: New York.

Marsden, D. & Duff, E. (1975). *Workless: Some Unemployed Men and Their Families*. Penguin: Harmondsworth.

Marshall, J. R. & Funch, D. P. (1979). Mental illness and the economy: a critique and partial replication. *Journal of Health and Social Behavior* **20**, 282–289.

Marshall, J. R. & Funch, D. P. (1980). Reply to Ratcliff. *Journal of Health and Social Behavior* **21**, 391–393.

Ratcliff, K. S. (1980). On Marshall and Funch's critique of 'Mental illness and the economy'. *Journal of Health and Social Behavior* **21**, 389–391.

Schlossberg, N. K. & Leibowitz, Z. (1980). Organizational support systems as buffers to job loss. *Journal of Vocational Behavior* **17**, 204–217.

Sinfield, A. (1981). *What Unemployment Means*. Martin Robertson: Oxford.

Stafford, E. M., Jackson, P. R. & Banks, M. H. (1980). Employment, work involvement and mental health in less qualified young people. *Journal of Occupational Psychology* **53**, 291–304.

Swinburne, P. (1981). The psychological impact of unemployment on managers and professional staff. *Journal of Occupational Psychology* **54**, 47–64.

Wall, T. D. (1978). Job redesign and employee participation. In *Psychology at Work* (second edition) (ed. P. B. Warr), pp. 264–285. Penguin: Harmondsworth.

Wall, T. D. (1980). Group work redesign in context: a two-phase model. In *Changes in Working Life* (ed. K. Duncan, M. Gruneberg and D. Wallis), pp. 329–350. Wiley: New York.

Warr, P. B. (1978). A study of psychological well-being. *British Journal of Psychology* **69**, 111–121.

Warr, P. B. (1981). Some studies of psychological well-being and unemployment. SAPU Memo 431. (Available on request.)

Warr, P. B. & Parry, G. (1981). Paid employment and women's psychological well-being. SAPU Memo 435. (Available on request.)

Psychological Medicine, 1983, **13**, 721–725

Neuropsychological studies of callosal agenesis[1]

A developmental error or arrest during the foetal growth of the telencephalic midline can lead to partial or complete agenesis of the corpus callosum. A person who is born with no corpus callosum at all is likely also to lack the hippocampal commissure, but unlikely to lack the anterior commissure (Loeser & Alvord, 1968*a*). Indeed, some congenitally acallosal individuals appear to have an enlarged anterior commissure (Bossy, 1970; Loeser & Alvord, 1968*b*). Their other commissures, as far as is known, do not differ appreciably from those of a normal brain. Against this background, behavioural investigations of totally acallosal subjects have been largely directed towards answering three neuropsychological questions. First, is an intact corpus callosum necessary for cerebral dominance to be established? Secondly, given that in most respects the 'disconnection syndrome' well known in patients who have undergone surgical section of the cerebral commissures (Sperry, 1974) is absent in cases of agenesis, how does the brain compensate for such a drastic structural deficiency? And, thirdly, what are the limits of compensation, both in regard to the cross-integration of sensory information and in relation to behavioural capacities which may depend in a less obvious way upon interhemispheric collaboration? In recent years some progress has been made towards answering all three of these questions, although complete answers are still not available.

The first question relates to the ontogeny of cerebral dominance. Some theorists (e.g. Kinsbourne & Hiscock, 1977) have argued that dominance may essentially be wired-in at birth, and that there is no good evidence that the degree of functional asymmetry between the cerebral hemispheres grows with age. Others (Selnes, 1974; Moscovitch, 1977; Denenberg, 1981) have argued that, even if there is the seed of cerebral asymmetry present at birth, this can only develop into the normal adult pattern through an inhibitory callosal interaction, by which one side can dominate and suppress the other. In support of their argument such theorists cite what they take to be evidence of weak or even non-existent lateralization of cerebral function in the acallosal brain. In particular, they cite small behavioural asymmetries in three types of test: tachistoscopic recognition (of words, letters and pictures), tactual naming of objects, and dichotic listening (to digits, syllables or words). It is true that following surgical callosal section in adulthood, even when the anterior commissure is spared, extreme asymmetries in these tasks are found (Sperry, 1974; McKeever *et al.* 1981).[2] However, the fact that congenital absence of the callosum does not have these consequences could be fully explained by the compensatory development of other commissures, decussations, and/or ipsilateral sensory projections. Such re-wirings might easily co-exist with normal degrees of *cerebral* lateralization in callosal agenesis (Milner & Jeeves, 1979, 1981). That some such development of neural pathways must have occurred is demonstrated by the existence of visual and tactile cross-matching abilities in acallosal subjects which are not present in patients with callosal section. These abilities (e.g. Ettlinger *et al.* 1972) cannot be explained by incomplete cerebral lateralization.

The question as to whether acallosal brains are incompletely lateralized cannot therefore be answered by comparing acallosal with callosotomized patients and demonstrating smaller behavioural asymmetries. On the other hand, it can be demonstrated that *some* asymmetry of function is present in acallosal brains. For example, there generally seems to be better tachistoscopic recognition of verbal and pictorial items presented in the right visual field which projects to the left hemisphere (Ettlinger *et al.* 1972; Jeeves *et al.* 1983). Furthermore, vocal responses to a photic stimulus have

[1] Address for correspondence: Dr David Milner, Psychological Laboratory, University of St Andrews, St Andrews, Fife KY16 9JU.

[2] The reported exceptions are the anterior-commissure-spared patients D.S., S.P. and D.H. (Risse *et al.* 1978) and the completely sectioned patient L.B. (Sperry, 1974). Of these, the first has long-standing left-hemisphere damage and also may not have a total callosal section (Wilson *et al.* 1982) and the last three were operated upon at the ages 13, 15 and 13 respectively.

been found to be consistently faster (by about 17 ms) in the right than in the left visual field in the acallosal K.C. (Milner, 1982). Although the evidence from dichotic listening studies (Chiarello, 1980; Jeeves *et al.* 1983) is less clear, it is compatible with a normal degree of cerebral dominance along with a non-suppressed left ear–left hemisphere ipsilateral projection (Chiarello, 1980; Milner & Jeeves, 1979). It is further worth pointing out that, despite claims to the contrary, acallosal patients are usually right-handed (Chiarello, 1980; Milner & Jeeves, 1979), so that asymmetry of motor control can certainly develop without a corpus callosum. (There is a slightly increased incidence of non-right handedness, but that is typical of neurological populations.) Finally, there have been two references in the literature to direct speech lateralization tests using the sodium amytal test, and one reported exclusive left-hemisphere control (Gazzaniga, 1970, p. 138, citing a personal communication from B. Milner). The other (on the left-handed patient S.K.) reported apparently bilateral control of speech (Gott & Saul, 1978); however, about 15% of left-handed people with intact commissures also apparently possess such dual control (Rasmussen & Milner, 1977).

Perhaps the most prudent conclusion would be that there may be greater differences in brain lateralization among acallosal individuals than among normal people. But there only needs to be *one* clear case of unilateral speech control for the question 'Is a corpus callosum necessary for cerebral dominance to be established?' to be answered in the negative. If the case of B. Milner (above) can be taken as one such example, then that is the end of the matter.

Nonetheless, the quest for bilateral control of speech in acallosals has yielded some intriguing information, by the use of a simple test in which subjects are shown tachistoscopically a word which spans the point of visual fixation. Sperry (1968) reported that the above-mentioned patient S.K., unlike the commissurotomized patients (Gazzaniga *et al.* 1965), could read such words completely and unhesitatingly. Yet if she were separately using both the left- and right-hemisphere speech mechanisms that she evidently possesses, some pronunciation errors would be expected in reading even such simple words as BEEN as against BEST. It seems instead that only one hemisphere is formulating and producing the spoken word. Perhaps the anterior commissure, for which there is radiological evidence in this patient (Gott & Saul, 1978), is providing the speaking hemisphere with the complete visual information, and the weaker speech mechanism is being consistently over-ridden. In contrast, the acallosal B.F. (Jeeves *et al.* 1983), who would seem on tachistoscopic and dichotic evidence to have a reliable and normal functional lateralization, has been found to read words presented across the point of fixation with less fluency than words presented to the left or right. His performance with central presentation is characterized by hesitations and letter-by-letter reading, providing behavioural evidence for two separate and simultaneously functioning speech control mechanisms (Jeeves *et al.* 1983). The acallosal K.C. (Reynolds & Jeeves, 1974; Milner, 1982), on the other hand, behaves essentially like S.K. It should be noted that some acallosals (e.g. Lassonde *et al.* 1983) have difficulty in maintaining ocular fixation. However, our patients K.C. and B.F. seem not to, since lateral differences persist, despite the use of very small visual angles (see Lines, 1983, and below). It is possible that both K.C. and S.K. have a dynamically-dominant speech mechanism on one side, which controls all spoken behaviour except in very exceptional circumstances.

The second question concerns the mechanisms of functional compensation in the brain. There are several possibilities, but little evidence to help one choose between them. The first line of evidence concerns the somatosensory system. Several investigators, though not all (e.g. Jeeves, 1979), have found that tactile integration between the hands, although sufficiently good for matching or identifying objects, is relatively impaired where cross-localization of stimulated points on the fingers is required (Gazzaniga, 1970; Ettlinger *et al.* 1972; Dennis, 1976; Reynolds & Jeeves, 1977). But Dennis (1976) has shown that an equal impairment is present where no cross-integration is required, but a similar cognitive demand is made. This strongly suggests that tactile localization is intrinsically poor, and Dennis argues that this is a consequence of an overdeveloped ipsilateral sensory pathway, which permits cross-integration (through a single hemisphere) at the cost of reduced sensory acuity. A lower somatosensory acuity is also manifest in a tendency to make errors when asked to report how many fingers apart two stimulated fingers are (Dennis, 1976).

If a sensory projection rather than a commissural one has developed to permit tactile cross-integration, the reverse seems likely to be the case in the visual domain. The capacity to name or cross-match lateralized visual stimuli would seem very likely to be mediated by a visual commissure. However, it would be possible in theory for the normal nasotemporal segregation of retinal ganglion cell fibres to be partially lost such that there was some input from each half of the visual field to the ipsilateral visual system. Furthermore, the acallosal subject's ability to make quick 'crossed' visuomotor responses (e.g. left visual field, right index finger) could be due to either of these two possibilities, or a third, namely the use of the ipsilateral motor projection (Kinsbourne & Fisher, 1971) which in normals is incapable of precise motor control (Brinkman & Kuypers, 1973). All these possibilities would be compatible with the observation that those acallosal subjects who have been extensively tested have been found to make 'crossed' responses in the visual simple-reaction-time (RT) task about 20 ms slower than uncrossed responses (Jeeves, 1969; Reynolds & Jeeves, 1974; Milner *et al.* 1983). However, certain variations of the task help to eliminate the options. The acallosals K.C. and B.F. have recently been found to maintain their large crossed–uncrossed difference (CUD) at a variety of stimulus eccentricities, even down to $\frac{1}{2}°$ (K.C.) and $\frac{1}{4}°$ (B.F.) (Lines, 1983; and unpublished). Yet if there were any useful ipsilateral visual projection, it would be expected to be clearly present at these small distances from the vertical meridian of the visual field; in that case the stimulus should no longer be lateralized to the contralateral cerebral hemisphere alone and hence no CUD should be observed.

Both of these acallosals have been tested in the same RT task, using different levels of stimulus luminance. Both have been found to generate clear and statistically reliable increases in CUD at low stimulus levels (Milner, 1982; Milner *et al.* 1983). These data are difficult to explain in terms of the theory that crossed RTs are mediated by ipsilateral motor pathways, but instead seem to implicate a commissural pathway coded for elementary visual stimulus characteristics. This relationship between stimulus intensity and size of the CUD is not found in normal subjects (Milner & Lines, 1982) whose brains evidently send a more abstract or response-related message across the corpus callosum in this task. It is also possible to exclude spatial compatibility *v.* incompatibility as a determinant of the acallosal's CUD (cf. Kinsbourne & Fisher, 1971), since B.F. shows an unchanged CUD, even when the responding arm is maintained in an extreme contralateral location during the task (Milner *et al.* 1983). On the basis of these various results, it seems most reasonable to implicate either the anterior commissure (or perhaps a midbrain commissure) in crossed visual reactions in acallosal patients, rather than the alternatives of ipsilateral visual or motor transmission.

This brings us to the final question, since although there may be normally no *efficient* ipsilateral motor control of the fingers, it has been argued (Dennis, 1976) that ipsilateral control nonetheless develops by default in the absence of callosal influence, to the detriment of fine contralateral control. Certainly, synkinesic 'unintended' movements do occur in acallosal patients, and a general clumsiness in skilled movement has often been reported (e.g. Jeeves, 1965; Reynolds & Jeeves, 1977). Synkinesias also occur in other pathological conditions (Abercrombie *et al.* 1964; Schott & Wyke, 1981) where callosal pathology is generally absent, but where it may still be true that normal suppressive or inhibitory processes are not fully functional. An absence of such processes more generally in acallosal brain development would also account for the finger-localization deficiencies described above, if it can be assumed that fine tactual distinctions also require that ipsilateral pathways be suppressed.

Limits on visual cross-integration in callosal agenesis are less clear, but seem likely to exist. In particular, the normal visual input to the primate anterior commissure emphasizes information about pattern at the expense of information about location (Jouandet & Gazzaniga, 1979; Ungerleider & Mishkin, 1982). Although the neocortical field of origin of the anterior commissure in the acallosal brain may be less restricted than normal (Bossy, 1970), possibly through the retention of connections otherwise lost during callosal development (Auroux & Roussel, 1967), it will be interesting to determine whether spatial cross-matching will be impaired, as it is following callosal section (Holtzman *et al.* 1981). In one acallosal patient location in the right half of the visual field has been found to be poor (Martin, 1981); however, this is not so in our patient B.F. and so may not be generalizable.

Intellect is generally underdeveloped in callosal agenesis, but whether this should be attributed to reduced interhemispheric communication or to other brain abnormalities is unknown. The most frequent description is of poor showing on 'performance' tests (e.g. Sperry, 1968), but Dennis (1977) has argued that there is just as likely to be a large difference in favour of Wechsler Performance over Verbal IQ as vice versa, and Chiarello (1980) calculates the average discrepancy to be zero (mean Verbal IQ = 89, mean Performance IQ = 89 among the published cases, excluding retardates). Dennis (1981) has reported on a number of linguistic tests given to an acallosal (D.S.) with a lower Verbal than Performance IQ. The most pervasive difficulty for this patient seemed to be in syntactic comprehension, although a word-finding difficulty also emerged in certain tests. In similar tests given to three acallosals (B.F., K.C. and M.J.) we too have found some similar impairments, but in no instance where D.S. was impaired have we found all three of our patients to be impaired (Jeeves *et al.* 1983). One very marked difficulty for D.S. was in retrieving words in response to rhyming cues; we have found a comparable problem in K.C. and B.F., but not in M.J. (despite his being only 6 years old). Indeed, in most cases M.J. was the least (relatively) impaired of the three, and this probably reflects the fact that he has a positive Verbal–Performance IQ discrepancy while the other two, like D.S., have the reverse. Similarly, Dennis (1977) reported that her partially acallosal J.E., who had a higher Verbal than Performance IQ, performed well on a test of syntactic comprehension. It may be the case that in agenesis 'either a linguistic or a spatial capacity develops' (Dennis, 1977). However, it will not be possible to state with certainty that the pattern of performance found in the 'undeveloped' part of the intellect is abnormal until controls matched not only on overall cognitive level but also on Verbal–Performance IQ discrepancy are examined.

In summary, the following provisional answers may be given to the three questions posed at the beginning of this editorial. First, there is no good evidence that acallosal brains are any less laterally specialized than normal ones; so there is no compelling reason to argue that hemispheric specialization requires the corpus callosum to have been present in childhood. Secondly, there is evidence for the use of visually-coded commissural fibres in some tests of cross-integration, but also of ipsilateral sensory pathways (tactile, and possibly auditory) in others. Finally, it is likely that both cognitive and skilled performances suffer as a result of callosal agenesis; but there are great individual differences and the nature of the impairments remains unclear.

DAVID MILNER

REFERENCES

Abercrombie, M. L., Lindon, R. L. & Tyson, M. C. (1964). Associated movements in normal and physically handicapped children. *Developmental Medicine and Child Neurology* **6**, 573–580.

Auroux, M. & Roussel, C. (1967). Relations néocorticales assurées par la commissure blanche antérieure chez le foetus humain. *Comptes Rendus de l'Association des Anatomistes* **137**, 152–159.

Bossy, J. G. (1970). Morphological study of a case of complete, isolated and asymptomatic agenesis of the corpus callosum. *Archives d'Anatomie, d'Histologie et d'Embryologie* **53**, 289–340.

Brinkman, J. & Kuypers, H. G. J. M. (1973). Cerebral control of contralateral and ipsilateral arm, hand and finger movements in the split-brain rhesus monkey. *Brain* **96**, 653–674.

Chiarello, C. (1980). A house divided? Cognitive functioning with callosal agenesis. *Brain and Language* **11**, 128–158.

Denenberg, V. H. (1981). Hemispheric laterality in animals and the effects of early experience. *Behavioral and Brain Sciences* **4**, 1–49.

Dennis, M. (1976). Impaired sensory and motor differentiation with corpus callosum agenesis: a lack of callosal inhibition during ontogeny? *Neuropsychologia* **14**, 455–469.

Dennis, M. (1977). Cerebral dominance in three forms of early brain disorder. In *Topics in Child Neurology* (ed. M. E. Blaw, I. Rapin and M. Kinsbourne), pp. 189–212. Spectrum: New York.

Dennis, M. (1981). Language in a congenitally acallosal brain. *Brain and Language* **12**, 33–53.

Ettlinger, G., Blakemore, C. B., Milner, A. D. & Wilson, J. (1972). Agenesis of the corpus callosum: a behavioural investigation. *Brain* **95**, 327–346.

Gazzaniga, M. S. (1970). *The Bisected Brain*. Appleton-Century-Crofts: New York.

Gazzaniga, M. S., Bogen, J. E. & Sperry, R. W. (1965). Observations on visual perception after disconnexion of the cerebral hemispheres in man. *Brain* **88**, 221–236.

Gott, P. S. & Saul, R. E. (1978). Agenesis of the corpus callosum: limits of functional compensation. *Neurology* **28**, 1272–1279.

Holtzman, J. D., Sidtis, J. J., Volpe, B. T., Wilson, D. H. & Gazzaniga, M. S. (1981). Dissociation of spatial information for stimulus localization and the control of attention. *Brain* **104**, 861–872.

Jeeves, M. A. (1965). Psychological studies of three cases of congenital agenesis of the corpus callosum. In *Functions of the Corpus Callosum* (ed. G. Ettlinger), pp. 73–94. Ciba Foundation Study Groups No. 20. Churchill: London.

Jeeves, M. A. (1969). A comparison of interhemispheric transmission times in acallosals and normals. *Psychonomic Science* **16**, 245–246.

Jeeves, M. A. (1979). Some limits to interhemispheric integration in cases of callosal agenesis and partial commissurotomy. In *Structure and Function of the Cerebral Commissures* (ed. I. S. Russell, M. W. van Hof and G. Berlucchi), pp. 449–474. Macmillan London.

Jeeves, M. A., Milner, A. D. & Silver, P. H. (1983). Language in callosal agenesis: deficits and asymmetries. Manuscript in preparation.

Jouandet, M. L. & Gazzaniga, M. S. (1979). Cortical field of origin of the anterior commissure of the rhesus monkey. *Experimental Neurology* **66**, 381–397.

Kinsbourne, M. & Fisher, M. (1971). Latency of uncrossed and of crossed reaction in callosal agenesis. *Neuropsychologia* **9**, 471–473.

Kinsbourne, M. & Hiscock, M. (1977). Does cerebral dominance develop? In *Language Development and Neurological Theory* (ed. S. J. Segalowitz and F. A. Gruber), pp. 171–191. Academic Press: New York.

Lassonde, M. C., Laurencelle, L. & Geoffroy, G. (1983). Hemispheric specialization in callosal agenesis: evidence from a tachistoscopic study. Manuscript submitted for publication.

Lines, C. R. (1983). Nasotemporal overlap investigated in a case of agenesis of the corpus callosum. Manuscript submitted for publication.

Loeser, J. D. & Alvord, E. C. Jr (1968*a*). Agenesis of the corpus callosum. *Brain* **91**, 553–570.

Loeser, J. D. & Alvord, E. C. Jr (1968*b*). Clinicopathological correlations in agenesis of the corpus callosum. *Neurology* **18**, 745–756.

McKeever, W. F., Sullivan, K. F., Ferguson, S. M. & Rayport, M. (1981). Typical cerebral hemisphere disconnection deficits following corpus callosum section despite sparing of the anterior commissure. *Neuropsychologia* **19**, 745–755.

Martin, A. (1981). Visual processing in the acallosal brain: a clue to the differential functions of the anterior commissure and the splenium. Paper presented at the 9th Annual Meeting of the International Neuropsychological Society.

Milner, A. D. (1982). Simple reaction times to lateralized visual stimuli in a case of callosal agenesis. *Neuropsychologia* **20**, 411–419.

Milner, A. D. & Jeeves, M. A. (1979). A review of behavioural studies of agenesis of the corpus callosum. In *Structure and Function of the Cerebral Commissures* (ed. I. S. Russell, M. W. van Hof and G. Berlucchi), pp. 428–448. Macmillan: London.

Milner, A. D. & Jeeves, M. A. (1981). Commentary: The functions of the corpus callosum in infancy and adulthood. *Behavioral and Brain Sciences* **4**, 30–31.

Milner, A. D. & Lines, C. R. (1982). Interhemispheric pathways in simple reaction time to lateralized light flash. *Neuropsychologia* **20**, 171–179.

Milner, A. D., Lines, C. R., Jeeves, M. A. & Silver, P. H. (1983). Reaction times to lateralised visual stimuli in callosal agenesis: stimulus and response factors. Manuscript in preparation.

Moscovitch, M. (1977). Development of lateralization of language functions and its relation to cognitive and linguistic development: a review. In *Language Development and Neurological Theory* (ed. S. J. Segalowitz and F. Gruber), pp. 193–211. Academic Press: New York.

Rasmussen, T. & Milner, B. (1977). The role of early left-brain injury in determining lateralization of cerebral speech functions. *Annals of the New York Academy of Sciences* **299**, 355–369.

Reynolds, D. M. & Jeeves, M. A. (1974). Further studies of crossed and uncrossed pathway responding in callosal agenesis – reply to Kinsbourne and Fisher. *Neuropsychologia* **12**, 287–290.

Reynolds, D. M. & Jeeves, M. A. (1977). Further studies of tactile perception and motor coordination in agenesis of the corpus callosum. *Cortex* **13**, 257–272.

Risse, G. L., Le Doux, J., Springer, S. P., Wilson, D. H. & Gazzaniga, M. S. (1978). The anterior commissure in man: functional variation in a multisensory system. *Neuropsychologia* **16**, 23–31.

Schott, G. D. & Wyke, M. A. (1981). Congenital mirror movements. *Journal of Neurology, Neurosurgery and Psychiatry* **44**, 586–599.

Selnes, O. A. (1974). The corpus callosum: some anatomical and functional considerations with special reference to language. *Brain and Language* **1**, 111–139.

Sperry, R. W. (1968). Plasticity of neural maturation. *Developmental Biology Supplement* **2**, 306–327.

Sperry, R. W. (1974). Lateral specialization in the surgically separated hemispheres. In *The Neurosciences Third Study Program* (ed. F. O. Schmitt and F. G. Worden), pp. 5–19. MIT Press: Cambridge, Mass.

Ungerleider, L. G. & Mishkin, M. (1982). Two cortical visual systems. In *Analysis of Visual Behavior* (ed. D. J. Ingle, M. A. Goodale and R. J. W. Mansfield), pp. 549–586. MIT Press: Cambridge, Mass.

Wilson, D. H., Reeves, A. G. & Gazzaniga, M. S. (1982). 'Central' commissurotomy for intractable generalized epilepsy: series two. *Neurology* **32**, 687–697.

EPIDEMIOLOGY

Psychological Medicine, 1978, **8**, 1–4

Trends in the epidemiology of alcoholism[1]

A Symposium of the epidemiology of alcoholism was held in London in January 1977 – at a time when theories about the aetiology and prevalence of alcoholism had reached a crossroads.

The epidemiological approach has continually been at odds with the mainstream of theories about alcoholism. The traditional disease theory perceived alcoholics to have certain psychological or physiological idiosyncrasies which rendered them unable to control their drinking. The most popular explanations were that either some personality defect predisposed them to become alcoholics, or else some biochemical abnormality made them physiologically allergic to alcohol. As Davies (1977) noted at the Symposium 'there is little or no evidence to support any of these constitutional views' and, for some years, the epidemiological study of alcoholism has been suggesting an alternative perspective to these aetiological theories of psychological or physiological predisposition. Epidemiology has linked the prevalence of alcoholism with *per capita* consumption, i.e. the total amount of alcohol consumed in a society divided by the adult population. Whenever *per capita* consumption rises, so do all the rates of alcohol-related problems such as alcoholic mortality, liver cirrhosis mortality, arrests for drunkenness and for drunken driving, and hospital admissions of persons diagnosed as alcoholics. The strength of this relationship between the level of consumption and the level of alcohol-related problems can be traced in the national statistics of England and Wales, for example, as far back as World War I (Wilson, 1940). The years in which alcohol consumption increased the most were invariably the same years in which the prevalence of alcohol-related problems also increased the most. The consistency of this relationship implied that the number of people diagnosed as suffering from alcoholism – conceptualized by the disease theory as a permanent affliction – actually rose and fell with the amount of alcohol consumed by the total population. This suggested that the size of the problem should not therefore be conceived in terms of the number of people who were in some way pathologically inclined to become alcoholics. Whereas the disease theory presumed the causes of alcoholism to lie in traits internal to the drinker, the epidemiology of alcoholism was suggesting the causes lay not in the drinker, but in the drink.

Ledermann (1964) incorporated the evidence of this relationship into a theory which claimed that the level of *per capita* consumption actually determined the prevalence of alcoholism. He asserted that the frequency distribution of drinkers according to their individual consumption will always be highly skewed, with a majority of the population drinking relatively small amounts and successively smaller proportions drinking increasingly heavier amounts. In mathematical terms this distribution would always conform to the characteristics of a logarithmic normal curve. He further asserted that the end point of the upper distribution of individual consumption must be fixed at a point of one litre of absolute alcohol per day, on the grounds that drinking any more than this would be fatal. Usually a lognormal curve has 2 parameters – the standard deviation and the mean. By fixing the upper limit, the 'Ledermann distribution' allows only 1 parameter – the mean. Therefore, as this mean, i.e. *per capita* consumption, rises, the frequency of drinkers will always be smoothly and continuously redistributed so that predictable proportions of drinkers move into higher consumption categories. According to Ledermann, any increase in *per capita* consumption must represent a general move towards heavier drinking throughout the population. Since he also showed that societies with a higher *per capita* consumption also had the highest rates of alcohol-related problems such as cirrhosis of the liver, then a movement of a society to a higher overall consumption must inevitably lead to a higher rate of alcohol-related problems within that society. At the Symposium, De Lint (1977) concurred that the distribution curve is typically continuous, unimodular and positively skewed, and

[1] Address for correspondence: Mr A. K. J. Cartwright, Maudsley Alcohol Pilot Project, 113 Denmark Hill, London SE5.

he believed 'the gradual transition from moderate to excessive consumption agrees very well with the failure thus far to discover real differences in the personality and physiology of the so-called social drinker and the so-called "alcoholic"'. His work over the years with Schmidt has led them to conclude that 'the prevalence of alcoholism is invariably determined by the overall level of consumption in the population' (De Lint & Schmidt, 1971). They have also been influential in demonstrating that *per capita* consumption was in turn related to the price and availability of alcohol. This phenomenon had been observed for many years (Wilson, 1940), but the Ledermann-based theory seemed to go further by explaining why reducing alcohol availability would reduce *per capita* consumption and thus also reduce the risk of people becoming alcoholics. A similar view was propounded in 1975 by a group of international experts headed by Bruun (1975), who propounded that alcohol-related health problems were concentrated among heavier drinkers and that the greater the average consumption the greater the number of heavy drinkers. They too suggested that the number of heavy drinkers, and consequently the number of alcohol-related problems, could both be reduced by restricting the availability of alcohol.

Prior to the Symposium, this consensus view had been somewhat disturbed by Miller & Agnew (1974) who queried Ledermann's manipulation of the lognormal distribution curve. They maintained that the fixed end point of one litre of absolute alcohol was just an arbitrary choice, and they cast doubts on the validity of the characteristics of a lognormal curve which had such a parameter artificially fixed. These criticisms were endorsed by statisticians at the Symposium, and Duffy (1977) added that surveys of the consumption of general population samples have produced distributions which did not correspond to a Ledermann distribution, or even a straightforward lognormal distribution. He therefore concluded that, despite the evidence of a strong relationship between consumption and problems, the explanations of this relationship reached by Brunn *et al.* 'are unjustified by their data', and that 'to reproduce the distribution of alcohol consumption on the basis of mean consumption alone' is 'illogical and contradicted by empirical evidence'.

Such a critique undermines many popular assumptions about the epidemiology of alcoholism. Ledermann's theory suggested that when *per capita* consumption rises the population moves towards generally heavier drinking; a much simpler explanation might be that there has just been a reduction in the number of abstainers. It has been assumed that consumption has increased because its real price has fallen, yet little data have been produced to show that groups whose disposable income has increased the most have also increased their alcohol consumption the most. Neither is there much good evidence that groups such as young people and women who have recently figured particularly in increased rates of alcohol problems were also the same groups who had most increased their consumption. In short, once the theories explaining the relationship between consumption and prevalence were exposed as equivocal, there was clearly very little data available to suggest any alternative mechanisms which might explain this relationship. The most blatant deficiency was the lack of data on relationships over time between consumption and problems within particular groups and individuals.

Three papers presented at the Symposium attempted to remedy this situation. Cartwright *et al.* (1977), Sulkunen (1977), and Makela (1977) all considered the potential importance of the stability of drinking patterns in determining how increased consumption was distributed. In 1974 Cartwright *et al.* replicated some measures of consumption in a London suburb previously made in 1965 (Edwards *et al.* 1972). Over the nine years *per capita* consumption increased 47 % and, as the Ledermann theory predicted, proportions of individual drinkers were smoothly redistributed into higher levels of consumption. Cartwright *et al.* felt that Ledermann's predictions had held pragmatically because there had been relatively little overall change in drinking patterns. The percentage of abstainers remained constant at 11 % and people did not drink on any more days of the week than previously. Rather, the major change was that on a drinking day in 1974, 'average drinkers' consumed 56 % more alcohol than they would have done in 1965. This fitted in with the theoretical framework suggested in papers by Sulkunen and Makela which hypothesized that increases in *per capita* consumption did not usually create new drinking patterns but were usually superimposed on existing patterns.

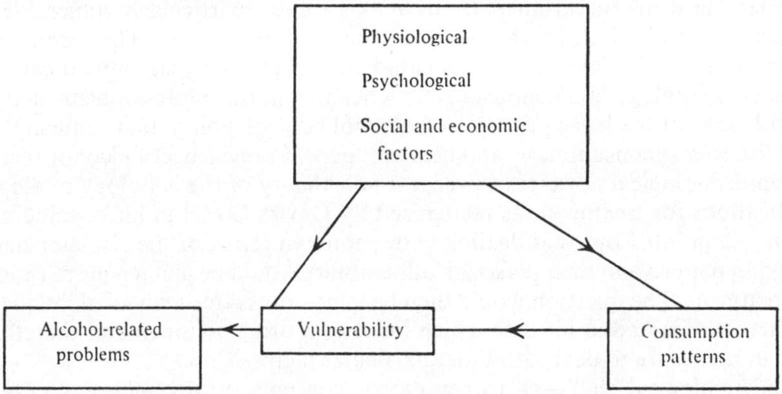

FIG. 1.

Makela's 'addition hypothesis' implies that new ways of drinking do not displace old ones but rather add new elements to them. Makela supported this conclusion with examples from Finland. Sulkunen stated that similar observations could be made in other countries. He pointed out that these additions to the existing drinking patterns comprised new consumer groups, new drinking situations, and new ways of drinking.

Cartwright *et al.* also replicated measures of some alcohol-related problems of individual drinkers. While there was a consistent correlation between consumption and problems in the population in 1965 and in 1974, there was considerable variation between different groups of drinkers within these populations. Groups reporting similar consumption levels reported different numbers of alcohol-related problems. The relationship between consumption and problems seemed to be mediated by two major factors – the drinking pattern and personal characteristics.

When two groups drank the same amount, the group who consumed more *per drinking day* reported more problems. Although this suggests that spreading consumption over more days of the week may carry less risk of experiencing some problems, other studies have shown that high-frequency moderate consumption is more likely than occasional heavy drinking to cause cirrhosis of the liver (Rankin *et al.* 1975). The data, however, show that there are probably relationships between types of drinking patterns and the development of specific alcohol-related problems.

The second intermediary factor between the level of consumption and the prevalence of problems appeared to be personal characteristics which made some people more vulnerable to experiencing problems than other people whose consumption and drinking pattern were the same. Physical, social and psychological factors must explain why one person is more likely than another to experience more problems from the same level of consumption consumed in the same way. For example, young males were more likely than any other demographic group to get into fights after drinking, but this would have to be explained as much in terms of the behaviour of young males as by their alcohol consumption.

This interpretation would comply with other well-known socio-cultural factors which seem to protect certain groups against developing alcohol-related problems while making others vulnerable. For example, Davies (1977) quoted one paper (Glad, 1948) which contrasted the rates of arrest and conviction for inebriety in one American city as 7876 per 100000 people of Irish ethnicity compared with only 27 per 100000 of Jewish ethnicity.

Nevertheless, the intermediary role of drinking patterns and vulnerability factors does not obviate the conclusion that an overall increase in consumption in a population is still likely to lead to more problems in that society. Although we cannot say that if any individual drinks a certain amount a day he will definitely suffer specific problems, we can say that if an individual increases his consumption, he is at a greater risk of experiencing alcohol-related problems. We can also say that his risk is probably greater if he drinks in certain patterns or if he appears particularly vulnerable to developing problems because of his physical, psychological or social characteristics. The reconceptualized view of the aetiology of alcohol-related problems could be represented diagrammatically as in Fig. 1.

Although the epidemiology of alcoholism is now heading in this more sophisticated direction, the current data still reaffirm the basic principle of alcohol control policy that reducing alcohol availability is likely to decrease consumption, and hence reduce the prevalence of alcohol-related problems. However, the epidemiological advances towards a new theory of the aetiology of alcohol problems also have implications for treatment, as recognized by Davies (1977) in his concluding remarks on the Symposium. He pointed out that dealing with people in terms of the risk associated with their particular drinking pattern and their personal vulnerability would be a much more rational approach to individual treatment. The question would then become not 'is this man an alcoholic or not?', but rather 'what factors operated in his case which made him drink so much and therefore what can I do to help him in the future to deal with those particular factors?'.

Thus the epidemiological challenge to traditional concepts of alcoholism is developing into a rationale for alternative approaches to conceptualization and treatment. To realize the potential of this new direction, there is a need for much closer investigation of the relationships between an individual's consumption pattern, his vulnerability and the development of alcohol-related problems.

A. K. J. CARTWRIGHT AND S. J. SHAW

REFERENCES

Bruun, K. (1975). *Alcohol Control Policies in the Public Health Perspective*. Finnish Foundation for Alcohol Studies.

Cartwright, A. K. J., Shaw, S. J. & Spratley, T. A. (1977). Changing consumption patterns and their relationship to the prevalence of alcohol related problems in a London suburb 1965–1974. In *The Ledermann Curve*, pp. 58–69, Report of Symposium held in London, January 1977 (Chairman: D. D. Reid). Alcohol Education Centre: London.

Davies, D. L. (1977). The epidemiology of alcoholism. In *The Ledermann Curve*, pp. 70–77, Report of Symposium held in London, January 1977 (Chairman: D. D. Reid). Alcohol Education Centre: London.

De Lint, J. (1977). The frequency distribution of alcohol consumption: an overview. In *The Ledermann Curve*, pp.1–10, Report of Symposium held in London, January 1977 (Chairman: D. D. Reid). Alcohol Education Centre: London.

De Lint, J. & Schmidt, W. (1971). Consumption averages and alcoholism prevalence: a brief review of epidemiological investigations. *British Journal of Addiction* **66**, 97–107.

Duffy, J. C. (1977). Estimating the proportion of heavy drinkers. In *The Ledermann Curve*, pp. 11–24, Report of Symposium held in London, January 1977 (Chairman: D. D. Reid). Alcohol Education Centre: London.

Edwards, G., Chandler, J. & Hensman, C. (1972). Drinking in a London suburb. I. Correlates of normal drinking. *Quarterly Journal of Studies on Alcohol* **6**, 69–93.

Glad, D. D. (1948). Attitudes and experiences of American Jewish and American Irish male youths as related to differences in adult rates of inebriety. *Quarterly Journal of Studies on Alcohol* **8**, 406–472.

Ledermann, S. (1964). *Alcool-Alcoolisme-Alcoolisation; Mortalité, Morbidité, Accidents du Travail*. Institut National d'Etudes Demographiques, Travaux et Documents, Cahier no. 41. Presses Universitaires de France.

Makela, K. (1977). Consumption level and cultural drinking patterns as determinants of alcohol problems. Previously published in *Journal of Drug Issues* **5**, 344 (1975).

Miller, C. H. & Agnew, N. (1974). The Ledermann model of alcohol consumption: description, implications and assessment. *Quarterly Journal of Studies on Alcohol* **35**, 877–898.

Rankin, J. G., Schmidt, W., Popham, R. E. & De Lint, J. (1975). Epidemiology of alcoholic liver disease – insights and problems. In *Alcoholic Liver Pathology* (ed. J. M. Khanna), pp. 31–41. International Symposium on Alcohol and Drug Addiction series. Alcoholism and Drug Addiction Research Foundation of Ontario: Toronto.

Sulkunen, P. (1977). Behind the curves. On the dynamics of rising consumption level. In *The Ledermann Curve*, pp. 44–57, Report of Symposium held in London, January 1977 (Chairman: D. D. Reid). Alcohol Education Centre: London.

Wilson, G. B. (1940). *Alcohol and the Nation*. Nicholson & Watson: London.

Psychological Medicine, 1979, **9**, 207–215

Epilepsy: some epidemiological aspects[1]

The epilepsies have been subject to effective chemical control for a good half century longer than the functional psychoses. Phenobarbitone, which was preceded by over 50 years by bromides, came into use in 1913, dilantin in 1938. Perhaps this early advent of successful pharmacological control of the epilepsies, as compared with that of the functional psychoses, damped epidemiological research into the subject. We venture that there is less epidemiological knowledge about the distribution and aetiology of the epilepsies than about the psychoses. This neglect of the epidemiology of seizure disorders has left fallow a most intriguing psychiatric issue, namely, the association of temporal lobe epilepsy with psychiatric disorders, and with schizophrenia in particular. We shall concern ourselves here with the more general epidemiological background of the epilepsies.

Anticonvulsants permit the control of seizures in 60–80 % of epileptic patients (Rodin, 1972). After a 20-year follow-up, some 70 % of patients have been found free of seizures for 5 years (Annegers *et al.* 1979). Still, as a recent review in this journal suggested, long-term use of anticonvulsants may produce mental deterioration (Trimble & Reynolds, 1976). Experiments on preweanling and postweanling rats also suggest, alarmingly, that phenobarbitone given during the brain growth spurt, or even during the subsequent deceleration, retards brain growth and disturbs behaviour (Diaz *et al.* 1977; Diaz & Schain, 1977). In addition, many persons with seizures go undiagnosed and untreated or improperly medicated. A recent report has drawn attention to under-medication and over-medication that is widespread and substantial in certain institutionalized settings (Murphy & D'Souza, 1977). Primary prevention is surely what we must aim for in the long run – an aim which can only be achieved by a search for causes. This goal is ambitious. At present, about 70 % of seizures identified in population surveys are ascribed to unknown causes (Hauser, 1978). Even this figure is an underestimate, since the environmental and genetic 'causes' often cited are best treated as hypothetical rather than established.

The search for causes begins with a quest for variations in the frequency of the disorder. Since 1950, at least 36 surveys – whether concerned exclusively with seizure disorders in particular or with neurological disorders in general – have been conducted in various settings around the world (see bibliography). Fourteen of these deal exclusively with infants and children. Worldwide, the reported incidence rates of the epilepsies for all ages combined range from 0·173 per 1000 in Niigata City, Japan (Sato, 1964) to 1 per 1000 in Australia (Crombie *et al.* 1960). Within England itself, the reported rates vary from 0·30 per 1000 in Carlisle (Brewis *et al.* 1966) to 0·73 per 1000 in 14 general practices in southeast England (Pond *et al.* 1960). Prevalence rates for all ages combined range from 1·50 per 1000, again in Niigata City, Japan (Sato, 1964), to 20 per 1000 among the Wapogoro tribe in Tanzania (Jilek & Jilek-Aall, 1970). In England, prevalence rates have varied from 3·33 (Logan & Cushion, 1958) to 7·90 per 1000 (Pond *et al.* 1960).

For many conditions true variation of this order is not beyond the limits of credibility, but the data to hand for the epilepsies conflate the contributions of research methods and those of morbidity. Studies employ non-comparable definitions, a variety of ways of finding and ascertaining cases, and different measures of frequency. At one extreme, Hauser & Kurland (1975) restrict epilepsy to recurrent seizures occurring in the absence of identifiable cause. At the other extreme, Gudmundsson (1966) includes isolated afebrile seizures, and Pond *et al.* (1960) include febrile seizures as well. Inclusion of isolated and/or febrile seizures can inflate estimates of incidence or prevalence anywhere from 1·7 (Hauser & Kurland, 1975) to 37 times (Lessell *et al.* 1962). Most surveys rely on medical

[1] Address for correspondence: Professor Mervyn Susser, The Gertrude H. Sergievsky Center, Faculty of Medicine, Columbia University, 630 West 168th Street, New York, NY 10032, USA.

records for case finding, a practice which inevitably results in under-estimation. The potential magnitude of such errors is suggested by an Eastern European and by an Israeli study. In Warsaw, 27 % of epileptic persons identified by means of a general population survey were unknown as seizure cases in medical records (Zielinsky, 1974*a*). In Beer-Sheva, Israel, a study of seizures among children in the first 5 years of life reported that 48 % of the cases had never been previously brought to the attention of medical personnel (Costeff, 1965).

Frequency measures of the epilepsies are different from those obtained with apparently comparable developmental disorders. For instance, with mental retardation, often an associated developmental disorder, incidence is difficult to measure and even to grasp conceptually (Stein & Susser, 1974). The expression of retarded mental growth must await the subtle unfolding of psychological and social development. On the other hand, the prevalence of mental retardation at a given age or point in time is readily determined; the classifying and labelling process so central to the educational systems of all developed societies yields both the numerator of the rate and a constantly enumerated, captive population as denominator. In contrast, the frank and usually explosive onset of the epilepsies poses fewer difficulties for the satisfactory measurement of incidence. With the epilepsies, it is the determination of prevalence that is more problematic. In industrial societies a large proportion of cases is adequately controlled by medication. Does a patient on anticonvulsants, who has been seizure free for 5 years, constitute a case? Shall we say 'once an epileptic, always an epileptic' (Kurtzke, 1972)? These questions are of pressing concern, not only in the context of frequency measures, but because of the social stigma and negative self-concept carried by the diagnosis of epilepsy.

We turn now to consider the variations in incidence and prevalence that exist in the literature. There is probably some excess of the epilepsies among males. Among incidence studies reporting rates for the epilepsies at all ages, only 7 provide usable sex ratios. The ratio is virtual unity in 1 (Juul-Jensen & Ipsen, 1975); males are in slight excess in 4 (Crombie *et al.* 1960; Sato, 1964; deGraaf, 1974; Hauser & Kurland, 1975); and in modest excess in another (Gudmundsson, 1966). In the remaining study the rate among females was somewhat higher than that among males (Pond *et al.* 1960). The 3 incidence studies reporting rates specifically for recurrent afebrile seizures all show higher rates for males.

Among 15 prevalence studies that report rates by sex for all ages combined, the ratios in 11 reflect a generally slight excess for males (Logan & Cushion, 1958; Crombie *et al.* 1960; Lessell *et al.* 1962; Sato, 1964; Gudmundsson, 1966; Wajsbort *et al.* 1967; Leibowitz & Alter, 1968; Mathai *et al.* 1968; Levy, 1970; Zielinski, 1974*b*; Hauser & Kurland, 1975); in 2, a slight excess for females (Pond *et al.* 1960; Juul-Jensen & Ipsen, 1975); and in another 2 they approach unity (Brewis *et al.* 1966; deGraaf, 1974). Eight studies give prevalence rates separately for recurrent afebrile seizures. Six of these report higher rates for males; 2, equal rates. None of the 15 studies finds a substantial difference in rates.

The higher prevalence rate among males may result from higher incidence, less successful seizure management, or greater duration of the disorder among males, or all three. Further, these studies may reflect differential help-seeking behaviour as much as seizure morbidity. The majority generated their data exclusively from medical records rather than from general population surveys. Because of the minor or negligible differences in the sex ratios of incidence studies, and the non-causal factors which contribute to the differences in the sex ratios of prevalence studies, strong aetiological hypotheses do not emerge from these studies.

Eight studies addressed the issue of the social class distribution of the epilepsies. Their conclusions are widely different and sometimes internally contradictory. One might anticipate that seizure disorders would be inversely related to social class because of so-called 'downward drift'. This model of social mobility would predict an accumulation of seizure cases at the bottom of the social order. Like other chronic disorders, seizures are bound to interfere, in varying degrees, with social and economic functioning. If inadequate prenatal, perinatal or postnatal care plays a role in the aetiology of seizures, that would lead to a similar prediction.

The prediction is supported by the prevalence survey of 67 general practices in England and Wales conducted by Crombie *et al.* (1960) in the late 1950s, and also by the more detailed survey of 14 of these practices by Pond *et al.* (1960). In these overlapping data, both groups of investigators report an impression of an inverse relationship between the frequency of seizure disorders and social class.

Rather different associations emerge from a Scandinavian survey and from another conducted several years earlier in England. Gudmundsson's data (1966) point to a curvilinear relationship between social class and the prevalence of the epilepsies in Iceland. Rates were higher in the middle class and lower at each end of the social spectrum. Gudmundsson dismissed these findings as unrelated to an aetiological factor. He explained the higher rates in the middle class as an artefact of the manner in which he obtained a denominator for this rate, and the lower rates in the upper class as a product of downward drift. The 1950s survey of 106 general practices in England by Logan & Cushion (Logan & Cushion, 1958; Logan, 1962) has often been cited as demonstrating an inverse relationship between social class and the epilepsies. In fact, to the extent that any relation is discernible in the data, it is curvilinear, but in a reverse direction from that reported by Gudmundsson.

The prevalence studies of seizure disorders for all ages combined discussed above do not present findings for specific seizure subtypes by social class. For such analyses we must turn to studies of birth cohorts, most of them followed into middle childhood. Their results afford a complex and provocative picture. In these studies, the social class of the cohort is derived from parental attributes recorded before the child's birth, and they are less vulnerable to artefacts of misclassification posed by phenomena such as downward drift.

In the Newcastle-upon-Tyne 1947 '1000 family' cohort, the incidence rate in the first 5 years of life among surviving children was higher the lower the class for all seizure types, except for those associated with infective illnesses such as gastro-enteritis, rubella and meningitis (Miller *et al.* 1960). The incidence rate also increased with increasing deficiency in the physical care parents gave their children. The results from the 1946 British national cohort of some 5000 children are at first sight paradoxical. In this cohort, children from higher social classes had experienced idiopathic seizures more frequently in the first 2 years of life than children from the lower classes. When homes were rated on the basis of standards of parental care and interest rather than by occupational class, however, lower standards of care were associated with higher rates of idiopathic seizures – a finding which parallels that of the Newcastle study. Also, as in the Newcastle cohort, the distribution of seizures arising from evident precipitating causes or illnesses was unrelated either to social class or to standards of care. Paradoxes are added by 2 other cohort studies: the Collaborative Perinatal Project in the United States (1959–63), which comprised more than 50000 births; and the 1958 British National Child Development Study about 17000 births. Preliminary analyses for the first year of life in the United States cohort (Myrianthopoulos, 1972), and in the first 11 years in the British cohort (Ross, 1973), failed to uncover straightforward or discernible associations between social class and the incidence of either febrile or afebrile seizures.

Those social class differences that do emerge from these studies could reflect true variation in the frequency of the epilepsies among groups enjoying widely different levels of health care, nutrition, and hygiene. Ascertainment biases constitute a serious potential source of error in these investigations, however, since so much depends on the responses of parents to illness. Whether they perceive infant convulsions as illness, the degree of alarm that attends such perceptions, and their propensity to call on medical services for help in such circumstances, may all vary with social class and all may colour their reports on interview.

There has been interest in cross-cultural research on the epilepsies for many years. Epidemiological surveys of varying quality exist for a number of ethnic and racial groups. A review of ethnic variations, however, soon runs up against the decisive influence of study methods on reported rates. For this reason, legitimate ethnic and racial comparisons can only be made within studies.

In a literature search on racial variation in the epilepsies, Rodin (1972) failed to locate any studies reporting rates for more than one race or ethnic group. As a second best strategy for addressing this research question, he calculated the mean prevalence of seizure disorders reported in 10 North American and European studies (4·5 per 1000) and compared this with the mean based upon 10

African studies (4·4 per 1000). This apparent convergence of rates cannot simply be dismissed, but it is a brave assumption that broad and narrow definitions of epilepsy are equally distributed across the African, North American and European research projects, and that the communities surveyed on these continents were randomly selected or representative.

Results from the Columbia University sector of the Collaborative Perinatal Project suggest that ethnic differences in the frequency of seizure disorders may, in fact, exist. In this cohort, comprised of approximately 625 White, 850 Black and 600 Puerto Rican children, the incidence rate, in the first 7 or 8 years of life both for febrile and afebrile seizures, was much the highest among Puerto Rican children. The incidence rate of febrile seizures among Whites exceeded that for Blacks, whereas for afebrile seizures the reverse was true (Gates, 1972). While one of these findings may be an ascertainment phenomenon, the other cannot be accounted for by the same logic.

A different picture emerges from the entire US Collaborative Perinatal Project data for incidence among Blacks and Whites in the first year of life. Among infants of all birth weights taken together, the total incidence of seizures did not differ between Blacks and Whites. Among low birth weight infants of less than 2500 g, however, the rate of afebrile seizures among Blacks was about twice as high as that among Whites, and of febrile seizures about 20 % higher (Myrianthopoulos, 1972). No test was performed to show whether these differences were independent of social class. These preliminary findings, which involve relatively small numbers, must be treated with caution.

Two other projects in the United States, the first in Washington County, Maryland (Rose *et al.* 1973), the second in Multnomah County, Oregon (Meighan *et al.* 1976), raise further intriguing questions about the possibility of true ethnic or geographic variations in the frequency of seizure disorders. These studies, although undertaken by separate teams, utilized nearly identical case finding methods involving mailed questionnaires. In Maryland the overall rate for all types of seizures in 1900 3rd grade children was 18·6 per 1000; in Oregon among 5300 3rd graders the rate was 9·7. Such a two-fold difference deserves further scrutiny and replication of the study design at other sites. Although neither group of investigators specified the exact ethnic composition of the target populations, US census data for Multnomah County (US Dept. of Commerce, 1973) and statistics supplied by Rose *et al.* (1973) indicate that the general population of both counties was over 95 % White.

The pattern of age-specific incidence rates, reported by many surveys, provides one consistent vein among the many inconsistencies to which we have alluded (Crombie *et al.* 1960; Brewis *et al.* 1966; Mathai *et al.* 1968; deGraaf, 1974; Hauser & Kurland, 1975; Juul-Jensen & Ipsen, 1975). Rates are highest among neonates, decline steadily until the end of the second decade, and then level off or continue to decline more gradually for the remainder of the life span. The Rochester, Minnesota, study of Hauser & Kurland (1975) is unique in showing an upswing in later life, starting approximately at age 60. Although an increased incidence with advancing age might be expected, given the link between age and organic cerebral disorder, this curvilinear relationship with age remains to be replicated elsewhere. Bea van den Berg and the late Jacob Yerushalmy, using a 1960–7 cohort of 18 500 births in Oakland, California, report to date the most refined age-specific incidence rates for infants and children. Afebrile seizures occurred in 0·76 per 1000 neonates, then in the second month of life dropped to less than half that rate, 0·33 per 1000. The rate for the remainder of the first year stabilized at a monthly rate of about 0·20 per 1000 and continued to decline unevenly thereafter. By the age of 5, about 10 per 1000 of the cohort had had at least one afebrile fit (Van den Berg & Yerushalmy, 1969).

With regard to the absolute values of the age-specific rates that comprise this regular pattern, however, we find the familiar wide range of variation. Only by the age of 10 did the Rochester, Minnesota, rates reach the cumulative incidence for isolated and recurrent seizures of 10 per 1000 reached by age 5 in Oakland (Hauser & Kurland, 1975). Other incidence rates, including those from 2 British studies which include all types of fits of whatever origin, are much higher than either of these: an estimated 25 per 1000 in the first 2 years of life in the 1946 British national birth cohort (Cooper, 1965), approximately 61 per 1000 in the first 5 years in the Newcastle-upon-Tyne 1000 family study (Miller *et al.* 1960), and an extraordinary cumulative rate of 192 per 1000 to age 5 in an Israeli study

(Costeff, 1965). From the data at hand, we are free to choose between true variation, under-reporting with many false negatives, over-reporting with many false positives, or all three.

Nonetheless, all studies agree upon the high rates of afebrile seizures in the early months and years of life. Many afebrile seizures may represent failures of inhibitory mechanisms in the immature brain. It is plausible to view these failures as caused by specific prenatal, perinatal or early postnatal factors. Several kinds of evidence support this view. Studies of extensive clinical series have implicated a wide variety of prenatal and perinatal factors in the causes of seizures appearing in early life. These investigators are usually limited to causal inferences drawn from internal comparisons among cases or from implicit comparisons with general population rates. Among prenatal conditions, maternal bleeding, infections and toxaemia are suspected of causal involvement in the early epilepsies. Prematurity, prolonged labour, forceps delivery, neonatal hypoxia and low birthweight have all been mentioned as possible peripartum aetiological factors (Ounsted *et al.* 1966; Lier & Zachau-Christiansen, 1970; Bergamini *et al.* 1977; Chevrie & Aicardi, 1977). Two intensive, controlled studies have demonstrated associations between transient metabolic disturbances, such as hypocalcaemia and hypoglycaemia, and neonatal seizures (Brown *et al.* 1972; Keen & Lee, 1973).

If these factors are at work, it is a reasonable hope that advances in obstetrics and neonatology would be reflected in a reduced incidence of seizures, especially those of early onset. And indeed, this hope appears to be realized in the Rochester, Minnesota, data. For the period 1965–74, as compared with the 2 preceding decades, these data suggest that there was a decline in the incidence of recurrent seizures in infants under age 1 (Annegers *et al.* 1977). This reduced incidence could be the result of changing childbearing patterns or even of the better management of single seizure patients. More likely, it is a genuine consequence of the interruption by improved medical care of the causal pathways between noxious prenatal or perinatal factors and subsequent infantile seizures.

The possible role of prenatal and perinatal factors in the epilepsies has been explored in 2 case control studies in the USA in the 1950s and 1960s. Lilienfeld & Pasamanick (1954) compared the perinatal and prenatal records of 564 epileptic children with the records of matched controls selected, from birth registers. Among the epileptic children they found an excess of complications of pregnancy and delivery, and of abnormal neonatal conditions such as cyanosis. The findings among Blacks were similar to those among Whites, but the differences between Black cases and controls were not statistically significant. Henderson *et al.* (1964) replicated this study using a larger sample to test the findings among Blacks specifically, but also failed to find statistically significant associations between epilepsy and various prenatal and perinatal factors.

These hypotheses need further testing. There are 2 obvious weaknesses in these enterprising early controlled studies: first, an unavoidable crudeness in the prenatal and perinatal independent variables, and secondly a similar lack of precision in the dependent variable, the diagnosis of epilepsy. Advances in the years intervening since those studies permit refinement in both the independent and dependent variables, and thus an enhanced power to detect an effect. Neonatal care has become greatly sophisticated in the past decade, and data can be compiled on the physiological state of the infant, for instance in terms of blood sugar, electrolytes, body temperature and infant behaviour. Even the simple Apgar score was not available to the earlier studies. On the diagnostic side, the changes are no less dramatic, although they involve classification more than technology.

The prospects for precision in the matter of classification have been greatly improved by the recent emphasis on the clinical phenomenology of seizures, an approach reflected in the classification adopted in 1970 by the International League Against Epilepsy (Gastaut, 1970). One consequence of this new classification has been the greater recognition of seizures with focal or partial onset. The Lilienfeld & Pasamanick work of the 1950s, for example, confined its seizure types to grand mal, petit mal, 'other' and combinations of the three (Pasamanick & Lilienfeld, 1954). Focal seizures were not discussed explicitly, although abnormal EEG recordings with localization were distinguished in 27 % of available materials. In Hauser & Kurland's paper of 1975, which relied on the new classification, seizures of focal origin constituted more than 60 % of all recurrent seizure types. This dramatic shift is essentially the result of a revised nosology. The Rochester, Minnesota, data used by Hauser & Kurland extended through the 3 decades beginning in 1935. What changed were not the data, but the use made of them. Focal seizures, it must be added, are those most likely to be the consequence of perinatal factors.

In the current classification offered by the International League Against Epilepsy, seizures of focal origin are termed partial seizures, and described as having either elementary or complex symptomatology. In prior classifications, partial seizures with complex symptomatology were referred to as 'psychomotor' or 'temporal lobe' seizures. In the Rochester, Minnesota, study these constituted at least 40 % of partial seizures and more than 25 % of all recurrent seizures generally (Hauser & Kurland, 1975). These seizures are particularly resistant to medication and comprise the group in which surgery is resorted to most often. The possibility of primary prevention of this seizure type deserves further study.[1]

In 1953 Earle, Baldwin and Penfield (Earle *et al.* 1953) put forward a hypothesis which linked temporal lobe epilepsy with birth trauma. The mesial temporal sclerosis they had observed in the excised brains of temporal lobe epileptics, they suggested, was the consequence of herniation of the temporal lobe through the incisura of the tentorium, produced by mechanical compression of the head at birth. Falconer *et al.* (1964), noting high frequency of febrile convulsions in the histories of persons coming to surgery with intractable temporal lobe epilepsy, and Ounsted *et al.* (1966), observing a similar history in their series of temporal lobe epileptics, have argued the alternative hypothesis that the mesial sclerosis results from anoxia and cerebral oedema produced by prolonged febrile convulsions in childhood.

We know of no published study which has made an unbiased test of the association of temporal lobe epilepsy with febrile convulsions. P. West, E. M. Ross and N. R. Butler (personal communication), in a careful unpublished analysis of the 1958 British national birth cohort, have not found an association of febrile convulsions with temporal lobe epilepsy. This result emphasizes the fierce bias that can arise from the study among hospital cases alone of associations between different disorders.

While a specific association of childhood febrile seizures with temporal lobe epilepsy remains to be established, there is little doubt that early febrile seizures are associated with an excess risk of subsequent recurrent afebrile seizures generally (Van den Berg & Yerushalmy, 1969; Hauser & Kurland, 1975; Nelson & Ellenberg, 1976). The aetiological question is whether febrile seizures 'kindle' later seizures, whether they indicate an epileptic predisposition, or whether both processes are involved. The intriguing kindling hypothesis provides one justification for the current prophylactic use of anti-convulsants in treating children who have experienced febrile seizures. Although several controlled trials have demonstrated that phenobarbital can reduce the recurrence of febrile seizures (Faerø *et al.* 1972; Wallace, 1975; Wolf *et al.* 1977), the larger question of the contribution of febrile seizures to subsequent afebrile seziures remains unanswered. For the present, the hypothesis rests on the demonstration of kindling in animal experimental studies, and on suggestive data on the evolution of epilepsy after head injury (Jennett, 1965).

Predisposition is almost certainly a factor in the association of febrile and afebrile seizures. A familial history of febrile seizures has been found in association with certain recurrent afebrile seizure types (Ounsted *et al.* 1966; Hauser & Kurland, 1975; Tsuboi & Endo, 1977). Recurrent afebrile seizures too have been found to have a familial distribution (Kimball & Hersh, 1954; Metrakos & Metrakos, 1961; Tsuboi & Christian, 1973). Among these reports, variation and conflict about familial distributions is hardly less than about the frequencies described above. Undoubtedly, every individual has a threshold above which an appropriate stimulus will produce a seizure. A rigorous effort by Anderson (1978) has brought a degree of order out of chaos. In his review, he took care to specify the type of seizure, and also to distinguish between seizures and electro-encephalographic patterns.

[1] Temporal lobe seizures are also of special interest to psychiatry because of the suspected link between temporal lobe epilepsy and 'functional' psychoses. This research area has wide implications for the biological bases of functional psychiatric disorders, and deserves review in its own right. We would contend that few investigators have employed appropriate study designs or samples of sufficient size to which to address their hypotheses.

The most provocative result comes from the Rochester, Minnesota, studies. Three decades of accessible records in a single community enabled the research team to follow the offspring of the probands. Annegers *et al.* (1976) found an excess of recurrent afebrile seizures in offspring of 183 epileptic mothers, but none among the offspring of 108 epileptic fathers. (This excess was particularly striking for mothers with seizures of focal, as compared with generalized, onset.) The finding is probably not aberrant. Close examination of other family studies reveals a similar bias towards maternal transmission (Tsuboi & Christian, 1973; Gerken *et al.* 1977; Tsuboi & Endo, 1977). In these studies, the possibility of an artefact cannot be excluded, since a history of epilepsy in mothers is almost always easier to obtain than in fathers. The Rochester cohort study averts this difficulty.

Genetic hypotheses could explain this maternal bias with a modest degree of contortion. Thus, the Rochester team cites Carter's suggestion that, in diseases which affect males more frequently than females, transmission is likely to be biased towards females, since females presumably have a higher threshold and require a heavier dose of genes to produce the given disease (Carter, 1969). Thus, females would transmit a heavier dose than males. Other hypotheses are simpler and more appealing. Maternal transmission might be induced by exposure to the intra-uterine environment, or the cytoplasm might be the vehicle (Fine, 1977). Mitochondria could be the maternal cytoplasmic carriers, since certain animal spermatozoa do not carry mitochondria and in all probability they are not carried in human sperm.

From this brief conspectus of variation in the epilepsies, we do not hesitate to make one contention. It is time for epidemiologists, epileptologists and other interested parties to set their sights on causal factors, and to begin to gather and to generate testable causal hypotheses. In the United States, this effort has been stimulated recently by publication of the *Plan for Nationwide Action on Epilepsy* (1978), a report by the Commission for the Control of Epilepsy and Its Consequences. While drawing public attention to the medical and social problems of epileptics and suggesting remedial policies, the report also summarizes present knowledge about frequency and aetiology. The Commission's work should contribute new energy and impetus to epidemiological research on aetiology.

RICHARD NEUGEBAUER AND MERVYN SUSSER

REFERENCES

Anderson, V. E. (1978). Genetic counseling for epilepsy. *Plan for Nationwide Action on Epilepsy*, Vol. II, Part 1. Sections I–VI, pp. 141–162. The Commission for the Control of Epilepsy and Its Consequences. US Department of Health, Education and Welfare.

Annegers, J. F., Hauser, W. A., Elveback, L. R., Anderson, V. E. & Kurland, L. T. (1976). Seizure disorders in offspring of parents with a history of seizures – a maternal–paternal difference? *Epilepsia* **17**, 1–9.

Annegers, J. F., Hauser, W. A. & Kurland, L. T. (1977). Secular changes in the incidence of seizure disorders in Rochester, Minnesota, 1935–1974. Paper presented at the American Epilepsy Society 1977 Annual Meeting. Abstract. *Epilepsia* (in the press).

Annegers, J. F., Hauser, W. A., Elveback, L. R. & Kurland, L. T. (1979). Remission and relapse of seizures in patients with epilepsy. In *Epilepsy: The Tenth International Symposium* (in the press). Raven Press: New York.

Bergamini, L., Bergamesco, B., Benna, P. & Gilli, M. (1977). Acquired etiological factors in 1785 epileptic subjects: clinical–anamnestic research. *Epilepsia* **18**, 437–444.

Brown, J. K., Cockburn, P. & Forfar, J. O. (1972). Clinical and chemical correlates in convulsions of the newborn. *Lancet* i, 135.

Carter, C. O. (1969). Genetics of common disorders. *British Medical Bulletin* **25**, 52–57.

Chevrie, J. J. & Aicardi, J. (1977). Convulsive disorders in the first year of life: etiologic factors. *Epilepsia* **18**, 489–498.

The Commission for the Control of Epilepsy and Its Consequences (1978). *Plan for Nationwide Action on Epilepsy*.

Diaz, J. & Schain, R. J. (1977). The effects on behavior and brain growth of chronic phenobarbital administered to young post-weanling rats. Paper presented at the American Epilepsy Society 1977 Annual Meeting.

Diaz, J., Schain, R. J. & Bailey, B. G. (1977). Phenobarbital-induced brain growth retardation in artificially reared rat pups. *Biology of the Neonate* **32**, 77–82.

Earle, K. M., Baldwin, M. & Penfield, W. (1953). Incisural sclerosis and temporal lobe seizures produced by hippocampal herniation at birth. *AMA Archives of Neurology and Psychiatry* **69**, 27–42.

Faerø, O., Kastrup, K. W., Lykkegaard, N. E., Melchior, J. C. & Thorn, I. (1972). Successful prophylaxis of febrile convulsions with phenobarbital. *Epilepsia* **13**, 279–285.

Falconer, M. A., Serafetinides, E. A. & Corsellis, J. A. N. (1964). Etiology and pathenogenesis of temporal lobe epilepsy. *Archives of Neurology* **10**, 233–248.

Fine, P. E. M. (1977). Analysis of family data for evidence of non-Mendelian inheritance resulting from vertical transmission. *Journal of Medical Genetics* **14**, 399–407.

Gastaut, H. (1970). Clinical and electroencephalographical classification of epileptic seizures. *Epilepsia* **11**, 102–113.

Gerken, H., Kiefer, R., Doose, H. & Völzke, E. (1977). Genetic factors in childhood epilepsy with focal sharp waves. 1. Clinical data and familial morbidity for seizures. *Neuropaediatrie* **8**, 3–9.

Hauser, W. A. (1978). Epidemiology of epilepsy. In *Neuroepidemiology* (ed. B. Schoenberg). Advances in Neurology Series (in the press). Raven Press: New York.

Henderson, M., Goldstein, H., Pogot, E., Goldberg, I. D. & Entwisle, G. (1964). Perinatal factors associated with epilepsy in negro children. *Public Health Reports* **79**, 501–509.

Jennett, W. B. (1965). Predicting epilepsy after blunt head injury. *British Medical Journal* ii, 1215–1216.

Keen, J. H. & Lee, D. (1973). Sequelae of neonatal convulsions: a study of 112 infants. *Archives of Disease in Childhood* **48**, 542–546.

Kimball, O. P. & Hersh, A. H. (1954). The genetics of epilepsy. *Acta Geneticae Medicae et Gemellologiae* **4**, 131–142.

Kurtzke, J. F. (1972). Discussion. In *The Epidemiology of Epilepsy: A Workshop* (ed. M. Alter and W. A. Hauser), p. 156. US Dept. of Health, Education and Welfare, NINDS Monograph No. 14.

Lier, L. & Zachau-Christiansen, B. (1970). Pre- and perinatal etiological factors in children with epilepsy and other convulsive disorders. A prospective study. *Acta Pediatrica Scandinavica* Suppl. 206, 27–29.

Lilienfeld, A. M. & Pasamanick, B. (1954). Association of maternal and fetal factors with the development of epilepsy. I. Abnormalities in the prenatal and paranatal periods. *Journal of the American Medical Association* **155**, 719–724.

Metrakos, K. & Metrakos, K. (1961). Genetics of convulsive disorders. *Neurology* **11**, 471–483.

Murphy, J. V. & D'Souza, B. J. (1977). Seizure control in mentally retarded, institutionalized patients: a pre-intervention survey. Paper presented at the American Epilepsy Society 1977 Annual Meeting.

Myrianthopoulos, N. C. (1972). Discussion in Gates, M. J. Age: risk of seizures in infants. In *The Epidemiology of Epilepsy: A Workshop* (ed. M. Alter and W. A. Hauser), pp. 79–80. US Dept. of Health, Education and Welfare, NINDS Monograph No. 14.

Nelson, K. B. & Ellenberg, J. H. (1976). Predictors of epilepsy in children who have experienced febrile seizures. *New England Journal of Medicine* **295**, 1029–1033.

Ounsted, C., Lindsay, J. & Norman, R. (1966). *Biological Factors in Temporal Lobe Epilepsy*. W. Heinemann Medical Books: London.

Pasamanick, B. & Lilienfeld, A. M. (1954). Maternal and fetal factors in the development of epilepsy. 2. Relationship to some clinical features of epilepsy. *Neurology* **5**, 80–83.

Rodin, E. A. (1972). Medical and social prognosis in epilepsy. *Epilepsia* **13**, 121–131.

Stein, Z. A. & Susser, M. (1974). The epidemiology of mental retardation. In *Child and Adolescent Psychiatry, Sociocultural and Community Psychiatry* (ed. Gerald Caplan), pp. 464–491. Vol. II of *American Handbook of Psychiatry* (2nd edn). Basic Books: New York.

Trimble, M. R. & Reynolds, E. H. (1976). Anticonvulsant drugs and mental symptoms: a review. *Psychological Medicine* **6**, 169–178.

Tsuboi, T. & Christian, W. (1973). On the genetics of the primary generalized epilepsy with sporadic myoclonias of impulsive petit mal type. *Humangenetik* **19**, 155–182.

Tsuboi, T. & Endo, S. (1977). Incidence of seizures and EEG abnormalities among offspring of epileptic patients. *Human Genetics* **36**, 173–189.

US Department of Commerce, Social and Economics Statistics Administration, Bureau of the Census (1973). *Country and City Data Book 1972*. Government Printing Office: Washington, D.C.

Wallace, S. (1975). Continuous prophylactic anticonvulsants in selected children with febrile convulsions. *Acta Neurologica Scandinavica* **60** (Suppl.), 62.

Wolf, S. M., Carr, A., Davis, D. C., Davidson, S., Dale, E. P., Forsythe, A., Goldenberg, E. D., Hanson, R., Lulejian, G. A., Nelson, M. A., Treitman, P. & Weinstein, A. (1977). The value of phenobarbital in the child who has had a single febrile seizure: a controlled prospective study. *Pediatrics* **59**, 378–385.

Zielinski, J. J. (1974*a*). Epileptics not in treatment. *Epilepsia* **15**, 203–210.

EPIDEMIOLOGICAL SURVEYS OF THE EPILEPSIES

Baldwin, R., Davens, E. & Harris, V. G. (1953). The epilepsy program in public health. *American Journal of Public Health* **43**, 452–459.

Baumann, R. J., Marx, M. B. & Leonidakis, M. G. (1977). An estimate of the prevalence of epilepsy in a rural Appalachian population. *American Journal of Epidemiology* **106**, 42–52.

Bongers, E., Coppoolse, J., Meinhardi, H., Posthuma, E. P. S. & Van Zyl, C. H. W. (1976). *A Survey of Epilepsy in Zeeland, the Netherlands*. Published by Institut Voor Epilepsiebestrijding 'Meer en Bosch' – 'De Crucuiushoeve': Heemstede, The Netherlands.

Brewis, M., Poskanzer, D. C., Rolland, C. & Miller, H. (1966). Neurological disease in an English city. *Acta Neurologica Scandinavica* **42** (Suppl. 24), 1–89.

Chen, K., Brody, J. A. & Kurland, L. T. (1968). Patterns of neurologic diseases on Guam. I. Epidemiologic aspects. *Archives of Neurology (Chicago)* **19**, 573–578.

Cooper, J. E. (1965). Epilepsy in a longitudinal survey of 5000 children. *British Medical Journal* i, 1020–1022.

Costeff, H. (1965). Convulsions in childhood. Their natural history and indications for treatment. *New England Journal of Medicine* **273**, 1410–1413.

Crombie, D. L., Cross, K. W., Fry, J., Pinsent, R. J. F. H. & Watts, C. A. H. (1960). A survey of the epilepsies in general practice: a report by the Research Committee of the College of General Practitioners. *British Medical Journal* ii, 416–422.

Dada, T. O. (1970). Epilepsy in Lagos, Nigeria. *African Journal of Medical Science* **14**, 161–184.

Gates, M. (1972). Age: risk of seizures in infants. In *The Epidemiology of Epilepsy: A Workshop* (ed. M. Alter & W. A. Hauser), pp. 75–81. US Dept. of Health, Education and Welfare. NINDS Monograph No. 14.

deGraaf, A. S. (1974). Epidemiological aspects of epilepsy in northern Norway. *Epilepsia* **15**, 291–299.

Gudmundsson, G. (1966). Epilepsy in Iceland. A clinical and epidemiological investigation. *Acta Neurologica Scandinavica* **43** (Suppl. 25), 4–124.

Hauser, W. A. & Kurland, L. T. (1975). The epidemiology of epilepsy in Rochester, Minnesota, 1935 through 1967. *Epilepsy* **16**, 1–66.

Jilek, W. G. & Jilek-Aall, L. M. (1970). The problem of epilepsy in a rural Tanzanian tribe. *African Journal of Medical Science* **1**, 305–307.

Juul-Jensen, P. & Ipsen, J. (1975). Praevalens og incidens af epilepsi i Stor-Århus. *Ugeskrift for Laeger* **137**, 2380–2388.

Krohn, W. (1961). A study of epilepsy in northern Norway, its frequency and character. *Acta Psychiatrica et Neurologica Scandinavica* **36** (Suppl. 150), 215–225.

Kurland, L. T. (1959/60). The incidence and prevalence of convulsive disorders in a small urban community. *Epilepsia* **1**, 143–161.

Leibowitz, U. & Alter, M. (1968). Epilepsy in Jerusalem, Israel. *Epilepsia* **9**, 87–105.

Lessell, S., Torres, J. M. & Kurland, L. T. (1962). Seizure disorders in a Guamanian village. *Archives of Neurology (Chicago)* **7**, 53–60.

Levy, L. F. (1970). Epilepsy in Rhodesia, Zambia and Malawi. *African Journal of Medical Science* **1**, 291–303.

Logan, W. P. D. (1962). *Morbidity Statistics from General Practice*. Volume III. *Disease in General Practice*. Studies on Medical and Population Subjects, No. 14. HMSO: London.

Logan, W. P. D. & Cushion, A. A. (1958). *Morbidity Statistics from General Practice*. Volume I. *General*. Studies on Medical and Population Subjects, No. 14. HMSO: London.

Mathai, K. V., Dunn, D. P., Kurland, L. T. & Reeder, F. A. (1968). Convulsive disorders in the Mariana Islands. *Epilepsia* **9**, 77–85.

McDonald, A. D. (1961). Maternal health in early pregnancy and congenital defect. Final report on a prospective inquiry. *British Journal of Preventive and Social Medicine* **15**, 154–166.

Meighan, S. S., Queener, L. & Weitman, M. (1976). Prevalence of epilepsy in children of Multnomah County, Oregon. *Epilepsia* **17**, 245–256.

Miller, F. J. W., Court, S. D. M., Walton, W. S. & Knox, E. G. (1960). *Growing up in Newcastle upon Tyne. A Continuing Study of Health and Illness in Young Children within their Families*. Oxford University Press: New York.

Parry Jones, A. (1958). Epilepsy in Cardiff school children. *The Medical Officer* 21 March, 164–166.

Pond, D. A., Bidwell, B. H. & Stein, L. (1960). A survey of epilepsy in fourteen general practices. Part 1. Demographic and medical data. *Psychiatria, Neurologia, Neurochirurgia (Amst.)* **63**, 217–236.

Rose, S. W., Penry, J. K., Markush, R. E., Radloff, L. A. & Putnam, P. L. (1973). Prevalence of epilepsy in children. *Epilepsia* **14**, 133–152.

Ross, E. M. (1973). Convulsive disorders in British children. *Proceedings of the Royal Society of Medicine* **66**, 702.

Rutter, M., Graham, P. & Yule, W. (1970). *A Neuropsychiatric Study in Childhood*. Clinics in Developmental Medicine, Nos. 35/36. J. P. Lippincott: Philadelphia.

Sato, S. (1964). The epidemiological and clinico-statistical study of epilepsy in Niigata City. Part 1. The epidemiological study of epilepsy in Niigata City. *Clinical Neurology (Tokyo)* **4**, 413–424.

Stanhope, J. M., Brody, J. A. & Brink, E. (1972). Convulsions among the Chamorro people of Guam, Mariana Islands. Part 1. Seizure disorders. *American Journal of Epidemiology* **95**, 292–298.

Van den Berg, B. J. & Yerushalmy, J. (1969). Studies on convulsive disorders in young children. I. Incidence of febrile and nonfebrile convulsions by age and other factors. *Pediatric Research* **3**, 298–304.

Wajsbort, J., Haral, N. & Alfandary, I. (1967). A study of the epidemiology of chronic epilepsy in northern Israel. *Epilepsia* **8**, 105–116.

Wishik, S. M. (1956). Handicapped children in Georgia: a study of prevalence, disability, needs and resources. *American Journal of Public Health* **46**, 195–203.

Zielinski, J. J. (1974*b*). *Epidemiology and Medico-Social Problems of Epilepsy in Warsaw*. Final report on research program No. 19-P-58325-F-01. The Social and Rehabilitation Service, Department of Health, Education and Welfare: Washington, D.C.

Psychological Medicine, 1980, **10**, 5–10

Methodological issues in psychiatric case-identification[1]

The use of the term 'case' in clinical psychiatric research implies that the investigator wishes to identify the presence or absence of some clinically relevant disorder or disorders in a human population; for example, to distinguish X from non-X, Y from non-Y, and X from Y. The main reasons for making such identifications are to clarify or refine the descriptive features of the disorder, to calculate an incidence or a prevalence rate, and to test hypotheses concerning, for example, causes, treatments or outcomes. Many of the ideas used in the research are derived from clinical practice and it is usually hoped that the results will, in turn, be found clinically useful.

The simplest technique of case-identification, therefore, is for a well-trained psychiatrist to interview all the members of the population under review and to 'make a diagnosis'. A substantial proportion of the research literature has been, and still is, based upon this technique. Its advantages are that it is simple, it has achieved (particularly in Scandinavian epidemiological studies of the functional psychoses) some remarkably replicable results, and there is no question as to its clinical reference. The disadvantages are also considerable. The well-known differences between the way 'schizophrenia' is diagnosed in various parts of the world, even by experienced psychiatrists, illustrate the major problem (Cooper *et al.* 1972; WHO, 1973). Less severe disorders give rise to greater differences, even among the Scandinavian investigators, and it is difficult to say how far these are due to different methods of reaching a diagnosis rather than to variations in true incidence or prevalence.

The central methodological issue in case-identification is how, in the absence of simple physiological or biochemical indices, to construct techniques which will ensure a useful degree of comparability between studies. This is not just a matter of achieving 'reliability' between a few close collaborators, but the much more difficult task of ensuring that teams working independently, perhaps in different countries and using different languages, can replicate each others' studies, thus adding to the stock of knowledge available to investigators all over the world.

The problems involved in achieving this kind of comparability can conveniently be reviewed by considering the information collected by a psychiatrist in order to make a diagnosis. This includes a knowledge of which out of a range of possible symptoms and signs are present, how severe (i.e. intense and continuous) they are, their time relationships, the extent to which they cluster together to form syndromes, and the relative diagnostic weighting of each syndrome. Symptom episodes in the recent, and perhaps the more distant, past, and the presence or absence of pathological indices and possible causative factors, are also considered. Kendell (1973) showed that a decision approximating to the final diagnosis could be reached quite quickly but this does not mean that the process can easily be standardized. It is not, of course, implied that any technique can achieve perfect standardization. Nor is it necessary, in most investigations, to try to standardize everything. Specific scales can be constructed for limited purposes (e.g. to measure improvement following treatment for a phobia of flying), or one of the useful schedules available for measuring change in conditions such as depression (Beck *et al.* 1961; Hamilton, 1960; Zung, 1965) or general anxiety (Taylor, 1953) can be used. It should be recalled, however, that the criteria for entry into the study also need specification and that this always includes an element of differential diagnosis.

Several factors which could be used as indirect measures of the severity of the effects of disorder are best kept separate, as far as possible, from the diagnostic elements mentioned so far. These include decline in social performance or status, degree of personal distress or dissatisfaction, and amount of contact with medical or social services. As we shall see, confusion between such factors

[1] Address for correspondence: Professor J. K. Wing, MRC Social Psychiatry Unit, Institute of Psychiatry, De Crespigny Park, Denmark Hill, London SE5 8AF.

and symptoms makes it difficult to test hypotheses about aetiology, treatment or course. The advantage of introducing standardization into the diagnostic process is that each element can be specified separately and various combinations of elements can then be investigated.

For many investigators, standardization begins and ends with symptoms. The simplest technique is to construct a set of questions, each representing a symptom, which can be answered by the respondent filling in a form, or giving his or her answers to an interviewer. The latter situation allows other observations to be made and provides for a limited degree of clarification if the subject asks what a question means. In general, however, the question is left for the respondent to interpret. One of the first such questionnaires was the Neuropsychiatric Screening Adjunct (Stouffer *et al.* 1950). Scores on the NSA differentiated quite well between groups of American soldiers and neurotic inpatients and between individuals who were judged by psychiatrists to be suitable or not suitable for army service. The most useful sections were concerned with so-called 'psychosomatic' items (mostly autonomic symptoms, insomnia and nervousness) and 'personal adjustment' (including depression, self-pity, worries and self-confidence).

Many such scales have been developed since, two early and much-used examples being the Cornell Medical Index (Brodman *et al.* 1952) and the Health Opinion Survey (Macmillan, 1957). Similar (though unfortunately not identical) instruments were used in the Stirling County and Midtown Manhattan projects (Leighton *et al.* 1963; Srole *et al.* 1962). The investigators adopted a unidimensional concept of mental disorder – an amalgam of symptoms and disability which was regarded as being quantitatively reactive to the degree of social stress. 'Social stress' was conceptualized in somewhat different ways in the two studies but it included adverse life events, disadvantage, low prestige and difficulty in maintaining 'a place in the social system.' The opportunities for contamination between social and clinical measures are evident.

Many authors (e.g. Dohrenwend & Dohrenwend, 1969) have pointed out that disorders defined through the use of such questionnaires cannot directly be related to the disorders diagnosed by psychiatrists in hospital practice. The fact that the latter tend to have high scores on the questionnaires does not give much information as to the nature of the condition measured. Tyhurst (1957) argued that transient stressful situations could produce transient psychological responses which need not be regarded as abnormal. By the same token, longer-term difficulties might be expected to produce more chronic distress and dissatisfaction without a psychiatric diagnosis being called for.

Recent work with the General Health Questionnaire (Goldberg, 1972) has confirmed the value of a simple self-rating instrument for detecting people in a state of personal distress and dissatisfaction. Such people are often socially disadvantaged or physically impaired. The GHQ can be used to monitor the effects of various kinds of intervention, such as extra counselling by a general practitioner (Johnstone & Goldberg, 1976). A simple cut-off score allows 'cases' to be differentiated, for screening purposes, from 'non-cases', but no suggestion is made that disorders thus defined are equivalent to any particular psychiatric diagnosis.

More comprehensive checklists of symptoms have been devised, with the twin characteristics of ease of administration and lack of control over the responses (Lorr *et al.* 1963; Overall & Gorham, 1962; Wittenborn, 1955). Foulds (1965) pointed out that the Minnesota Multiphasic Personality Inventory (MMPI) (Hathaway & McKinley, 1951) and other schedules contain items representing psychological symptoms mixed with others representing personality traits. He could have added that yet other items represent attitudes. His own checklists have the merits of keeping symptoms and traits separate and of basing the symptom scales firmly on psychiatric experience. The latter is not true of most of the other scales, perhaps because of Lorr's judgement that 'in much of American psychiatry, formal diagnosis is actually ignored as relatively unimportant and outmoded, or disparaged as nondynamic and useless' (Lorr, 1966).

The situation in the USA has changed a good deal since Lorr made this statement and it could not, even at that time, have been applied with the same force to European diagnostic practices. Foulds (1965), who reviewed the evidence concerning the reliability with which psychiatrists classified mental disorders, pointed out that there was very little evidence in the few, mostly inadequate, studies then published, to justify the wholesale condemnation often made, whereas there were studies indicating a useful degree of reliability (Kreitman, 1961). Further work has shown how psychiatric nosology, particularly in the relevant sections of the International Classification of Diseases, can be improved by providing more precise definitions for use by clinical psychiatrists (Feighner *et al.* 1972; Scharfetter, 1971; Spitzer *et al.* 1978; WHO, 1974). This practical line of development has been paralleled by attempts to standardize more of the elements of the diagnostic process in order to be able to make the diagnoses used in scientific research more comparable.

Again, these efforts had to begin with symptoms. The Present State Examination (PSE), for example, is based on a glossary of differential definitions derived from the clinical practice taught in one particular school of British psychiatry. Apart from a few items, social elements are excluded from the definitions. Rules are laid down for rating the presence or absence of symptoms during the month before interview and, if present, their intensity and stability. The interviewer is free to ask further questions, beyond those laid down in the schedule, in order to elicit sufficient detail from the subject to allow an adequate decision to be made. Ratings on the 140 items allow the calculation of sub-scores and a total score and clustering in order to provide a syndrome profile which can be used as a descriptive summary of the clinical condition (Wing *et al.* 1967, 1974; Wing & Sturt, 1978).

The PSE is intended to cover the whole range of symptoms found in the functional neuroses and psychoses. The fact that it is based on the month before interview and excludes possible aetiological factors means that certain diagnoses (e.g. personality disorders, mental retardation and alcoholic hallucinosis) cannot be derived from the PSE alone. An Aetiology Schedule can be used to help codify the presence or absence of possible causal factors. During acute episodes of disorder sufficient symptoms are usually present to allow a clinical diagnosis to be made, but in a small proportion of cases additional information is required about symptoms present more than a month previously (Simon *et al.* 1971; Sartorius *et al.* 1970). This restriction on clinical diagnosis applies *ipso facto* to any technique designed to simulate it. Extra data are therefore extracted from contemporary case-records on a Syndrome Check List. Reliability is quite reasonable but obviously depends on the quality of the records (Wing *et al.* 1974, p. 106). If good records are not available, it is possible to ask informants, but memory, even for acute and severe episodes, may well be unreliable.

The other major element needed to simulate a diagnosis is a set of rules, laid down sufficiently precisely to obviate the necessity for further subjective interpretation, for differentiating between clinical classes. This is provided by the CATEGO computer program (Wing *et al.* 1974; Wing & Sturt, 1978). The procedures used are clinical throughout. Obviously, no higher claim is made for the validity of the classes produced than for the clinical diagnostic groups they simulate, and the system is explicitly not intended to be used clinically as a substitute for a diagnosis (Wing *et al.* 1974, p. 136). Many clinicians do find it useful to know the outcome of a standard procedure but the use they make of it still depends on their clinical judgement. It is also found useful in teaching. But the chief value is in research, since it allows comparability in the testing of hypotheses. A useful degree of concordance between CATEGO classes and broad clinical diagnoses has been observed, and studies of the small proportion of discrepancies has led to suggestions for improving both types of classification (Scharfetter *et al.* 1976; WHO, 1973, p. 243; Wing & Nixon, 1975; Wing *et al.* 1977*a*).

This system is firmly grounded in the clinical experience of psychiatrists examining patients with acute disorders. A further element of incomparability needs to be eliminated, as far as possible, before it can be used with samples of people from a general population. This is the threshold at which it can be said that sufficient key symptoms are present to allow the recognition of a disorder. The question rarely arises when examining recently admitted in-patients, since most are suffering from severe disorders. Recalling the earlier discussion about case-identification, it is clear that the procedure governing the determination of a threshold must be clinical, specifiable and replicable.

One such technique is the Index of Definition (Wing *et al.* 1977*b*, 1978; Wing & Sturt, 1978). The solution adopted is to lay down, on the basis of clinical experience, rules determining a number of levels of certainty that sufficient PSE symptoms are present to allow recognition of a 'disorder'. The threshold is, of course, defined separately for each major type of symptom, since no single criterion could be applied to all the possible combinations of symptoms found in a population survey. The extent of the problem can be understood if it is recalled that a total PSE score of 1 can indicate the presence of any one of more than 120 symptoms, ranging from a moderate degree of muscular tension to a first-rank symptom of schizophrenia.

The Index of Definition allows 8 different levels of certainty as to the presence of a recognizable functional disorder. Level 5 indicates that certain minimal criteria have been met and levels 6–8 indicate more definite disorders. Disorders at or above the threshold can be classified using the CATEGO program. Thus, the PSE–ID–CATEGO system can be used to classify the conditions found in people admitted to hospital, referred to out-patient clinics, or interviewed in general population surveys. The Syndrome Check List can be used to provide a degree of standardization of the symptoms present in previous episodes of disorder in subjects interviewed in population surveys but detailed case-records are rarely available and the subject's memory is an unreliable guide. The Index of Definition cannot be applied. Estimates of incidence or descriptions of 'disorders' not present at the time of examination must therefore be regarded as very approximate. This is, of course, even more true of any less specified judgement about past episodes.

One test of the distinction between 'cases' and 'non-cases' as defined by the Index of Definition is to compare it with an independent clinical judgement. Two published series allow such a comparison. The first was the 'second Camberwell survey' in which a team of sociologists from Bedford College interviewed a sample of 237 women aged 18–65 (Brown *et al.* 1975). Three psychiatrists (J. P. Leff, S. A. Mann and J. K. Wing) interviewed 95 of these women, using the ninth edition of the PSE and rated tapes of the Bedford interviews with a further 28. They made global clinical judgements of 'caseness' and compared these with the distinction based on the subsequently developed Index of Definition. The concordance (level 5 and above) was 90% (Wing *et al.* 1978). The second survey was carried out by Orley, who used the PSE to interview the adult population of two small Ugandan villages. The concordance with the Index of Definition was 91% (Orley & Wing, 1979).

The global clinical judgement in these studies is therefore likely to have been based mainly on the presence or absence of key symptoms. The non-medical interviewers in the second Camberwell survey were trained by members of the MRC Social Psychiatry Unit to use the short form of the PSE (the first 40 of the 140 items) and were able to do so with fair reliability (Wing *et al.* 1977*b*). The training technique used was to provide experience with rating severe disorders in in-patients (see also Cooper *et al.* 1977). Whether the criteria used by such interviewers are likely to 'drift' after a period of time without further training has yet to be established. The Index of Definition and the CATEGO program can be applied to PSE ratings with absolute reliability. The system can therefore be used wherever teams of trained investigators are available. (Problems of translation are discussed elsewhere: Orley & Wing, 1979; WHO, 1973.) The same cannot be said of a global judgement. Members of a team often come to achieve very close agreement on such judgements but other teams may reasonably adopt different, though equally reliable, criteria. Moreover, the threshold may be affected by the setting in which the interviews are undertaken. Urwin & Gibbons (1979) found that level 5 (the threshold level) of the Index of Definition could be divided into two roughly equal sub-levels, the lower one (5*a*) approximating to what they regarded, clinically, as 'not a case', the upper one (5*b*) approximating to their judgement of a 'case'. In studies of a population in North Uist, conducted by the Bedford College team (Brown *et al.* 1977), we have suggested that the psychiatrist adopted a somewhat similar threshold (i.e. somewhere in the middle of level 5) to that used by the Southampton investigators (R. Prudo, unpublished; Brown & Harris, 1978, p. 580). These differences in private clinical judgement can only be made manifest in comparison with the more detailed and public standards of a more standardized system.

The same must be true, *a fortiori*, when comparing 'cases' detected in a general population with severe depressive or other disorders in in-patients. It is only when this problem of methodological comparability is solved that the clinical nature of 'psychiatric disorders' found in the general population can be investigated. The familiar method of working from the known to the unknown can then be used (Wing *et al.* 1978).

One further common misunderstanding of standardized techniques needs to be considered. This is that standardization is unnecessarily arbitrary or rigid. It is true that *all* standardization requires a degree of rigidity, in the sense that the techniques can only be used if the rules are adhered to.

However, the advantages of the techniques stem from these restrictions. The more precisely and communicably the limits are laid down, the greater is the value of the technique to research workers, who can then criticize and improve it. The criticisms, however, must be specified in just as precise and communicable a manner.

We return now to the starting point of this review. All the techniques discussed are 'clinical', in the sense that they are more or less based on the experience of clinical psychiatrists and are intended, in the longer or shorter run, to be of use to people with psychiatric disorders. There is no point in using a sledgehammer to crack a nut. The simplest technique that will serve the purposes of the study is the most efficient one to use. But many of the problems of concern to contemporary psychiatrists are highly complex; for example (*a*) the nature of the relationship between the severe affective disorders observed in in-patients and the less severe conditions found in some members of general population samples, and (*b*) the comparison of disorders found in samples of people living under different social and cultural conditions. The more complex the theories under test, the more important it is to be sure that the techniques used are open to scrutiny by the scientific community.

J. K. WING

REFERENCES

Beck, A. T., Ward, C. H., Mendelson, M., Mock, J. & Erbaugh, J. (1961). An inventory for measuring depression. *Archives of General Psychiatry* **4**, 561–571.

Brodman, K., Erdman, A. J. & Lorge, I. (1952). The Cornell Medical Index Health Questionnaire: the evaluation of emotional disturbance. *Journal of Clinical Psychology* **8**, 119–124.

Brown, G. W. & Harris, T. (1978). Social origins of depression: a reply. *Psychological Medicine* **8**, 577–588.

Brown, G. W., Bhrolchain, M. & Harris, T. (1975). Social class and psychiatric disturbance among women in an urban population. *Sociology* **9**, 225–254.

Brown, G. W., Davidson, S., Harris, T., Maclean, U., Pollock, S. & Prudo, R. (1977). Psychiatric disorder in London and North Uist. *Social Science and Medicine* **11**, 367–377.

Cooper, J. E., Kendell, R. E., Gurland, B. J., Sharpe, L., Copeland, J. R. M. & Simon, R. (1972) *Psychiatric Diagnosis in New York and London*. Maudsley Monograph no. 20. Oxford University Press: London.

Cooper, J. E., Copeland, J. R. M., Brown, G. W., Harris, T. & Gourlay, A. J. (1977). Further studies on interviewer training and inter-rater reliability of the PSE. *Psychological Medicine* **7**, 517–523.

Dohrenwend, B. P. & Dohrenwend, B. S. (1969). *Social Status and Psychological Disorder: A Causal Enquiry*. Wiley: New York.

Feighner, J. P., Robins, E., Guze, S. B., Woodruff, R. A., Winokur, G. & Munoz, R. (1972). Diagnostic criteria for use in psychiatric research. *Archives of General Psychiatry* **26**, 57–63.

Foulds, G. A. (1965). *Personality and Personal Illness*. Tavistock: London.

Goldberg, D. P. (1972). *The Detection of Psychiatric Illness by Questionnaire*. Oxford University Press: London.

Hamilton, M. (1960). A rating scale for depression. *Journal of Neurosurgery and Psychiatry* **23**, 56–62.

Hathaway, S. R. & McKinley, J. C. (1951). *The Minnesota Multiphasic Personality Inventory Manual (Revised)*. Psychological Corporation: New York.

Johnstone, A. & Goldberg, D. (1976). Psychiatric screening in general practice: A controlled trial. *Lancet* i, 605–608.

Kendell, R. E. (1973). Psychiatric diagnoses: a study of how they are made. *British Journal of Psychiatry* **122**, 437–445.

Kreitman, N. (1961). Reliability of psychiatric diagnosis. *Journal of Mental Science* **107**, 876.

Leighton, D. C., Harding, J. S., Macklin, D. B., Macmillan, A. M. & Leighton, A. H. (1963). *The Character of Danger: Psychiatric Symptoms in Selected Communities*. Basic Books: New York.

Lorr, M. (ed.) (1966). *Explorations in Typing Psychotics*. Pergamon: New York.

Lorr, M., Klett, C. J., McNair, D. M. & Lasky, J. (1963). *Inpatient Multidimensional Psychiatric Scale (Manual)*. Consulting Psychologists Press: Palo Alto.

Macmillan, A. M. (1957). The health opinion survey: technique for estimating prevalence of psychoneurotic and related types of disorder in communities. *Psychological Reports* **3**, 325–329.

Orley, J. & Wing, J. K. (1979). Psychiatric disorders in two African villages. *Archives of General Psychiatry* **36**, 513–520.

Overall, J. E. & Gorham, D. R. (1962). The brief psychiatric rating scale. *Psychological Reports* **10**, 799–812.

Sartorius, N., Brooke, E. & Lin, T. Y. (1970). Reliability of psychiatric assessment in international research. *Psychiatric Epidemiology* (ed. E. H. Hare and J. K. Wing), pp. 138–148. Oxford University Press: London.

Scharfetter, C. (1971). *Das AMP-System: Manual zur Dokumentation psychiatrischer Befunde*. Springer-Verlag: Berlin.

Scharfetter, C., Moerbt, H. & Wing, J. K. (1976). Diagnosis of functional psychoses: comparison of clinical and computerized classification. *Archiv für Psychiatrie und Nervenkrankheiten* **222**, 61–67.

Simon, R. J., Gurland, B. J., Fleiss, J. L. & Sharpe, L. (1971). Impact of a patient history interview on psychiatric diagnosis. *Archives of General Psychiatry* **24**, 437–440.

Spitzer, R. L., Endicott, J. & Robins, E. (1978). Research diagnostic criteria: rationale and reliability. *Archives of General Psychiatry* **35**, 773–782.

Srole, L., Langer, T. S., Michael, S. T., Opler, M. K. & Rennie, T. A. C. (1962). *Mental Health in the Metropolis: The Midtown Manhattan Study*. McGraw-Hill: New York.

Stouffer, S. A., Guttman, L., Suchman, E. A., Lazarsfeld, P. F., Star, S. A., & Clausen, J. A. (1950). *Measurement and Prediction*. Studies in Social Psychology in World War II, Volume IV. Princeton University Press: Princeton.

Taylor, J. A. (1953). A personality scale of manifest anxiety. *Journal of Abnormal and Social Psychology* **48**, 285–290.

Tyhurst, J. S. (1957). The role of transition states – including disasters – in mental illness. In *Symposium on Preventive and Social Psychiatry* pp. 149–169. Government Publishing Office: Washington, D.C.

Urwin, P. & Gibbons, J. L. (1979). Psychiatric diagnosis in

self-poisoning patients. *Psychological Medicine* **9**, 501–507.
Wing, J. K. & Nixon, J. (1975). Discriminating symptoms in schizophrenia. *Archives of General Psychiatry* **32**, 853–859.
Wing, J. K. & Sturt, E. (1978). *The PSE–ID–CATEGO System: A Supplementary Manual.* Institute of Psychiatry, Mimeo: London.
Wing, J. K., Birley, J. L. T., Cooper, J. E., Graham, P. & Isaacs A. (1967). Reliability of a procedure for measuring and classifying 'present psychiatric state'. *British Journal of Psychiatry* **113**, 499–515.
Wing, J. K., Cooper J. E. & Sartorius, N. (1974). *Measurement and Classification of Psychiatric Symptoms.* Cambridge University Press: London.
Wing, J. K., Nixon, J., von Cranach, M. & Strauss, A. (1977*a*). Further developments of the PSE and CATEGO system. *Archiv für Psychiarie und Nervenkrankenheiten* **224**, 151–160.
Wing J. K., Nixon, J. M., Mann, S. A. & Leff, J. P. (1977*b*). Reliability of the PSE (ninth edition) used in a population survey. *Psychological Medicine* **7**, 505–516.
Wing, J. K., Mann, S. A., Leff, J. P. & Nixon, J. N. (1978). The concept of a 'case' in psychiatric population surveys. *Psychological Medicine* **8**, 203–217.
Wittenborn, J. R. (1955). *Wittenborn Psychiatric Rating Scales.* Psychological Corporation: New York.
World Health Organization (1973). *Schizophrenia: Report of an International Pilot Study.* WHO: Geneva.
World Health Organization (1974). *Glossary of Mental Disorders and Guide to their Classification.* WHO: Geneva.
Zung, W. W. K. (1965). A self-rating depression scale. *Archives of General Psychiatry* **12**, 63–70.

Psychological Medicine, 1981, **11**, 1–8

The epidemiology of life stress[1]

Different contemporary societies, different historical periods in the same societies, and different strata within the same societies, produce different patterns of health disorders. At the ecological level, there can be no dispute that particular social structures generate particular patterns of health disorder. To put it another way, the distribution of health in a society is one dimension of the social structure and an indicator of its nature and impact on people's lives (Susser & Watson, 1971).

When we turn to the individual level, however, and to the question of how the impact of the social structure is translated into pathology, much that is said must rest on assertions of authority and faith. It is about 40 or 50 years since the 'stress' hypothesis gathered momentum and began to displace the fashionable hypothesis of that time, which attributed a gallimaufry of obscure ills to foci of infection. Many excellent sets of teeth and many pairs of tonsils were sacrificed to that hypothesis. We can count ourselves fortunate that the stress hypothesis does not require surgical intervention.

The starting point for social scientists is concern with society, and hence with total populations, both the healthy and unhealthy, rather than with disordered segments of populations. They thereby gain breadth. Social scientists extend our vision also because they tend to begin with the independent variable – a social factor – and seek out its many effects, rather than begin with the dependent variable – a health disorder – and seek out what impinges on it. To start with health disorders is a narrowing view that is the norm in medicine, since its concerns arise there. Multifaceted society leads social scientists quickly and naturally to multivariate paradigms, rather than to the specificity of one-to-one relationships.

Much of my own endeavour has been to bring the concepts and the methods of the social sciences into medicine and epidemiology. I shall here reverse myself and try and bring out for social scientists the notions and emphases of epidemiologists. One of these is the notion of the triad, agent–host–environment, and the need, in analysing the problems of health disorders and in constructing research designs, to segregate these three interdigitating elements. This triad is entrenched in epidemiology. Indeed, the triad appeared at last to have become an impediment to flexible multivariate analysis, to the extent that the subject needed to be freed from its tyranny.

In counterpoint, the literature of 'stress' disorders shows that many investigators could have benefited from familiarity with the concept. There has been a lack of differentiation among the components of the triad: some studies concentrate on agents, namely stressful events; others on the environment, namely situations; while the characteristics of the host have been virtually ignored, and we know little of susceptibilities and resistance.

In classifying *agents*, researchers conscious of the triad might less often have lumped stimuli indiscriminantly together, irrespective of force and direction. Stress disorders can be construed in the manner of Hans Selye as the intermediate result of some final common pathway, analogous to inflammation, which is a general pathological response to many agents and the antecedent of a variety of specific manifestations of disorder. Understanding of inflammation was much advanced when the agents were sorted one from another: chemicals, heat, ultraviolet and ionizing radiation, bacteria, viruses, protozoa and multicellular parasites all cause inflammation. In the field of stress, it is clear that specified events yield more convincing evidence than do undifferentiated ones: 'loss' emerges as the particular antecedent of depression (Paykel *et al.* 1969).

In describing *hosts*, researchers conscious of the triad might have paid more attention to the varying susceptibility and immunity of individuals with different constitutions and experiences, including variability denoted by 'simple' indices like age, sex and other statuses and roles. No disease is uniform in all these respects.

[1] Address for correspondence: Dr Mervyn Susser, Gertrude H. Sergievsky Center, Columbia University, 630 West 168 Street, New York, NY10032, USA.

In specifying *environments*, it might quickly have become obvious that the action of any agent or stimulus cannot meaningfully be considered free of context and situation. A social variable like population density will have different meanings for crowding and its effects when measured in terms of persons per room, or per household, or per area. Within families the likelihood of common respiratory infections, for instance, is quite altered by the presence of children of school-going age. Likewise, with recurrent psychotic episodes, family environment must be expected to cushion or exacerbate the impact of stressful events (Brown *et al.* 1972).

Secondly, the problems of disease that confront epidemiologists present themselves in many guises, in a great variety of circumstances, and with varying degrees of urgency. Health disorders may be acute, recurrent, or chronic; they may be mild or severe; they may be of abrupt or insidious onset; they may be distinctive or shade gradually in a continuum in which it is difficult to tell health from disease; they may be rare or common. To cope with this variability has required many approaches to research design. Epidemiology is best pursued with the largest possible arsenal of designs and strategies at hand. Social epidemiology is not less in need of flexible and complementary approaches.

Thirdly, as noted, the concerns of medicine and of epidemiology arise from the primary source of manifest health disorders and pathology in individuals. If the response to these problems is to be effective, then the realities of the biological, genetic and demographic substrate which carries the imprint of disease cannot be bypassed or ignored.

Fourthly, the history of the explosive advance of biomedical knowledge in the nineteenth and the first half of the twentieth century was the history of a search for highly specific causal relationships, to the point of gross distortion when single causes were sought for each disease. Nonetheless, this history has its dialectic: it is also the history of the continuous refinement and specification of relationships, of the dogged elimination of alternative hypotheses, of the increasing specificity and 'testability' of hypotheses, and the resultant strengthening of inference.

The best and most active researchers are not in need of sermons from the side-lines: they are already testing many of these ideas. The care that has gone into recent reports and the rigorous critical effort that characterizes recent reviews augurs well (Dohrenwend & Dohrenwend, 1974; Rabkin & Struening, 1976; Brown & Harris, 1978*a*, *b*, 1979; Tennant & Bebbington, 1978; Shapiro, 1979). But a reading of the mass of the literature suggests that discussion is needed nonetheless. The themes fall under the heads of (A) Instruments, (B) Design, (C) Analysis and hypothesis testing, (D) Control and prevention of pathology.

INSTRUMENTS

Reviews by others of efforts to measure the cumulative impact of stressful life events point to serious shortcomings of a popular instrument (Dohrenwend & Dohrenwend, 1974; Rabkin & Struening, 1976). The readily used approach of Holmes & Rahe (1967) produced a great spurt of studies about the impact of life events. Scientific advance has regularly followed from the development and accessibility of new techniques, whether the microscope or the randomized clinical trial, and now in the study of stressors too we may be hopeful. Typically with new techniques a hundred flowers bloom, but much weeding and culling must usually be done to refine them before notable advance can follow.

Researchers have come to recognize and correct for a number of obvious problems with the technique. If we aim to separate cause from consequence, a single scale that combines events, many of which are not certainly antecedent to the manifestations under study, is disqualified. For instance, many of the supposed stressors are transitional events. For any one such event, say divorce or any other, the task of separating a stress reaction to an event from self and social selection for exposure to that event has proved difficult. The history of studies in the area makes this plain. Divorcees may not only become divorced and confound inference because they are physically or mentally sick; like the single, they may remain unmarried for that reason.

A further intractable problem in establishing the criterion of time-order to secure causal inference is the possibility of predisposition in the host. Predisposition conceived as an independent variable and controlled from the outset is manageable; predisposition conceived *post hoc* as a latent manifestation of the dependent variable and left uncontrolled is less amenable to firm inference (Susser, 1973).

The instruments in use have obviously needed considerable refinement. Magnitude, direction and familiarity of stressors should not be neglected. Categorization of events can help to define both host susceptibility and context. Susceptibility varies with stage in the life-cycle which differentiates certain universal transitions, *rites de passage*, and normal role changes as incremental or decremental. Context and situation are bound to be important. Animal experimenters teach us that the social context determines the impact of a biological insult; for instance, nutritional deprivation has no detectable effects on associative learning in rhesus monkeys or in rats when they are not socially isolated (Zimmerman *et al.* 1975; Levitsky & Barnes, 1970). Finally, since psychosocial stressors of necessity are mediated by the psyche, we need to find the means to take into account the perception or denial of stress by the subject, as Brown (1974), Cobb (1974) and others have emphasized.

These are problems of logical construction. Dangers also arise from the fundamental technical difficulty of establishing validity. The basic problem which these instruments have shared with many other social instruments is their weakness as measures of reality. The simple danger is that if the instrument fails to measure the hypothetical causal variable, no association (causal or otherwise) can be demonstrated. One must, therefore, be ready to accept the social costs of a false negative result.

Researchers have laboured with determination and good effect to perfect population survey instruments for the valid and reliable measurement of mental disorder, the dependent variable in a majority of previous studies (Srole *et al.* 1962; Leighton *et al.* 1963; Weissman *et al.* 1977). Equal attention needs to be given to the independent variable. Brown and his team have put effort and care into developing an instrument that takes account of both circumstances and perceptions in assessing events listed in a standardized dictionary; the gains in sensitivity must compensate for losses in simplicity and portability. Reliability studies are under way (Neugebauer, 1980). Compared with reliability, however, the validity of measures of stressors has had little attention. An effort has been made in one study to test whether the events reported did in fact happen, and as many as 80% could be confirmed. This indicates a degree of validity in measuring exposure to events, but whether they are in fact stressful events is another question. The discovery of an association tends to be taken as in itself a validation of an instrument. Where events that carry much freight besides affective stress are under study, this is not a safe assumption. For example, a change in marital state often implies marked changes in income, in diet, in exposure to infectious disease, in life style and habits, as well as in emotional state.

Validity needs to be tested, as difficult a task as this may be. For this purpose one might look to a marriage of social and psychological stress indicators with physiological indicators. In the almost equally difficult measurement area of nutritional intake, for example, measures are beginning to achieve a degree of validity in terms of changes in body weight and the excretion of nutrients in the urine. Stressors are surely mediated through the central nervous and the endocrine systems. Thus, several physiological indicators responsive to short-term emotional change are available for testing as potential indicators of longer-term stress. A start has been made by Cobb and his colleagues (1973), Theorell (1974), and others (Stevens, 1959).

With regard to measurement of the dependent variable, the problems are more tractable. Mental disorder is the most obvious and likely, if not the sole, outcome of stressful experience. In psychiatric epidemiology, where the definition of a case has been a central problem for decades, a good distance has been travelled. The unidimensional scales used in many prevalence surveys created problems that resemble those of undifferentiated lists of stressful life events. The differentiation in the diagnosis of mental state attained through the research of the past decade has made a distinct advance on the unidimensional approach (Wing *et al.*1974; Spitzer *et al.* 1975). Other workers have begun to exploit and develop these diagnostic instruments for population survey work. So long as we have had to acknowledge that a case of psychiatric illness was defined with difficulty, we have also had to acknowledge that we could not be precise about the effects of exposure to life stresses. We should do better on this score in the future.

DESIGN

Fortunately, social and psychiatric epidemiologists are no longer wedded to the prevalence survey as the only tactic for reaching out to populations. But a too ready commitment to cohort studies as the universal replacement for cross-sectional surveys, and the dismissal of case–control designs, would be an over-reaction. Major problems in the case–control design are to establish time-order, to recognize selective bias where there is a long time interval from exposure to manifestation, to select truly comparable controls, and to recognize the multiple outcomes of a single type of exposure.

In case–control studies of the effects of life events, the outstanding unsolved problem is the bias that is likely to inhere in the *post hoc* reports of events by the cases: their recollection is coloured by the outcomes that have befallen them and made them cases. A notorious, unwitting example was the demonstration of an association of Down's syndrome births with 'stressful' pregnancies. Another source of bias, contamination by the investigator's subjective judgement when either the potential stressors or the hypothesized effects are assessed or scored, is amenable to control by standard techniques which keep the assessors of the effects blind to knowledge of stressors and *vice versa.* In reports of even the best studies it is not always clear that such precautions have been rigorously applied.

On the other hand, the case–control design is efficient and parsimonious; it allows the estimate of the odds ratio as an equivalent of relative risk, even though it cannot yield a direct estimate of attributable risk; it permits the simultaneous study of several independent variables; and often it offers the only possible way to study rare diseases (MacMahon & Pugh, 1970; Susser, 1973; Fleiss, 1973; Ibrahim, 1979).

The cohort design is superior in theory with regard to establishing both time-order and the starting population. There is no problem of retrospective bias in eliciting exposure, and observer bias in making observations of outcome is amenable to control. One can also recognize the multiple outcomes of a single type of exposure, such as a psychosocial stressor, and the design is likely to be superior for the study of rare causal variables, for example war-time bombing or famines (Neel & Schull, 1956; Stein *et al.* 1975). In practice, the design may be less satisfactory than in theory. During years of laborious prospective observation, the nature of the problem may undergo change with the advent of new knowledge; expense may restrict observation to a single cohort or generation without the advantages of quick replication; rare outcomes may be impossible to study. Cohort studies tend to be most advantageous when cohorts can be reconstructed from existing historical data (Stein *et al.* 1975), or when they can exploit existing longitudinal data sets (Vaillant, 1979).

A cohort design, moreover, is not always essential to establishing time-order. Without benefit of cohort designs, Goldberg & Morrison (1963) fixed the phenomenon of downward drift in schizophrenia by comparing the social class of young schizophrenic men with that of their fathers recorded on their birth certificates. The difficult question of the effects of the loss of a spouse has also been clarified by a succession of studies using other types of research design. In trying to demonstrate assortative mating, Karl Pearson and his colleagues at the turn of the century found evidence, from studies of parish registers and tombstones, of an association of age at death among spouses (*Biometrika*, 1903). In the early 1940s, Anthony Ciocco (1940) followed this lead, meaning to counter Pearson's hereditarian bias. He linked the death certificates of spouses in a Maryland county, and demonstrated associations among them, not only for age at death but also specific for several causes of death. Later, Kraus & Lilienfeld (1959) showed that in national statistics the widowed, and especially the young widowed, had excessive death rates from several causes.

These early studies laid the ground for the testing of specific hypotheses. Thus, MacMahon & Pugh (1965) demonstrated the role of widowhood in suicide in a case–control study. They examined the death certificates of suicides and controls for the status of their spouses and, when deceased, the date of the loss, and showed a clustering of suicides following recent bereavement. Parkes (1964) indicated the possible further effect of recent widowhood on entry to psychiatric care by comparing the bereavement experience of Maudsley Hospital in-patients with that expected from the mortality rates of England and Wales applied to the age and sex distribution of the spouses of patients. This study was vulnerable to confounding, because lack of social support is associated with both widowhood and hospital admission, and because the national comparison was an imprecise control. Stein & Susser (1969) confirmed the result, however, by demonstrating the clustering of recent bereavement among inceptions of psychiatric care in a community register of all referred psychiatric disorder, as compared with all chronic psychiatric disability and with a local census population.

What is needed is a flexible approach and an arsenal of methods. Different approaches vary in their utility in different situations. They should be seen as complementary to each other. If we are fortunate, a variety of approaches will give a result the force of replication. If we are less fortunate and the results are contradictory, incoherence helps either to detect flaws in method or to generate new theory.

The Framingham study of coronary heart disease is one of the great exemplars of the cohort design (Dawber & Kannel, 1963) and it too has been put to use, although belatedly, to study the effects of psychological factors in coronary heart disease (Haynes *et al.* 1978*a*, *b*, 1980). But the case-series and time-series studies which preceded the Framingham study (for instance, the decline in heart disease in a war-beleagured and hungry Europe in the early 1940s) yielded the hypotheses to be tested. Many subsequent case–control studies have helped us follow leads generated by the Framingham study, and now the stage is set for efforts to control pathology through intervention studies. This is a natural sequence in epidemiological investigation.

In another example taken from one of our own series of studies, we sought to understand the socializing influence of family, class and culture on development. For this purpose we chose the symptom of enuresis as likely to be sensitive to such socializing influences. In order to explore this large range of influences, we found it necessary to carry out many complementary studies: a community prevalence survey established the distribution, variation and natural remission of the condition and the true scale of the problem; intensive family interviews with a case–control design differentiated the effects of socialization on sphincter control within family types; studies of populations in special institutions (reform schools, children's homes, foster homes, day-care centres) in which cohort, historical cohort and case–control designs were used to demonstrate that disruptions of socialization had adverse effects on the frequency of enuresis, and that restoration to family settings had reparative effects (Stein & Susser, 1967). In this series an intervention study, in the form of the first controlled trial of conditioning treatment, came early and with a practical objective rather than at the end, but that study too strengthened the plausibility of the hypothesis that nocturnal sphincter control could be seen as a learned behaviour. For excellent examples of the complementarity of several designs in the solution of specific problems, one can point to the studies of Cobb, Kasl and their colleagues on rheumatoid arthritis (Kasl & Cobb, 1969) and of the late John Cassel and his colleagues on the effects of culture change (Cassel & Tyroler, 1961).

ANALYSIS AND HYPOTHESIS-TESTING

Rigor in setting up hypotheses, and close scrutiny of underlying assumptions, accelerates the acquisition of new knowledge. This testing approach has been too little practised. For example, the effects of social mobility and resulting inconsistencies of status have long been favourite topics in the social sciences. Yet almost the only consistency that exists among the results of studies of the stressful effects of status inconsistency and social mobility is their inconsistency. In part this muddle arises from weak analysis and inference and, especially, from failures to control for statistical interaction and for status levels at the starting point of change (Blalock, 1967). While these problems have come to be better understood, ecological and individual levels of study and analysis are still often not differentiated. For instance, it is inviting fallacy to amalgamate without qualification, as examples of results of culture change, the studies of Cassel & Tyroler on individual adaptation to migration with their studies of the changes that occurred in populations as society changed around them in a given area (Cassel, 1971, 1974).

With regard to hypothesis testing, we have enough knowledge to generate concepts and broad theory, but too little knowledge at the specific level to enable us to examine the validity of such broad theories across many conditions. To achieve this we shall need to study specific stressors and specific outcomes. The Holmes & Rahe approach through a compendium of stressful events, it should be noted, is essentially a test of just one plausible hypothesis: namely, that stress is a response to the cumulation of events. There are as many other possible hypotheses as there are specifiable types of stressors and specific outcomes. The replication of studies addressing the same broad hypothesis seems endless. A close look at what has emerged from these explorations, combined with disciplined review of biomedical knowledge for given disorders, must yield new designs and more answers.

Strong inference demands the effort to eliminate alternative explanations. For example, with regard to the inconsistencies in the social class distribution of coronary heart disease that have been apparent for the past three decades, the difference in the spread of occupations nationally and within organizations has been no better an explanation than the misclassification of disease at death (Lilienfeld, 1956; Lehman, 1966; Antonovsky, 1968). Little effort was made to test these hypotheses against each other. However, neither of these hypotheses is the most likely explanation. It is slowly becoming apparent that secular change in the disease is probably affecting different social strata in different ways (Marmot *et al.* 1978; Susser & Watson, 1971). Such competing explanations can be examined in study designs that are capable of eliminating them.

CONTROL AND PREVENTION OF PATHOLOGY

Most observations relevant to controlling the effects of stress would require individual behaviour change. Aside from the difficulty, and sometimes the questionable desirability, of inducing such change, much current life stress research can add little to our ability to control health disorders. The demonstration that the cumulation of a wide array of undifferentiated stressful events can generate stressful states does not point to the means of prevention or treatment.

On the other hand, the study of *specific major events* can point the way to prevention. If the immediate aftermath of widowhood puts a person at risk for suicide (MacMahon & Pugh, 1965), death from cirrhosis of the liver (McNeil & Kelsey, 1974; Parkes *et al.* 1969) (presumably caused by alcoholism) and other causes (Ciocco, 1940; Kraus & Lilienfeld, 1959), as well as for entry to psychiatric care (Parkes, 1964; Stein & Susser, 1969), then a target group has been defined and various interventions can be tested.

Similar potential for intervention resides in demonstrating the effects of lack of *social support*, and possibly even those of malfunctioning social networks. Germane theory has long been available, from anthropology and sociology (Bott, 1957; Townsend, 1957; Young & Wilmott, 1957; Cobb, 1976; Susser & Watson, 1971), and attempts to apply it have begun (Raphael, 1977). The availability and effectiveness of the family networks of children can have crucial effects on their subsequent careers and behaviour (Goldfarb, 1943; Bowlby, 1952; Gregory, 1965, 1966; Stein & Susser, 1960; Skeels, 1966; Rutter, 1966). Recent attempts to apply theories of social support suggest that supportive networks may protect the health of adults as well as children (Nuckolls *et al.* 1972; Berkman & Syme, 1979). For specified vulnerable groups, it is not fanciful to think that health and social agencies could intervene effectively.

The detection and control of *harmful environments* is a classical public health strategy. The strategy can be applied to the social as well as to the physical or the biological environment. It can be objected that a health agency, which is necessarily an arm of established society, cannot itself be an instrument that overturns or even modifies the social structure created by that society, its productive relations, and its political forms. This objection does not rule out planned change within that structure of an order sufficient to benefit health.

It may be well in this instance to change the paradigm from the individual to the ecological level. The most powerful forces that effect change in the disease patterns of populations clearly operate at this level. If we take history as our guide, we can be sure that to eliminate poverty, and indeed to restructure ways of life, will change the health of populations.

We need not be overweening in our ideas. The example of smoking, the major specific health hazard demonstrated in the post-war era in developed countries, will serve. Successes in controlling smoking at the individual level seem minimal, and have rendered many health professionals pessimistic. At the ecological level, the picture is much more optimistic. There is little question that there has been a distinct decline in the smoking habit in successive cohorts, although the decline varies according to sex and social position (Hammond & Garfinkel, 1968; Moss, 1979). This is, I believe, the result of what amounts to a social movement that has grown powerful enough to counter the economic, social and psychological forces that have sustained the smoking habit. A social movement is constituted by groups that share social values and aim to transform the values of the society around them by example and private persuasion, and by education, political action and public policy: the groups themselves and the actions they pursue have both organized elements (with leaders, membership, and defined programmes) and unorganized ones (with informal interaction among partisans) (Herberle, 1967). In the light of this social movement model, epidemiologists might add a new set of social strategies for the control of pathology. Prevention and control constitute the ultimate business of health professionals. They must enlist a broad range of forces before they can hope to achieve them.

MERVYN SUSSER

Richard Neugebauer and Zena Stein were kind enough to read this script and enhance its rigor. Deborah Kayman helped with the references and Carol Giles with the typing. The paper had its origin in the Symposium on Psychosocial Epidemiology, organized by Saxon Graham for the American Sociological Association meeting in New York in 1976.

REFERENCES

Antonovsky, A. (1968). Social class and coronary heart disease. *Journal of Chronic Diseases* **21**, 65–106.

Berkman, L. F. & Syme, S. L. (1979). Social networks, hosts resistance, and mortality: a nine-year follow-up of Alameda County residents. *American Journal of Epidemiology* **109**, 186–204.

Biometrika (1903). Assortative mating in man; **2**, 481–498.

Blalock, H. M. (1967). Status and consistency: integration and structural effects. *American Sociological Review* **32**, 790–801.

Bott, E. (1957). *Family and Social Network*. Tavistock: London.

Bowlby, J. (1952). *Maternal Care and Mental Health*. World Health Organization Monograph Series, No. 2. WHO: Geneva.

Brown, G. W. (1974), Meaning, measurement, and stress of life events. In *Stressful Life Events: Their Nature and Effects* (ed. B. S. Dohrenwend and B. P. Dohrenwend), pp. 217-243. Wiley: New York.

Brown, G. W. & Harris, T. (1978*a*). *Social Origins of Depression: A Study of Psychiatric Disorder in Women*. Tavistock: London.

Brown, G. W. & Harris, T. (1978*b*). Social origins of depression: a reply. *Psychological Medicine* **8**, 577–588.

Brown, G. W. & Harris, T. (1979). The sin of subjectivism: a reply to Shapiro. *Behavior Research and Therapy* **17**, 605–613.

Brown, G. W., Birley, J. L. T. & Wing, J. K. (1972). Influence of family life on the course of schizophrenic disorders: a replication. *British Journal of Psychiatry* **121**, 241–258.

Cassel, J. C. (1971). Evans County cardiovascular and cerebrovascular epidemiologic study. *Archives of Internal Medicine* **128**, 883–986.

Cassel, J. (1974). Psychosocial processes and 'stress': theoretical formulation. *International Journal of Health Services* **4**, 471–482.

Cassel, J. & Tyroler, H. A. (1961). Epidemiological studies of culture change: I. Health status and recency of industrialization. *Archives of Environmental Health* **3**, 25–33.

Ciocco A. (1940). On the mortality in husbands and wives. *Human Biology* **12**, 508–531.

Cobb, S. (1974). A model for life events and their consequences. In *Stressful Life Events: Their Nature and Effects* (ed. B. S. Dohrenwend and B. P. Dohrenwend), pp. 151–156. Wiley: New York.

Cobb, S. (1976). Social support as a moderator of life stress. *Psychosomatic Medicine* **28**, 310–314.

Cobb, S., Kasl, S. V., Roth, T. L. & Brooks, G. W. (1973). Urinary norepinephrine in men whose jobs are abolished. *Psychosomatic Medicine* **35**, 459.

Dawber, T. R. & Kannel, W. B. (1963). An approach to longitudinal studies in a community: the Framingham study. *Proceedings of the New York Academy of Sciences* **107**, 539–556.

Dohrenwend, B. S. & Dohrenwend, B. P. (eds.) (1974). *Stressful Life Events: Their Nature and Effects*. Wiley: New York.

Fleiss, J. L. (1973). *Statistical Methods for Rates and Proportions*. Wiley: New York.

Goldberg, E. M. & Morrison, S. L. (1963). Schizophrenia and social class. *British Journal of Psychiatry* **132**, 785–802.

Goldfarb, W. (1943). The effects of early institutional care on adolescent personality. *Journal of Experimental Education* **12**, 106–126.

Gregory, I. (1965). Anterospective data following childhood loss of a parent: I. Delinquency and high school dropout. *Archives of General Psychiatry* **13**, 99–109.

Gregory, I. (1966). Retrospective data concerning childhood loss of a parent: II. Category of parental loss in decade of birth, diagnosis, and MMPI. *Archives of General Psychiatry* **15**, 362–368.

Hammond, E. C. & Garfinkel, L. (1968). Changes in cigarette smoking 1959–65. *American Journal of Public Health* **58**, 30–45.

Haynes, S., Levine, S., Scotch, N., Feinleib, M. & Kannel, W. B. (1978*a*). The relationship of psychosocial factors to coronary heart disease in the Framingham study. I. Methods and risk factors. *American Journal of Epidemiology* **107**, 362–383.

Haynes, S., Feinleib, M., Levine, S., Scotch, N. & Kannel, W. B. (1978*b*). The relationship of psychosocial factors to coronary heart disease in the Framingham study. II. Prevalence of coronary heart disease. *American Journal of Epidemiology* **107**, 384–402.

Haynes, S., Feinleib, M. & Kannel, W. B. (1980). The relationship of psychosocial factors to coronary heart disease in the Framingham study. III. Eight-year incidence of coronary heart disease. *American Journal of Epidemiology* **111**, 37–58.

Herberle, R. (1967). Social movements: types and functions. In *International Encyclopedia of the Social Sciences* (ed. D. Sills), pp. 201–208. Free Press: New York.

Holmes, T. H. & Rahe, R. H. (1967). The social readjustment rating scale. *Journal of Psychosomatic Medicine* **11**, 213–218.

Ibrahim, M. A. (1979). The case–control study: consensus and controversy. *Journal of Chronic Disease* **32**, 1–190.

Kasl, S. V. & Cobb, S. (1969). The intrafamilial transmission of rheumatoid arthritis. V. Differences between rheumatoid arthritis and controls on selected personality variables. *Journal of Chronic Diseases* **22**, 239–258.

Kraus, A. S. & Lilienfeld, A. M. (1959). Some epidemiologic aspects of the high mortality rate in the young widowed group. *Journal of Chronic Diseases* **10**, 207–217.

Lehman, E. W. (1966). Social class and coronary heart disease: a sociological assessment of the medical literature. *Journal of Chronic Diseases* **20**, 381–391.

Leighton, D. C., Harding, J. S., Macklin, D. B., MacMillan, N. M. & Leighton, A. H. (1963). *The Stirling County Study of Psychiatric Disorder and Socio-Cultural Environment.* Vol. 3: *The Character of Danger: Psychiatric Symptoms in Selected Communities.* Basic Books: New York.

Levitsky, D. A. & Barnes, R. H. (1970). Effects of early malnutrition on the reaction of adult rats to aversive stimuli. *Nature* **225**, 468–469.

Lilienfeld, A. M. (1956). Variation in mortality from heart disease. *Public Health Reports* **71**, 545–552.

MacMahon, B. & Pugh, T. F. (1965). Suicide in the widowed. *American Journal of Epidemiology* **8**, 23–31.

MacMahon, B. & Pugh, T. F. (1970). *Epidemiology: Principles and Methods.* Little, Brown: Boston.

McNeil, D. & Kelsey, J. L. (1974). Cirrhosis mortality among widows. Seventh International Meeting of International Epidemiological Association, August 17–21: University of Sussex, England.

Marmot, M. G., Adelstein, A. M., Robinson, N. & Rose, G. A. (1978). Changing social-class distribution of heart disease. *British Medical Journal* ii, 1109–1112.

Moss, A. J. (1979). Changes in cigarette smoking and current smoking practices among adults: United States, 1978. Advance data from *Vital and Health Statistics of the National Center Health Statistics*, No. 52. USDHEW.

Neel, J. V. & Schull, W. J. (1956). *The Effect of Exposure to the Atomic Bombs on Pregnancy Determination in Hiroshima and Nagasaki.* Atomic Bomb Casualty Commission: Washington.

Neugebauer, R. N. (1980). Reliability of life event reports. In *Stressful Life Events* (ed. B. P. Dohrenwend and B. S. Dohrenwend). In the press.

Nuckolls, K. B., Cassel, J. & Kaplan, B. H. (1972). Psychological assets, life crisis and the prognosis of pregnancy. *American Journal of Epidemiology* **109**, 186–204.

Parkes, C. M. (1964). Recent bereavement as a cause of mental illness. *British Journal of Psychiatry* **110**, 198–204.

Parkes, C. M., Benjamin, G. & Fitzgerald, R. G. (1969). Broken heart: a statistical study of increased mortality among widowers. *British Medical Journal* i, 740–743.

Paykel, E. S., Myers, J. K., Dienelt, M. N., Klerman, G. L., Lindenthal, J. J. & Pepper, M. P. (1969). Life events and depression: a controlled study. *Archives of General Psychology* **21**, 753–760.

Rabkin, J. G. & Struening, E. L. (1976). Life events, stress and illness. *Science* **194**, 1013–1020.

Raphael, B. (1977). Preventive intervention with the recently bereaved. *Archives of General Psychiatry* **34**, 1450–1454.

Rutter, M. (1966). *Children of Sick Parents.* Maudsley Monograph No. 16. Oxford University Press: London.

Shapiro, M. B. (1979). *The Social Origins of Depression* by G. W. Brown and T. Harris: its methodological philosophy. *Behavior Research and Therapy* **17**, 597–603.

Skeels, H. M. (1966). *Adult Studies of Children with Contrasting Early Life Experiences.* Monograph of Social Research and Child Development **51**, No. 3.

Spitzer, R. L., Endicott, J. & Robins, E. (1975). Clinical criteria for psychiatric diagnoses and DSM-III. *American Journal of Psychiatry* **132**, 1187–1192.

Srole, L., Langner, T. S., Michael, S. T., Opler, M. K. & Rennie, T. M. C. (1962). *Mental Health in the Metropolis: The Midtown Manhattan Study.* McGraw-Hill: New York.

Stein, Z. A. & Susser, M. W. (1960). The families of dull children: I. A classification for predicting careers. *British Journal of Preventive and Social Medicine* **14**, 83–88.

Stein, Z. & Susser, M. (1967). The social dimensions of a symptom. A socio-medical study of enuresis. *Social Science and Medicine* **1**, 183–201.

Stein, Z. & Susser, M. (1969). Widowhood and mental illness. *British Journal of Preventive and Social Medicine* **23**, 106–110.

Stein, Z., Susser, M., Saenger, G. & Marolla, F. (1975) *Famine and Human Development: Studies of the Dutch Hunger Winter of* 1944/45. Oxford University Press: New York.

Stevens, J. R. (1959). Emotional activation of the EEG in patients with convulsive disorder. *Neurology of Mental Disorders* **128**, 339–351.

Susser, M. (1973). *Causal Thinking in the Health Sciences: Concepts and Strategies in Epidemiology.* Oxford University Press: New York.

Susser, M. & Watson, W. (1971). *Sociology in Medicine* (2nd edn). Oxford University Press: London.

Tennant, C. & Bebbington, P. (1978). The social causation of depression: a critique of the work of Brown and his colleagues. *Psychological Medicine* **8**, 565–575.

Theorell, T. (1974). Life events before and after the onset of a premature myocardial infarction. In *Stressful Life Events: Their Nature and Effects* (ed. B. S. Dohrenwend and B. P. Dohrenwend), pp. 101–117. Wiley: New York.

Townsend, P. (1957). *The Family Life of Old People.* Routledge and Kegan Paul: London.

Vaillant, E. G. (1979). Natural history of male psychologic health: effects of mental health on physical health. *New England Journal of Medicine* **301**, 1249–1254.

Weissman, M., Sholomskas, D., Pottenger, M., Prusoff, B. & Locke, B. (1977). Assessing depressive symptoms in five psychiatric populations: a validation study. *American Journal of Epidemiology* **106**, 203–214.

Wing, J. K., Cooper, J. E. & Sartorius, N. (1974). *The Measurement and Classification of Psychiatric Symptoms.* Cambridge University Press: Cambridge.

Young, M. & Wilmott, P. (1957). *Family and Kinship in East London.* Routledge and Kegan Paul: London.

Zimmerman, R. R., Strobel, D. A., Steere, P. & Geist, C. R. (1975). Behavior and malnutrition in the rhesus monkey. *Primate Behavior* **4**, 241.

Psychological Medicine, 1984, **14**, 1–4

Psychogeriatrics and the neo-epidemiologists[1]

Almost 25 years ago a WHO Expert Committee produced a 50-page report on *Mental Health Problems of Aging and the Aged*, aiming

to place the mental health problems of aging and the aged in their demographic...social and medical setting as a preliminary to discussing the possible means of protecting and promoting mental health and mitigating or curing mental illness in the aged (WHO, 1959).

While acknowledging the various issues raised by the well-established associations between senescence and mental ill-health, the tenor of the report was broadly optimistic. Referring to the expectations in Sweden that 'the expected increase in the proportion of invalids in old age may have been more than offset by social and medical progress', it concluded that:

although the aging of populations creates certain serious problems, there has been a tendency to magnify the dangers that are like to arise. The approach to the problems created by the increasing proportion of old people in many populations should be informed by the fact that such aging is a part of social progress.

A generation later, this verdict is difficult to reconcile with the widespread concern aroused by the lengthening human life-span. In retrospect, it is significant that the WHO report barely mentioned the epidemiological contribution to its subject-matter. Times have changed. The epidemiological perspective has now become indispensable not only for the psychiatrist concerned with the assessment and management of mental illness in the senium, but also for workers in several related disciplines.

The descriptive epidemiologists, drawing on the techniques of demography and medical geography, have mapped the contours of a disturbing situation, based on an estimated increase in the global population of from 3·97 to 6·25 billion over the final quarter of the twentieth century. During this period, a reduced mortality in the early and late stages of the life-cycle will result in the achievement of their potential longevity by a much higher proportion of people so that the histogram of life-spans will become increasingly Gaussian about a mode of 75–80 years, with a shortening tail in the early years.

The trend is already one of acute concern to industrialized countries and is clearly discernible in the developing world (Kramer, 1980). It confronts the medical epidemiologist with a challenge which can be approached in one of two ways, depending on whether the senescent population be defined as an age-limited aggregate which is different from and contrasted with chronologically younger groups, or as the residuum of a total population which has survived the hazards of middle age to enter the senium. The objectives of the investigator may, accordingly, tend towards the study either of disease or of decrement.

The clearest example of the former outlook is that of the recently founded sub-discipline of 'neuroepidemiology', with its special focus on the dementias (Mortimer & Schuman, 1981; Capildeo *et al.* 1983). After a long period of neglect these conditions have recently reanimated the attention of neurologists because of the threat they pose as 'an approaching epidemic' (Plum, 1979). Their particular target is the Alzheimer–senile form of dementias because it accounts for more than 50% of dementia over the age of 65. To Plum this is

an increasingly prevalent neurological disease...an epidemic that can be prevented only by the successful attention of science and especially neurobiology to solving the problems that manifest themselves predominantly in the aging brain...Alzheimer disease, like Parkinsonism, may turn out to be a specific neurochemical system

[1] Based on a paper read at the Third European Symposium on Social Psychiatry, Helsinki, September 1982. Address for correspondence: Professor Michael Shepherd, Institute of Psychiatry, De Crespigny Park, Denmark Hill, London SE5 8AF.

degeneration, perhaps susceptible to at least temporary improvement with pharmacotherapy...fundamental neuroscience now shares responsbility to our future public health comparable to that shouldered by microbiology a half century ago.

The spectacularly successful elucidation of the pathogenesis of kuru by Gajdusek and his colleagues has encouraged the advancement of aetiological hypotheses in terms of neurochemistry, immunology, virology and genetics, but biologically-oriented neuroepidemiological research in this field is hampered by two clinical obstacles: first, dementia is a syndrome which results from several disease processes and, secondly, Alzheimer's disease remains a diagnosis by exclusion so that, as Gajdusek and his colleagues have pointed out (Masters *et al.* 1981):

Until criteria are established for diagnosis, it seems almost pointless to attempt an epidemiologic analysis...At this stage there does not even appear to be any reliable information on the accuracy of clinical diagnoses in a large enough series of patients with Alzheimer's Disease. Therefore, no estimate is available on the degree of case ascertainment that might be expected from population surveys.

In the present state of knowledge the development of longitudinal studies with case–controls designed to identify risk-factors represents perhaps the most promising approach to causation via epidemiology, but its potential must be severely limited until more diagnostic precision can be obtained (Sluss, 1980).

This observation may serve as a pointer to the need for an intensification of work in the important field of clinical epidemiology, especially in what Morris has called 'completing the clinical picture' (Morris, 1957). Some of this effort has been directed to the delineation of particular syndromes, which include the varieties of psycho-organic reactions, morbid preoccupations with the themes of decline and death, the psychiatric links with physical illness and the environmental strains of isolation. All these conditions, though not unknown among members of younger age-groups, present themselves more prominently by virtue of their efflorescence in the senium. One fundamental reason for expanding knowledge in this sphere is its significance for classification, a topic of particular concern to epidemiologists and one which is poorly developed in psychogeriatrics, as may be demonstrated by the differences between the schemata of the International Classification of Diseases (ICD-9) and the American Diagnostic and Statistical Manual (DSM-III). In addition, the prospects of clinical epidemiology have been extended by the study of the large captive populations of chronic psychiatric patients whose declining mortality-rate has enabled large-scale observations to be made on the later stages of the natural history of their disorders. Manfred Bleuler, for example, has pointed to the surprising improvement in his unique series of schizophrenics, suggesting that it may be associated with anoxic cerebral changes (Bleuler, 1978). Again, Ciompi has reported that patients with an earlier neurotic or depressive illness improve in their later years, a finding which appears to reflect primarily the influence of social or environmental factors (Ciompi, 1969).

Such factors also exercise a key role in the outcome of mental disorders arising in the senium. Although the 5-year prognosis of those conditions necessitating admission to hospital is poor (Whitehead & Hunt, 1982), the extra-mural milieu clearly plays a major role in both the patients' symptomatology and their capacity for adaptation.

So much for the institutionalized elderly. Community surveys, however, reveal a large extra-mural reservoir of all but the most severe degrees of mental disorders in old age (Magnussen *et al.* 1982). The key medical agent concerned with their care is the primary care physician, who may acknowledge the significance of psychosocial factors in the genesis of these conditions but all too often relies exclusively on medication in their management, so much so that the prescription of psychotropic drugs to the elderly has become one of the major aspects of another new sub-discipline, that of 'drug-epidemiology'. Population based figures show a seemingly universal picture. In a recent survey of the Canadian province of Saskatchewan, for example, the over-60s constitute some 16% of the population but receive 42% of all psychotropic drugs prescribed; more than half the people in this age-group were taking these drugs, twice the proportion for people of all ages (Saskatchewan Alcoholism Commission, 1981). In the United Kingdom the same trend affects the prescription of sedatives, hypnotics, neuroleptics and antidepressants, to which should be added the large array of 'cerebral vasodilators and activators', all of them scientifically dubious but widely employed (Swift, 1981).

The most striking effect of this therapeutic fashion has been an iatrogenically induced epidemic of adverse pharmacological effects, some more incapacitating than the disorder being treated. From a biological standpoint the increased susceptibility of the elderly to the unwanted effects appears to be related to a change in the pharmacokinetics and an impairment in the homeostatic mechanisms in old age. From an epidemiological standpoint it represents a major hazard to be weighed against the possible advantages of medication.

In the ascertainment of mental illness in the population at large epidemiologists are able to draw on their traditional techniques, laying particular emphasis on such issues as sampling and standardized methods of assessment. In disorders of the senium, however, a particular problem arises from the need to study decline or decrement as well as disease, for while the study of decline has to do with psychobiological variation, epidemiology *per se* deals only with the pathological part of that variation. The remainder is normal variation, in part a physiological adaptive response to environment, in part a failure of homeostasis. In operational terms, therefore, as several workers have acknowledged, a dimensional rather than a categorical model of dysfunction becomes imperative in distinguishing between mental health and ill-health in the aged by means of the epidemiological method.

The methodological problems of this task have been analysed by Cooper & Schwarz (1982), who point out that 'mental health must...be defined in terms of psychological rather than of physiological functioning'. They stop short, however, of extending their discussion to the sphere of yet another new sub-discipline, that of 'psychosocial epidemiology'. Thus, while drawing attention to the 'shortage of accurate reliable measures' they make no mention of intelligence, though the borderlands between decrement and disease are sharply illuminated by recent developments in psychology. Here the a-theoretical psychometric mode of enquiry, based on statistical theory, has been superseded by modern cognitive psychology which favours a more active concern with functional mechanisms. According to this approach, whereas the fluid, and to some extent the crystallized, cognitive abilities developing in the early years represent a genetically regulated process of maturation, aging is not so much an orderly, uni-directional process of decline as a disorderly, multi-directional process resembling, in military terms, a rout rather than a retreat. The end-state of later years thus becomes dependent on the stability of the psychobiological systems underlying intellectual performance, which in turn is subject to a variety of environmental influences, including disease and dysfunction. In these circustances psychometrics are less useful than the concept of intelligence developed by Welford as an extension of Bartlett's work on the analysis of skills in real-life situations, where performance is affected by not only bodily changes but also by such forces as motivation, social prestige and expectations, and the development of methods of coping with situations and problems.

This view leads naturally from the psychological to the social component of psychosocial epidemiology. Here the emphasis is on what, over and above the formal increase in failing faculties, has been called 'the real pathology of old age...pain, disablement, frustration, boredom, lack of purpose, and loss of identity and self-respect, all of which lead to dissatisfaction with the quality of life' (Tulloch & Moore, 1979). Most of these features have been confirmed by recent surveys of old people, and many of the problems are summarized in the so-called 'environmental docility' hypothesis, according to which: 'As the competence of the individual decreases, the proportion of behaviour attributable to environmental as compared with personal characteristics increases' (Amann, 1982). This is not, . owever, to demean the role of those personal attributes, among which the subject's sense of well-being emerges as the most important (Garritt *et al.* 1978). And it is via the concept of self-rated health status that the interests of social gerontologists and epidemiologists overlap most closely, as a number of studies on elderly populations have shown (Tissue, 1972). The evidence makes it clear that the subject's state of health, as assessed by medical examination, is related to the level of the percept but that this in turn is an essentially subjective response, related more to general health than to verifiable criteria of the physical and mental condition. Such findings constitute the twin basis of Mark Abrams' (1978) conclusion, based on a detailed survey of a group of 1600 individuals over 65, that

any substantial progress in raising the life satisfaction of elderly people depends largely upon providing better and more extensive health services for them and upon providing them with equivalents of the support already available to many through proximity to good neighbours and friends.

Already, therefore, a variety of separate disciplines – demography, neuropsychiatry, genetics, psychology, sociology, pharmacology, gerontology – are all employing the epidemiological method to study the aetiology, clinical features and management of mental disorder in old age. It is to be hoped that their joint efforts will contribute to knowledge and to effective action.

MICHAEL SHEPHERD

REFERENCES

Abrams, M. (1978). *Beyond Three-Score and Ten*, p. 23. Age Concern Research Publication. The Trinity Press: Worcester and London.

Amann, A. (1981). *The Status and Prospects of the Aging in Western Europe*. Occasional Paper No. 8. European Centre for Social Welfare Training and Research: Vienna.

Bleuler, M. (1978). *The Schizophrenic Disorders*. Yale University Press: New Haven and London.

Capildeo, R., Haberman, S., Benjamin, B. & Rose, F. C. (1983). Why neuroepidemiology? *Psychological Medicine* **13**, 15–16.

Ciompi, L. (1969). Follow-up studies on evolution of former neurotic and depressive states in old age: clinical and psychodynamic aspects. *Journal of Geriatric Psychiatry* **3**, 90–106.

Cooper, B. & Schwarz, R. (1982). Psychiatric case-identification in an elderly urban population. *Social Psychiatry* **17**, 43–52.

Garritt, T. F., Somes, G. W. & Marx, M. B. (1978). Factors influencing self-assessment of health. *Social Science and Medicine* **12**, 77–81.

Kramer, M. (1980). The rising pandemic of mental disorders and associated chronic diseases and disabilities. In *Epidemiological Research as Basis for the Organization of Extramural Psychiatry* (ed. E. Strömgren, A. Dupont and J. A. Nielsen), pp. 382–397. *Acta Psychiatrica Scandinavica* **65**, Suppl. 28.

Magnussen, G., Nielsen, J. & Buch, J. (1982). Epidemiology and prevention of mental illness in old age. *Nordisk Gerontologisk Tidskrift*. Supplement.

Masters, C. L., Gajdusek, D. C. & Gibbs, C. J. (1981). Problems of case ascertainment and diagnosis in the epidemiology of dementia occurring in geographic isolates and worldwide. In *The Epidemiology of Dementia* (ed. J. A. Mortimer and L. M. Schuman), pp. 155–170. Oxford University Press: New York.

Morris, J. N. (1957). *Uses of Epidemiology*. Livingstone: Edinburgh and London.

Mortimer, J. A. & Schuman, L. M. (eds.) (1981). *The Epidemiology of Dementia*. Oxford University Press: New York.

Plum, F. (1979). Dementia: an approaching epidemic. *Nature* **279**, 372–373.

Saskatchewan Alcoholism Commission, Research Division (1981). Central nervous system prescription drugs and elderly people: an overview of issues and a Saskatchewan profile. Final report.

Sluss, T. K. (1980). A method for investigating risk factors for senile dementia – Alzheimer's type in the Baltimore longitudinal study. Doctoral Thesis. The Johns Hopkins University: Baltimore.

Swift, C. G. (1981). Psychotropic drugs and the elderly. In *Epidemiological Impact of Psychotropic Drugs* (ed. G. Tognoni, C. Bellantuono and M. Lader), pp. 325–338. Elsevier: Amsterdam.

Tissue, T. (1972). Another look at self-rated health among the elderly. *Journal of Gerontology* **27**, 91–94.

Tulloch, A. J. & Moore, V. (1979). A randomized controlled trial of geriatic screening and surveillance in general practice. *Journal of the Royal College of General Practitioners* **29**, 733–742.

Whitehead, A. & Hunt, A. (1982). Elderly psychiatric patients: a 5-year prospective study. *Psychological Medicine* **12**, 149–157.

World Health Organization (1959). *Mental Health Problems of Aging and the Aged*. Technical Report Series No. 171. WHO: Geneva.

Psychological Medicine, 1983, **13**, 1–8

Clinical trials in psychiatry[1]

Clinical trials were introduced as a method of scientific investigation before 1945 (Bull, 1959) and have been used extensively since, but it is only recently that publications devoted entirely to their management (design, conduct and analysis) have appeared (Controlled Clinical Trials, 1980; Friedman *et al.* 1981; Harris & Fitzgerald, 1970; Johnson & Johnson, 1977; Schwartz *et al.* 1980). Indeed, the methodology of clinical trials has developed to such an extent that their management is now highly complex (Peterson & Fisher, 1980), and the number of criteria to be satisfied in their design is formidable (Chalmers *et al.* 1981; Gore, 1982). In psychiatry many clinical trials conducted during the past twenty years have incorporated such important features of design as the inclusion of adequate controls, random and blind allocation of treatments, and blind assessment of 'objective' response. This editorial considers other equally important, though neglected, aspects of the design of clinical trials in psychiatry and re-emphasizes some notable aspects of their conduct and analysis.

OBJECTIVES

The objectives of a clinical trial, first, should be simple and specific and, secondly, should seek to answer a question of importance to medical science or patient welfare within a reasonable period. Clinical trials, which should be designed for the efficient comparison of treatments, are not suitable vehicles for other investigations such as constructing, testing or validating rating scales or biochemical studies of the effects of a particular drug treatment on key metabolites. Identifying subgroups of patients who respond favourably to treatment, for example, those with particular combinations of features characteristic of illness in a clinical trial comparing treatments for neurotic disorders or for whom a particular treatment is indicated or contra-indicated, for example, one anti-depressant in a clinical trial comparing response to several, is difficult and nebulous, and such vague objectives should be avoided (see below – Analysis). Of course, a comparison of response to treatment in two separate subgroups of patients (for example, unipolar depressives and bipolar manic-depressives) may be made, but preferably in a trial specifically designed with such an objective.

PROTOCOL

A detailed protocol should be prepared and piloted as part of the design of a clinical trial. Ideally, this document should provide a complete specification of the management of the trial from its objectives to the reporting of results (Chaput de tonge, 1977), together with specimen copies of forms and rating scales. Instructions for the completion and scoring of rating scales should also be included. It is particularly important in psychiatry that the protocol specifies the methods of data handling since large quantities of both baseline and response data are frequently collected, and imperative that it describes the methods of analysis. The preparation of such protocols can be tedious and exacting, and may take several months of discussion but it does focus thought about the trial wonderfully. Obviously, it is better to spend time preparing and piloting a protocol than to be forced into abandoning or fundamentally changing the management of a trial before its scheduled termination.

[1] Address for correspondence: Dr Anthony L. Johnson, Medical Research Council Biostatistics Unit, Medical Research Council Centre, Hills Road, Cambridge CB2 2QH.

CRITERIA FOR ENTRY

Patients entered in a clinical trial should preferably be representative of a much larger patient population so that the results from the trial are of potential application to many patients. In psychiatry, where diagnosis may be both difficult and diffuse, the criteria for patient entry to a clinical trial should be assessed critically. They may require standardization – for example, in terms of the presence of specific Schneiderian first-rank symptoms in schizophrenia, the attainment of a minimal score on the Hamilton or some other rating scale for depression, or particular categorization by an instrument such as the Present State Examination – so that the implications for treatment deduced from a clinical trial in one centre or region can be extrapolated to the treatment of patients elsewhere.

PATIENT ACCRUAL

Overestimation of patient entry to a clinical trial occurs so frequently that it has been (whimsically) expressed in Lasagna's Law: once a trial begins the number of suitable patients dwindles to a tenth of what was calculated before the trial began (Harris & Fitzgerald, 1970). Consequently, it is important to monitor the overall rate of patient accrual, especially during the early stages of recruitment, and compare it with the rate estimated during planning. Serious discrepancy between the two may then be corrected either by extending the recruitment period of the trial or by extending the trial itself to other clinicians and/or hospitals; alternatively, the trial may be abandoned before the commitment of many patients and extensive resources.

Patients treated at a particular location or by a particular clinician will fall into two groups: namely, those who satisfy the clinical and demographic conditions for entry to a clinical trial and are therefore 'eligible' for entry, and those who are ineligible; some of the 'eligible' patients will enter the trial, others will not. It is important to record demographic and clinical details of *all* 'eligible' patients, together with reasons for non-entry of those who are not included; these may indicate that some factor important in the logistics of the trial such as increased workload on busy psychiatrists or other clinical staff, or inadequate clerical assistance has been overlooked. This is particularly true of clinical trials recruiting patients at more than one clinic or hospital (multi-centre trials). The monitoring of non-eligible patients may also be useful both to highlight unnecessary restrictions in entry criteria at the pilot stage and to indicate the appropriate proportion of some target population to which the results of the trial are applicable.

TYPE OF CLINICAL TRIAL

In psychiatry clinical trials may be broadly divided into those comparing the therapeutic efficacy of two or more treatments (drugs, therapies, doses) in relieving symptoms, and those comparing prophylactic treatments which prevent the recurrence of symptoms or episodes; these are discussed separately. In addition, clinical trials comparing different durations of therapy, especially prophylaxis, are also considered for, although such trials have been rarely performed, they are likely to become of increasing importance.

(a) Trials of therapeutic efficacy

Trials of therapeutic efficacy are usually of short duration (less than two months) and frequently conducted at a single centre; patients either receive one of several treatments in a fixed-size comparative trial, sometimes called a parallel group study, or, less frequently, two treatments in a crossover trial. In psychiatry, crossover trials with more than two treatments are rare. Symptoms of the disease or psychiatric state are recorded by observers and/or the patients themselves, and the response to treatment is assessed by the changes in symptom rating on appropriate scales.

An example of the fixed-size comparative trial is the Northwick Park trial of electroconvulsive therapy (ECT) (Johnstone *et al.* 1980), in which 70 patients with endogenous depression were allocated randomly to a course of 8 simulated ECTs or a course of 8 real ECTs, all other aspects of ECT being identical in the two groups; depression was assessed using rating scales by a psychiatrist, the nursing staff and the patients themselves at weekly intervals up to 4 weeks from trial entry and again at 1 month and 6 months following the course of ECT. The principal aim of this trial was to assess the role of the convulsion in the efficacy of ECT. A second example is the comparison of flupenthixol and amitriptyline in the treatment of mild or moderately severe depression not requiring ECT in 60 out-patients (Young *et al.* 1976); the two treatments were prescribed using flexible dose schedules for a period of 6 weeks and assessed using observer-rated and self-rated scales at initial examination and after 1, 3 and 6 weeks of treatment. The aim of the study was a controlled comparison of flupenthixol against a standard tricyclic compound in depressed out-patients.

Two-period crossover trials (Grizzle, 1965; Wallenstein & Fisher, 1977; Hills & Armitage, 1979; Barker *et al.* 1982) in which patients receive two treatments, sometimes separated by a 'washout period', in random order are used in the study of acute conditions in chronic illness, for example Parkinsonism (Godwin-Austen *et al.* 1970; Hughes *et al.* 1971); the self-limiting nature of many psychiatric episodes restricts their use in psychiatry. They have been used in studies of the alleviation of side-effects from anti-psychotic or neuroleptic medication – for example, the effects of lithium carbonate on established tardive dyskinesia were compared with placebo in 11 psychiatric patients who had been treated with neuroleptics for at least two years (Mackay *et al.* 1980). Patients received 5 weeks' treatment with either lithium or placebo followed by a 6 week 'washout' and 5 weeks of the alternative treatment; dyskinesia was rated by observers, nurses and the patients themselves.

Studies of the types described above may be complicated by patients who do not comply with the treatment regimes under investigation – for example, because of failure to tolerate side-effects of treatment, failure to respond to treatment (usually styled 'withdrawn because of treatment failure'), or simply failure to 'cooperate'. In addition, 'ratings' may be missing from patients who are too ill to be evaluated by the chosen scales, who have been discharged well, who are under treatment elsewhere for concurrent illnesses, or who simply decide not to attend. The exclusion from analysis of patients in any of these categories *may* lead to a biased comparison of treatments. In trials where the amount of 'missing' information is too large to permit legitimate substitution by standard statistical techniques the analysis of the rating scale data themselves may have to be abandoned. An analysis of the proportions of patients who recover – measured in a clinical trial of anti-depressant therapy by a score on the Hamilton Rating Scale below a pre-defined threshold, for example, or of the times from randomization to recovery may be used instead.

(b) Trials of prophylaxis

Trials of prophylaxis are usually conducted over a long period (greater than 6 months) and frequently involve the participation of several hospitals in a multi-centre trial. On recovery from a psychiatric episode patients are randomly allocated to treatment and are followed up until relapse (the 'event' of interest), death, or the end of the stipulated 'follow-up' period, whichever is the shortest. All patients are followed up *irrespective* of additional treatment and side-effects of, or non-compliance with, prescribed trial treatment. The times from randomization to relapse are summarized for each treatment using actuarial 'life-table' methods which take account of the (censored) times in those patients who die without relapse or who complete the follow-up period, and the overall patterns of relapse on each treatment are compared. Some patients, inevitably, will be 'lost to follow-up' but the numbers of such patients may be reduced to a very small proportion of the total by special follow-up of patients who do not keep clinic appointments and by intensive tracing of patients who have migrated. Compliance with drug treatment regimes in such studies may be monitored through counts of tablets when relevant, the issue of prescriptions and the routine estimation of serum drug concentrations. The aim of such studies is usually to compare the *policy* of giving one treatment with the *policy* of giving another, in other words to compare the usefulness of treatments in routine clinical practice. An example is the trial of continuation therapy in unipolar depressive illness (Medical Research Council Drug Trials Subcommittee, 1981) in which 136 patients were randomly allocated to prophylactic treatment with lithium, amitriptyline or placebo on recovery from a depressive episode, and followed up for 3 years or until relapse. Only one patient who emigrated was lost to follow-up.

The management of trials involving the prolonged observation of each patient with special reference to cancer therapy has been described in two classic papers by Peto *et al.* (1976, 1977). In clinical trials comparing survival under different chemotherapy regimes in cancer the 'event of interest', namely death, is unambiguous, can be dated easily and, if necessary, monitored by national agencies such as the Office for Population Censuses and Surveys. By contrast, in clinical trials in psychiatry patients may be followed up until psychotic or depressive relapse or some other 'event' which cannot be diagnosed unambiguously and whose onset is difficult to date. Such complications are unimportant in the sense that they do not bias the comparison of treatments, provided that a practical and objective definition of the 'event of interest' can be devised. For example, in the MRC trial cited above, relapse was defined as an episode of affective illness requiring treatment other than the administration of a benzodiazepine and dated by the prescription of such treatment. The assessment of such 'events' should be made by a clinician who is unaware of the treatment randomly allocated to the patient on entry to the trial.

(c) Trials of duration of therapy

Clinical trials comparing different durations of therapy (especially prophylaxis) have rarely been conducted in psychiatry (Paykel *et al.* 1975), although they have been used in other areas of medicine such as the study of long-term (6 months, 1 year and 2 years) chemotherapy in the treatment of chronic pulmonary tuberculosis (Medical Research Council, 1962). Concern about dependence and other adverse effects of long-term use of psychotropic drugs (Williams *et al.* 1982) and lithium (*British Medical Journal*, 1977), for example, suggests that once prophylactic efficacy has been demonstrated, it is pertinent to enquire whether such treatment should be continued indefinitely or whether it can be discontinued without the risk of relapse after some further interval. In practice, decisions to terminate continuation therapy may involve careful balancing of the risks of relapse and the risks of adverse effects, especially if the latter involve cardiovascular, oncogenic or other severe toxic reactions. While the risks of adverse effects associated with continuation therapy can only be assessed from large monitoring or epidemiological studies, the risks of relapse associated with different durations of therapy can be compared in clinical trials similar to those used to study prophylaxis ((b) above). Thus, for example, patients may be randomly allocated to receive continuation therapy for one or two years and followed up from randomization to relapse, death or the end of the follow-up period (say 3 years). The aim of such a study would be to compare the policy of 1 year's continuation therapy with that of 2 years; in other words, to determine whether therapy for an additional year was efficacious in routine clinical use. While non-compliance with the prescribed treatment will reduce the difference in relapse rates between the two groups, especially when therapy is maintained over long periods, the increasing availability of depot and sustained release preparations should make such studies feasible.

CLINICAL TRIALS IN GENERAL PRACTICE

Following the development of effective psychotropic drugs and the increased availability of other forms of treatment such as supportive therapy, many patients who might otherwise have been referred to a psychiatrist are now treated in general practice. As a result, clinical trials of psychiatric treatment in general practice, which have been conducted only rarely (for example, Porter, 1970), are likely to become more common; some guidelines for their conduct have been published recently (Drug Trials in General Practice, 1981). However, a treatment known, from other studies, to be efficacious in the treatment of a particular disorder need not be re-evaluated by a controlled 'scientific' study in general practice. Essentially, the general practitioner or out-patient clinician will want to know which is the best treatment or dose in routine clinical use. Since lifestyle and attitude may interfere with the treatment prescribed, these effects should not be 'designed out' of clinical trials undertaken in general practice. For example, with two drugs, A and B, both known to be effective in the relief of anxiety, but with A more effective than B, it may nonetheless be better policy to prescribe B if it is associated with a lower non-compliance rate than A.

CLINICAL TRIAL SIZE

Many clinical trials are too small (*British Medical Journal*, 1978; Freiman *et al.* 1978; Tate *et al.* 1979) because they are conducted simply on the basis of the number of patients available at a particular clinic or to a particular clinician, instead of by anticipating the differences between treatments likely to be found and the methods of analysis to be employed. Subjecting patients to clinical trials which are likely to produce inconclusive results may be 'unethical' (Altman, 1980). Given any difference between treatments and a measure of its variability, then it is always possible to specify the number of patients required to be, say, 80 or 90% confident of detecting significance at a specified level (whether 5%, 1% or 0·1%). These numbers may, of course, run into hundreds, thousands or even more, especially if the specified treatment difference is extremely small. Essentially, clinical trials should be designed with a good chance, at least 75% and preferably more than 80%, of detecting an important clinical difference between treatments, so that a statistically non-significant result (at some specified level) is of clinical relevance and does not imply that the trial merely had little chance of detecting anything other than a large treatment difference. Quantifying the 'important clinical difference' is a difficult (and partly subjective) task but it must be done if a clinical trial is to be more than a serendipitous excursion into the unknown. Perhaps the greatest fallacy in scientific inference in the past twenty years has been the assumption that failure to detect a significant difference at 5% or any other level automatically implies no difference whatsoever.

In psychiatry the failure to consider clinical trial size at the design stage has led to a large number of trials with little or no prospect of detecting even a moderate difference between treatments (*Lancet*, 1981). Further, a significant difference between treatments reported in a small-sized trial must be interpreted cautiously since such results are often produced by selective effects or chance and are not reproducible. In clinical trials which employ rating scales the power of a statistical analysis, that is, its chance of detecting a difference between treatments, is dependent upon: first, the magnitude of the difference between treatments as measured by the rating scale; secondly, the variability of the rating scale itself; thirdly, the level of statistical significance at which this difference is to be detected; and, lastly, the number of patients entered in the trial. In designing such trials the number of patients necessary to achieve a given power, preferably greater than 80%, may be calculated from standard tables (Cohen, 1977; Lachin, 1981). While it is difficult to define sensible guidelines without resort to specific examples, experience suggests that fixed-size comparative trials with fewer than 30 patients per treatment are likely to be inconclusive. In crossover trials each patient receives both treatments and the treatment comparison is made within rather than between patients, as in a parallel group study. Since variation within patients is usually less than variation between patients, crossover trials are often thought to require fewer patients than comparable parallel group studies. Such a view is too simple; crossover trials should be conducted only with the anticipation that it may be necessary to use either an analysis of the data collected during the first treatment period only (Hills & Armitage, 1979) or an analysis based on multivariate methods (Zimmermann & Rahlfs, 1980; Poloniecki & Daniel, 1981).

As well as using rating scales to assess psychiatric state, clinical trials in psychiatry frequently elicit information on the side-effects of treatments, sometimes with the idea that, even if there is no demonstrable difference in efficacy, there may at least be a difference in the prevalence of undesirable side-effects. However, a clinical trial which is optimally designed to detect a clinically important difference between treatments using sensitive rating instruments is usually not well designed to detect differences in the prevalence of side-effects. Any trial using more than one method of assessing treatment differences should therefore be designed either to meet the size criterion determined by the least sensitive of these methods or, since side-effects are usually a secondary consideration, to exclude or reveal only gross disadvantages of treatment. No clinical trial, however large, can be sure of detecting an unexpected and rare side-effect; these should be sought through careful drug monitoring once efficacy has been established.

In clinical trials where more than a small proportion of patients do not complete the scheduled programme of assessment it may be necessary to abandon the original intention to analyse the rating scale data themselves and, instead, adopt an analysis based, for example, upon the proportion of patients who recover, the proportion of patients who achieve a specific target rating, or the times to such 'events'. Such changes to the methods of analysis should be anticipated at the design stage and followed by appropriate adjustment to the size of the clinical trial. In particular, the power of an analysis of times to some 'event', such as recovery from an episode in a trial of therapeutic efficacy or relapse as in a trial of prophylaxis, is dependent not so much upon the size of the trial but on the total number of 'events' that has occurred (for example, the number of patients who have recovered or the number of relapses) (Peto *et al.* 1976). The number of patients required to achieve a given power can again be calculated from standard tables (Lachin, 1981; Freedman, 1982). Analyses based on the observation of less than 70 'events' are insensitive to even moderate treatment differences.

ANALYSIS

The method of analysing data collected from a clinical trial should be anticipated during the design of the trial and should be outlined in the protocol. It must be appropriate to the type of data collected and should incorporate (in the initial stages at least) all features of the trial design, including matching and more complicated schemes of stratification.

It should be emphasized that for all clinical trials, irrespective of type or design, the only treatment comparison known to be unbiased is that based on the analysis of *all* randomized patients. To quote Friedman *et al.* (1981): 'If subjects are withdrawn (from analysis), the burden rests with the investigator to convince the scientific community that the analysis has not been biased.' The fate of all patients entered in a trial should therefore be summarized with special mention of the numbers lost to follow-up and deviating from prescribed treatment; reasons for the latter should also be summarized, and death and other untoward incidents reported in detail. An analysis based on intention to treat comparing treatment groups as randomized should always be given, irrespective of any other analyses of selected subgroups. The exclusion of patients who do not comply with, or respond to, treatment or for other reasons may lead to serious bias in treatment comparisons and inconclusive analyses (Gore, 1981*a*). In clinical trials recording the time to some 'event', and especially those involving long-term follow-up of patients (such as in prophylaxis), the analysis should be based on actuarial techniques and not on the presentation of results for patients followed for some arbitrary interval.

To aid the sensible interpretation of significance tests, and especially those reported as 'not significant', the power of the tests to detect appropriate differences between treatments should be quoted. Alternatively, a 95% confidence interval should be given (Gore, 1981*b*). Such information allows a realistic assessment of the usefulness of any clinical trial; this cannot be deduced from the reporting of the results of significance tests alone.

The objectives of many clinical trials in psychiatry include non-specific statements about identifying the characteristics of subgroups of patients who respond either favourably or unfavourably to a particular treatment. While it is difficult to curb the enthusiasm for such 'data fishing' expeditions, it must be stressed that they are of extremely limited value and may be counter-productive. In many clinical trials it is possible to identify specific subgroups of patients for whom one treatment is 'significantly' better than another as well as subgroups of patients who respond 'significantly' better than other subgroups to treatment. Since such 'significant' differences frequently arise by chance or result from selective effects, the conclusions drawn from analyses of subgroups of patients should be regarded with scepticism, and investigated further in other trials only when they are scientifically or clinically plausible.

MULTI-CENTRE TRIALS

As greater understanding of psychiatric disorders leads to improvements in the efficacy of, and compliance with, treatment, it is likely that clinical trials will be required to detect smaller differences between new and standard treatments. Unless there are simultaneous refinements in assessing the effects of treatment, the size of clinical trials must inevitably increase. When no single centre can recruit sufficient patients in a reasonable period, the collaboration of several centres in a multi-centre trial is desirable. Such trials are already used in the study of prophylaxis, where large numbers of patients are entered over an extended period.

Multi-centre trials are complex and require detailed planning, coordination and control both by central and local management. Experience with such trials in other areas of medicine, especially cancer, suggests that many multi-centre trials are conducted over long periods, entry plus follow-up in excess of 5 years (Pocock, 1978). This situation has arisen mainly because entry rates during the early stages of trials have been much too low; indeed, many trials may have been stopped not by a definite policy decision but simply because patient entry has declined. There is no reason to expect that the situation is any different in psychiatry. In the recent trial of continuation therapy with lithium and amitriptyline (Medical Research Council Drug Trials Subcommittee, 1981) 136 patients were recruited in a period of 54 months with one centre entering 53 patients (39% of the total) and four other centres less than 10 patients each. If these four centres had been replaced by other centres recruiting patients at the rate of one per month then this trial could either have been completed in half the time or could have achieved greater power to detect differences between treatments.

The organization of multi-centre trials in psychiatry through the collaboration of a small number of major treatment centres which are able to maintain a steady and appreciable recruitment rate would allow comparatively rapid assessment of therapies and would achieve a great advance in clinical trial methodology.

CONCLUSION

The management of any clinical trial involves an elaborate and complex interaction of several disciplines between which failure to establish or maintain adequate communication can be nothing but a recipe for disaster. Many difficulties arise in the conduct of trials, the collection of data and interpretation of results. Careful consideration of the issues discussed above may anticipate and resolve some of these problems before the recruitment of patients to clinical trials in psychiatry.

ANTHONY L. JOHNSON

I thank Laurence Freedman, Sheila Gore and Ian Sutherland for their helpful comments and suggestions.

REFERENCES

Altman, D. G. (1980). Statistics and ethics in medical research. Misuse of statistics is unethical. *British Medical Journal* ii, 1182–1184.

Barker, N., Hews, R. J., Huitson, A. & Poloniecki, J. (1982). The two period cross over trial. *Bulletin in Applied Statistics* **9**, 67–116.

British Medical Journal (1977). Leading article: Adverse effects of lithium treatment; ii, 346–347.

British Medical Journal (1978). Leading article: Interpreting clinical trials; ii, 1318.

Bull, J. P. (1959). The historical development of clinical therapeutic trials. *Journal of Chronic Disease* **10**, 218–248.

Chalmers, T. C., Smith, H., Blackburn, B., Silvermann, B., Schroeder, B., Rettman, D. & Ambroz, A. (1981). A method of assessing the quality of a randomized clinical trial. *Controlled Clinical Trials* **2**, 31–49.

Chaput de tonge, D. M. (1977). Aide-memoire for preparing clinical trial protocols. *British Medical Journal* i, 1323–1324.

Cohen, J. (1977). *Statistical Power Analysis for the Behavioural Sciences* (second edn). Academic Press: New York and London.

Controlled Clinical Trials. Design and Methods (1980). *Official Journal of the Society for Clinical Trials*. Elsevier/North Holland: Amsterdam.

Drug Trials in General Practice (1981). *Drug and Therapeutics Bulletin* **19**, 97–99.

Freedman, L. S. (1982). Tables of the number of patients required in clinical trials using the logrank test. *Statistics in Medicine* **1**, 121–129.

Freiman, J. A., Chalmers, T. C., Smith, H. & Kuebler, R. R. (1978). The importance of beta, the type II error and sample size in the design and interpretation of the randomized control trial. Survey of 71 'negative' trials. *New England Journal of Medicine* **299**, 690–694.

Friedman, L. M., Furberg, C. D. & DeMets, D. L. (1981). *Fundamentals of Clinical Trials*. John Wright: Bristol.

Godwin-Austen, R. B., Frears, C. C., Bergmann, S., Parkes, J. D. & Knill-Jones, R. P. (1970). Combined treatment of Parkinsonism with L-dopa and amantadine. *Lancet* ii, 383–385.
Gore, S. M. (1981*a*). Assessing clinical trials – rash adventures. *British Medical Journal* ii, 426–428.
Gore, S. M. (1981*b*). Assessing methods – confidence intervals. *British Medical Journal* ii, 660–662.
Gore, S. M. (1982). Statistics in question: assessing clinical trials. In *Statistics in Practice* (by S. M. Gore and D. G. Altman), pp. 27–63. British Medical Association: London.
Grizzle, J. E. (1965). The two-period change-over design and its use in clinical trials. *Biometrics* **21**, 467–480.
Harris, E. L. & Fitzgerald, J. D. (eds.) (1970). *The Principles and Practice of Clinical Trials.* Livingstone: Edinburgh and London.
Hills, M. & Armitage, P. (1979). The two-period crossover clinical trial. *British Journal of Clinical Pharmacology* **8**, 7–20.
Hughes, R. C., Polgar, J. G., Weightman, D. & Walton, J. N. (1971). L-Dopa in Parkinsonism and the influence of previous thalamotomy. *British Medical Journal* i, 7–13.
Johnson, F. N. & Johnson S. (eds.) (1977). *Clinical Trials.* Blackwell: Oxford.
Johnstone, E. C., Deakin, J. F. W., Lawler, P., Frith, C. D., Stevens, M., McPherson, K. & Crow, T. J. (1980). The Northwick Park Electroconvulsive Therapy Trial. *Lancet* ii, 1317–1320.
Lachin, J. M. (1981). Introduction to sample size determination and power analysis for clinical trials. *Controlled Clinical Trials* **2**, 93–113.
Lancet (1981). Leading article: Multicentre depression; ii, 563–564.
Mackay, A. V. P., Sheppard, G. P., Saha, B. K., Motley, B., Johnson, A. L. & Marsden, C. D. (1980). Failure of lithium treatment in established tardive dyskinesia. *Psychological Medicine* **10**, 583–587.
Medical Research Council (1962). A report by the Tuberculosis Chemotherapy Trials Committee. Long term chemotherapy in the treatment of chronic pulmonary tuberculosis with cavitation. *Tubercle* **43**, 201–267.
Medical Research Council Drug Trials Subcommittee (1981). Continuation therapy with lithium and amitriptyline in unipolar depressive illness: a controlled clinical trial. *Psychological Medicine* **11**, 409–416.
Paykel, E. S., DiMascio, A., Haskell, D. & Prusoff, B. A. (1975). Effects of maintenance amitriptyline and psychotherapy on symptoms of depression. *Psychological Medicine* **5**, 67–77.
Peterson, A. V. & Fisher, L. D. (1980). Teaching the principles of clinical trials design and management. *Biometrics* **36**, 687–697.
Peto, R., Pike, M. C., Armitage, P., Breslow, N. E., Cox, D. R., Howard, S. V., Mantel, N., McPherson, K., Peto, J. & Smith, P. G. (1976). Design and analysis of randomized clinical trials requiring prolonged observation of each patient. I. Introduction and design. *British Journal of Cancer* **34**, 585–612.
Peto, R., Pike, M. C., Armitage, P., Breslow, N. E., Cox, D. R., Howard, S. V., Mantel, N., McPherson, K., Peto, J. & Smith, P. G. (1977). Design and analysis of randomized clinical trials requiring prolonged observation of each patient. II. Analysis and examples. *British Journal of Cancer* **35**, 1–39.
Pocock, S. J. (1978). Size of cancer clinical trials and stopping rules. *British Journal of Cancer* **38**, 757–766.
Poloniecki, J. & Daniel, D. (1981). Further analysis of the Hills and Armitage data. *The Statistician* **30**, 225–229.
Porter, A. M. W. (1970). Depressive illness in a general practice. A demographic study and a controlled trial of imipramine. *British Medical Journal* i, 773–778.
Schwartz, D., Flamant, R. & Lellouch, J. (1980). *Clinical Trials* (transl. M. J. R. Healy). Academic Press: London.
Tate, H. C., Rawlinson, J. B. & Freedman, L. S. (1979). Randomized comparative studies in the treatment of cancer in the United Kingdom: room for improvement. *Lancet* ii, 623–625.
Wallenstein, S. & Fisher, A. C. (1977). The analysis of the two-period repeated measurements crossover design with application to clinical trials. *Biometrics* **33**, 261–269.
Williams, P., Murray, J. & Clare, A. (1982). A longitudinal study of psychotropic drug prescription. *Psychological Medicine* **12**, 201–206.
Young, J. P. R., Hughes, W. C. & Lader, M. H. (1976). A controlled comparison of flupenthixol and amitriptyline in depressed out-patients. *British Medical Journal* i, 1116–1118.
Zimmermann, H. & Rahlfs, W. (1980). Model building and testing for the change-over design. *Biometrical Journal* **22**, 197–210.

GENERAL PSYCHOPATHOLOGY AND CLINICAL ISSUES

Psychological Medicine, 1979, **9**, 409–415

The epistemology of normality[1]

'It does not seem a profitable procedure to make odd noises on the offchance that posterity will find a significance to attribute to them' (Eddington, 1928).

DETACHMENT AND SYMMETRY

The more a science deals with humanity, the less highly resolved it is, and the less its truths are susceptible of cogent proof. This principle is, I think, ascribable to Norbert Wiener, although it is difficult to document adequately. Thus, the 'exact' sciences, physics and chemistry, are also the most remote; scientifically, microbial genetics is much more satisfactory than human genetics; and of all topics of human genetics, the most distinctively human, behaviour and psychiatric disease, are in the most parlous state.

It is not difficult to see, in broad terms at least, why this should be so.

(1) Even the most extreme reductionist would agree that the structure and functioning of the human body is vastly more complex than that of the individual atom. Whether there is an *ensemble* effect, an *emergence*, ascribable to the complexity of the interactions and to be inferred with difficulty (or perhaps not at all) from the individual properties of the component parts, is a matter well known to the neurophysiologists. But the problem of finding an illuminating conceptualization of the whole pattern is open. The field is still in that somewhat naïve state which existed before Mendel and Galton in genetics and Clerk-Maxwell in physics perceived that the joint behaviour of a complex system may follow certain probabilistic patterns which can be conveniently and usefully studied even when no individual component could be scrutinized. The canons of rigour of such a representation certainly exist but are very different in type from those of classical Laplacian physics. The mere fact that no analogous paradigm has yet been found for human behaviour is no reason for assertive nihilism.

(2) There are many constraints on research in man: the relatively long life of the subject compared with that of the investigator; the ethical limitations on manipulation; the constraint of political freedom; the expense of human research; and many more.

(3) More than any other animal, man is self-conscious. The fact of being observed alters behaviour and in man the change may be deliberate or the result of suggestion. Those who do clinical trials are acutely aware of these problems: the need for the double blind, and the problems of maintaining it.

(4) Scientific experimentation on man (as distinct from passive observation) has a shorter history than comparable disciplines.

For these reasons (and doubtless many others) past accomplishments in human biology are meagre; and we look forward to future developments. But it would be foolish to underestimate the dimensions of the ultimate problems. We do not know enough about human biology to warrant any great precision for that statement; but, at least by analogy from other fields, one can see wherein one major problem lies: the difficulty of detachment. I cite analogies from 4 disciplines: physics, mathematics, psychiatry and epistemology.

In physics, the most explicit science of all, relativity theory has abandoned the facile separation of the observer from the observed, as Bronowski (1960) has pointed out. Into any equation for which invariance is to be claimed the observer himself must be incorporated. This involvement is not merely that invoked by pre-Einsteinian physicists to patch up the wounds of Newtonian mechanics, but a fundamental invasion of the sacred detachment of the observer. The observer is merely a part of the whole system, and (in a physical sense) neither a privileged nor a special part.

[1] Address for correspondence: Dr Edmond A. Murphy, Division of Medical Genetics, Johns Hopkins University School of Medicine, Baltimore, Maryland 21205, USA.

In mathematics even a steady retreat from physical reality, into a pure mathematics which owes allegiance to axiomatics alone, has proved no safeguard. Gödel's incompleteness theorem has shown in some generality that any finite set of axioms must, sooner or later, lead to problems, falling within their compass, to which no unambiguous answers can be given. Always, further axioms are needed. The mathematician is denied economy, his principal aesthetic criterion. Inasmuch as axioms are arbitrary, the mathematician cannot remain uninvolved. He is no more a detached and self-contained observer than the physicist is, but must personally invade his field from time to time.

To the psychiatrist, of course, this pattern of inexorable participation is a commonplace. The psychiatrist is not one class of being, the patient another. Analytical psychiatry has insisted, very rightly, on 2 key principles. First, the resources for solving the patient's problem must ultimately come from within: they cannot be manufactured by the psychiatrist, or quarried from the sacred writings of the masters. The second is the explicit recognition that the psychiatrist's own view of the world is personal, and that to foist it on the patient is prejudice. In the stricter schools, the psychiatrist is required to undergo analysis with the express aim of laying bare his own prejudices and making allowances for them in the interactions with his patients.

The philosopher has, of course, long recognized that, while epistemology cannot be constructed entirely from within the field of its application, neither can it afford to ignore that field. If it is not to be void, epistemology must appeal to empirical fact. Once this appeal is made, the philosopher is bound by the discipline he has embraced. But he remains a philosopher and is not to be treated democratically as merely one voice of no special importance. The impartiality of (say) physics does not lend itself to a theory of values or a quest for ultimate meaning; they can come only from a study of the relationship of physics to other knowledge and insights.

From these 4 examples I draw a general principle of the symmetry of the parts expressed somewhat crudely, as follows. In the domain of natural knowledge (that is, without appealing to revelation, mysticism or other transcendental forms), *a priori* every part of a system is as good, as important, as significant, as every other part. (I insert the term '*a priori*' because, if the symmetry were inalienable, no non-trivial conclusions at all could be reached by argument or by the pursuit of knowledge.) We always suppose that, ultimately, truth is more important than evidence and parity cannot be maintained between them.

I do not claim to have proved this principle of symmetry in general, or even in particular. But reflection on it in the light of the 4 examples persuades me that it is a sounder and safer viewpoint than, say Maritain's (1956) theory of knowledge, that philosophy has a special right to sit in judgement on science, a right which is asymmetrical because it is unreciprocated. If we believe that, in some sense, truth is homogeneous, then philosophy, theology, science and art must be *mutually* reconciled and reconcilable. Bad philosophy should be subject to condemnation by science, as bad science is condemnable by philosophy.

NORMALITY AND THE MEANING OF MEANING

It is commonly claimed that medicine is a science which is gaining strength as our understanding and knowledge progress. We are also often reminded that medicine is an 'art', a term used apologetically for jury-rigged solutions to problems, where current science falls short. But sound practitioners know that medicine is a 'full-thickness' slice of life, not merely an academic abstraction of certain points of interest. In the past, medical judgement drew on an education which was presumed to be broad; it could presume a largely unified social conscience; such judgements centred on immediate and urgent problems; and they were severely curtailed by the narrow scope of the possible. All 4 factors have been eroded in recent years: the surrender of at least the ideal of broad education to technical instruction; the half-informed turmoil and polarization of public opinion crudely manipulated by the demagogue; the technical successes which have shifted interest from acute to chronic disease; and the precipitous change in the scope of our diagnosis, prognosis and treatment. A need, and (in lesser degree) a demand, for a philosophy of medicine has surfaced; and despite the energies of a handful of scholars, the hiatus is wide, and growing. The difficulties are twofold. On the one hand, there is a shortage of philosophers who are really prepared to study the medical scene and of physicians with even the most rudimentary grasp of the nature and scope of philosophy. On the other hand, there is little recognition that the gap of communication exists: that neither Procrustian formulae a thousand years old, nor naïve common sense is sufficient to meet the need. At best, shallow solutions postpone the day of reckoning; at worst, they obscure, falsify, mislead.

There are a great many notions that have a crude utility which constitute what we call common sense. No doubt it is a good (if somewhat obvious) general principle that tall men should beware of bumping their heads going through doorways. It does not matter that doorways vary in size or that the notion of a 'tall man' is a vague one. The caution embodies, with logical precision, the peril of incompatibility. We might refine it somewhat by saying that the taller a man the fewer doors he can go through without stooping. It is a moot point as to whether any more precise distillation is possible or desirable. One might even say that the strength of the statement lies in its physical vagueness.

However, this is a quantitative age with a widespread implicit belief that 'precision' and 'reproducible measurement' are interchangeable terms. (And indeed 'precision' has come to have exactly that technical meaning in statistics.) Certainly, reproducible measurement is evidence of precision of a kind, although its predicate may be something of trivial import (as for instance the weight of Michaelangelo's *David* would be). It would be foolish either to suppose no other form of precision possible or that precision is the ineluctable metric of all profound surmise. That useless pain is undesirable and that it is the duty of the medical profession to relieve it are perfectly definite statements which cannot be eroded by the lack of a satisfactory measurement, the semantic problems of defining pain, or the formidable problems of deciding which pains are indeed useless. Nevertheless, this claim is not to say that these terms are not worthy of more profound exploration. Nor, on the other hand, does it mean that our craving for precision should let us settle for some measurement for no better reason than that it is highly reproducible. We have suffered more than enough from the heresies of both vague nihilism and untimely quantitation. Canonizing tentative measurement, especially of that which has not been subjected to profound reflection, is to be condemned. Yet there is a kind of naïve theory among medical scientists (which fortunately the practitioners do not take seriously) which dismisses as 'noise' everything which measurement does not comprise.

For a long time we have glorified 'fitness', 'health', 'normality', as ideals to be pursued by attacking their contraries. As they stand, these goals go scarcely beyond broad sentiment. But (as Adlai Stevenson remarked) slogans are designed to produce action, not thought. It is only from mobilizing concern that we may expect useful progress; but ill-directed motion can have devastating consequences. It is the traditional function of the philosopher, not to produce ideals out of thin air, but to help his fellow men to perceive the implications of their narrow analyses on the one hand and their broad enthusiasms on the other. But (with minor and often ignominious exceptions) the medical profession, for one, has floundered in vain with its weighty problems. A scholar's allegiance is a sacred matter which we cannot attack without imperilling academic freedom. But right and responsibility are inseparable; and whatever the individual philosopher may do, we are surely entitled to vest a corporate responsibility with philosophers to help us with our difficulties. Conversely we would not deny the physician the right to do research in some field perhaps remote from clinical practice; but the philosopher would have a grievance if he could find no physician to look after him when he is sick. A profession can fail as a whole even if no one person can be blamed.

It is not as if the issue is a trivial one. A large part of medical ethics and much of the whole underpinning of current medical policy, private and public, are squarely based on the notion of disease and normality. Left to himself the physician (whether he realizes it or not) can do very well without a formal definition of disease. Despite the clumsy nosology in which textbooks abound, he treats, not technical terms, but patients. The notorious debate about the nature of essential hypertension passes him by: what he does to patients is dictated by what the patient's state and needs are. Insofar as he makes any decision on the basis of blood pressure, he considers what the blood pressure reading actually is, not what it is called. Superficial thinkers mistake this policy for nominalism, supposing erroneously that the only form of scientific reduction is categorical. This naïve belief ignores everything in scientific and mathematical development since Descartes' fundamental work on continuous mathematical functions. The confusion of dimensionality with cardinality (Murphy, 1976) is a consequence of decadent neo-Aristotelianism from which medicine still suffers (Whitehead, 1925).

Unfortunately, the physician is not left alone to work his common sense. He is attacked from 2 angles: the predatory consumers and the pretentious advisors.

The predatory consumers are those who demand of him not merely a precisely reasoned answer to their questions (even their meaningless questions) but reserve the right to cross-question him, condemn his diffidence, and threaten him with malpractice. He will be expected to apply (with spurious exactitude) laws about mental deficiency which, by their very nature, can embody nothing more than broad sentiment. He is required to provide often meaningless detail on death certificates (from which in due course specious vital statistics will be compiled). He cannot give patients what he deems warranted reassurance but, in an increasing mania for disclosure (especially in the United States), must furnish, out of context, whatever raw data the patient demands. Whole areas of legislation on the pursuit, elucidation and prevention of disease are consigned to him for execution, however ill-considered, ambiguous or fanciful.

On the other hand, and much more damagingly, he is the victim of his advisors who more and more worship false gods. They suppose that measurement is always better than non-measurement. They do not grasp that there are hierarchies of precision and that, while they may have solved the purely metrical aspect of a subject, they have before them as great a task or greater in infusing precision into the *meaning* of the answer. A commonplace, if superficial, illustration is the investigator who will calculate a chi-square test to 4 significant figures, consult a set of tables with scrupulous attention to degrees of freedom, and publish a probability value; and then in his explanatory comments make it clear that he has a completely mistaken notion what the answer is the probability of. But this is a trivial illustration, 'pure ignorance', which could have been put right with a little more instruction. The real difficulties lie in those cases where no adequate interpretation of the highly precise measurement has been proposed, where there is even no assurance that it has any non-trivial meaning. This gap is rarely met by an honest avowal of ignorance or incompetence. Instead it is carelessly overlooked, glossed over, or handled with a little hasty addendum.

An admirable example is the XYY karyotype. The cytological aspects of this interesting condition were handled faultlessly. How the interpretation was handled is a standing disgrace to both medicine and the law. There was much more to these lapses than mere ignorance of the elementary techniques of inference (although one might have supposed that any scientist would know that one cannot do tests of association between karyotype and phenotype without serious attention to definition of the reference population and the sampling procedure). What is appalling is that the fruit of this insouciance has so much power to affect human lives: the suspicion it engenders; the false importance ascribed to it in legal defence; even, by implication, one more shallow attack on personal responsibility and freedom. There have been heroic, but not altogether successful, attempts to remedy, after the event, the lack of sound empirical information on the relationships between karyotype and phenotype (Borgaonkar & Shah, 1974; Hook, 1973; Hamerton, 1976). But they have been constrained by an atmosphere already biased and emotionally charged with militant concern for human freedom, which has hampered the collection of the facts necessary to clarify the issue.

However, let us suppose that the empirical evidence of the relationships were sound, that those with the XYY karyotype were convicted more often of crimes of violence; and, for simplicity, we will further suppose that the association is not due to more efficient policing (because of conspicuous height) or prejudice of juries against men with acne. What are we to make of the meaning of such an empirical association? There have been attempts to use the karyotype, as insanity is used, as a legal defence. But clearly empirical association is an insufficient argument. No doubt but that rape is much more commonly committed by men than by women: but, even in the midst of a furore against sexual discrimination, nobody would argue that possession of a Y chromosome is a defence against a charge of rape or any other crime to which adult males are disposed. Besides, no evidence whatsoever has been adduced that all XYY subjects commit acts of aggression; hence it is difficult to argue (in any deterministic sense) that this karyotype causes such crimes. Confused as the legal practice is on the use of insanity as a defence, it has never to my knowledge been ruled – even in the extreme *Durham* opinion (1954) – that no insane person can ever be found legally guilty of a crime.

What keeps it from being dismissed out of hand is an implicit appeal to normality. The principle would be somewhat as follows. Where a condition is so abnormal as to impose an extraordinary burden on the patient, we may invoke it as a defence. The law does not state it so; indeed, I have had the greatest difficulty in finding the word 'normal' used in any legal ruling; but without its unseen presence, any legal principle of defence for medical reasons would flounder. Acute alcoholism is as rational a defence as insanity. The main difference lies in the fact that acute alcoholism must be presumed culpable. But leaving this aspect aside, all the legal psychiatric principles of defence – nature-and-quality, uncontrollable impulse, product-disease – apply to drunkenness, as well as to schizophrenia.

THE DELIMITATION OF NORMALITY

Two of the main 'consumers' of the physician's opinions about normality, the surgeon and the criminal lawyer, have in common the need for a sharp endpoint. The patient is either operated on or not. The prisoner is either convicted or not. The details may modify the extent of the operation or mitigate the severity of the sentence, but there is no such outcome as being slightly operated on, or moderately convicted. Hence 3 questions arise:

(1) Do multiple states exist?
(2) How are they best distinguished?
(3) Which of them are to be designated abnormal?

In some very few areas the first 2 questions are easily dealt with. Sickle cell disease is clearly demonstrated at a chemical level, the most highly resolved we have. Precise distinction between it and the wild-type trait is available. Galactosaemia and haemophilia undoubtedly exist; diagnosis is almost foolproof, and reasonable criteria for resolving diagnostic (as distinct from ontological) doubt exist. In a great many cases – hypertension, diabetes, obesity – the answers to both questions are doubtful; but at least precise and well-established measurements provide data for speculation.

In some cases, most notably in disorders of behaviour, intellect and emotion, no such well-tried scales exist, although arbitrary scales have been devised. Now, of course, in the ultimate economy of things, these arbitrary scales are not necessarily inferior to the centimetre–gram–second scale of the physicist. Doubtless the measurements are more subject to spontaneous variation or observer error; but no scientist refuses to use the cgs scale in biochemistry on grounds of variance. The issue is not mainly the *statistical* but the *epistemological* properties of these scales of measurement. It is not at all easy to see wherein the difference lies except the ineluctably *reflexive* character of psychiatric scales of behaviour. Theoretically the problem could be approached by techniques of cluster analysis. There are, of course, well-known statistical problems in cluster analysis. The main epistemological difficulty is that the very choice of raw data introduces a bias which no system of scaling can correct *a posteriori*. (Some of the data may be discarded; but missing data cannot usually be recovered.)

In a trivial sense, of course, wherever there is variation in the characteristics, one can classify. One may divide patients into introverts and extroverts by some arbitrary point on an arbitrary scale. Invariance of order of magnitude may still be preserved even if absolute magnitude is not. But a classification in the face of a measurement seems to have warrant only if the classification *transcends* the measurement: if beneath the 'noise' of the measurement there is some significant state which is the real object of our enquiries. For instance, the valency of an element must be a whole number. If an experimental measurement gave the value 2·1, there is little doubt that '2' is a better estimate of the true value than '2·1' (which would be meaningless). In contrast, it seems doubtful that to say a man of 30 exhibits 'tallness' is ever a better estimate of any significant state than his actual height. In practice, it is by no means easy to identify how far the problem is one of discrimination (question 2) and how far it is to identify groups (question 1).

We have not entirely explicated the word 'significant' in the previous paragraph. What may be a scientifically significant grouping is not necessarily clinically significant: the Xg(a) blood type being a good example. Detailed analysis of an unselected population would doubtless turn up innocent haemoglobinopathies which might be of considerable interest to a geneticist. In such cases, the third question – which states are to be designated abnormal – is the point of dispute. Sometimes it is answered very easily: the state of one or more of the groups being grossly disruptive and leading perhaps to rapid death; or alternatively, the distinguishing characters of the groups may be subtle and the phenotypic differences slight or absent, so that by no contortions can it be regarded as an abnormal state. But the dictum 'hard cases make bad law' is readily reinterpreted to our purpose: a principle founded on these open-and-shut examples would be useless in many, perhaps most, adjudications. The more a conclusion is said to be 'obvious', the more we should have our suspicions awakened that the issue is being not solved, but evaded. It may be 'obvious' to a fashion designer whether a woman's hair is or is not red; there is much (probably unfounded) popular psychology about such people; admirers of Titian may discuss its aesthetic properties; but the evidence we have is that, scientifically, there is no such category as redheadedness (Reed, 1952). But, after all, it is rarely a hanging matter whether a person's hair is red or not: if Sherlock Holmes had been as astute as Watson thought he was, he would have seen through the story of the red-headed league (Doyle, 1930) from the start as something which could not be defined legally. Yet, wherever due legal process is denied, there is a tendency to pass laws which for lack of sound criteria cannot be applied except by abuse. A professional geneticist has the greatest difficulty over the notion of race. So far as one can define by gene frequencies, it has been established repeatedly that, on average, the so-called American Negro derives 30 % of his genes from 'White' North European ancestors; and this must mean that, by random variation, in many the proportions must be 50 % or over. If race has any meaning other than social, such people are White not Negro; for, if those with any genes which may be of Negro origin are to be called Negroes, almost the entire American population would fall into this group.

It is interesting to note that while, by the content of their field, psychiatrists are the least well equipped to confront the issue of defining normality, they are the only group of clinicians who have taken these problems with anything like the seriousness they merit. Many of these writings are penetrating (Cantor, 1941; Hacker, 1945; Reider, 1950; Offer & Sabshin, 1966; Sabshin, 1967). Some are radical, and that of Freides (1960) concisely and articulately makes a case for discarding the notion of normality as unworkable. It is perhaps even more remarkable that philosophers in their rare discussions on the idea of normality choose with a kind of perverseness this least well-defined of all fields of clinical medicine.

IMPLICATIONS

How far should it be the responsibility of the medical profession to become involved in these intricate issues? At first sight it might appear that lacking any formal training in the analysis of values the physician as a professional man had best leave the matter alone. There seem to be at least 4 reasons why this detachment is not to be recommended in practice.

First, the physician does have to make actual decisions. Doubtless it would be best if in seeking values he could appeal to a consensus; but the latter does not exist, and the views of the self-appointed spokesman must not be mistaken for it.

Secondly, supposed views of physicians and the supposed conclusions of medical science are commonly misrepresented, even by scholars from other fields, and such errors must be unmasked. It would be a distasteful exercise to list instances in the writings of distinguished philosophers, theologians, educationalists, politicians and even physicians themselves where totally unwarranted statements about what 'medical science has shown' are used as the bedrock of weighty discussions: as that emotional structure and behavioural disorders are inherited; that statistics has shown how the normal is to be defined; that the Kinsey reports have shown that such and such practices are not abnormal (despite the most explicit statement from the authors that they were attempting to make no normative inferences). Such statements can be authoritatively condemned only by those prepared and disposed to analyse the issues.

Thirdly, the physician, for all his limitations, is usually at least as well informed on the issues of normality and disease as the layman or most experts from other fields. One might wish that he had as much cultivated detachment, and as much insight into his own prejudices, as the psychiatrist. But an imperfect understanding of the implication of facts seems clearly better than an imperfect understanding of gossip or of nothing at all.

Finally, much as we may dislike the idea, patients expect their physicians to have views which they are ready to express. Many of us involved in genetic counselling set a goal of communicating fact and perspective, with compassion and concern, but in strictly non-directive fashion. But parents do not readily embrace the responsibility of making decisions; and if they must have prefabricated ideas they might as well come from the physician as from their neighbours (who are rarely so diffident about directiveness).

EDMOND A. MURPHY

The work in this paper is supported by NIH Grant No. GM 24736.

REFERENCES

Borgaonkar, D. S. & Shah, S. A. (1974). The XYY chromosome male or syndrome. *Progress in Medical Genetics* **10**, 135–222.

Bronowski, J. (1960). *The Common Sense of Science*. Penguin: Harmondsworth.

Cantor, N. (1941). What is a normal mind? *American Journal of Orthopsychiatry* **15**, 47–64.

Doyle, A. C. (1930). The Red-Headed League. In *The Adventures of Sherlock Holmes*. Harper and Row: New York.

Durham v. *The United States* (1954). 214: F 2nd 862–876.

Eddington, H. S. (1928). *The Nature of the Physical World*, p. 21. Cambridge University Press: London.

Freides, D. (1960). Towards the elimination of the concept of normality. *Journal of Consulting Psychology* **24**, 128–133.

Hacker, F. J. (1945). The concept of normality and its practical significance. *American Journal of Orthopsychiatry* **15**, 47–64.

Hamerton, J. L. (1976). Human population genetics: dilemmas and problems. *American Journal of Human Genetics* **22**, 107–122.

Hook, E. B. (1973). Behavioural implications of the human XYY genotype. *Science* **179**, 139–150.

Maritain, J. (1956). *General Introduction to Philosophy*. New York.

Murphy, E. A. (1976). *The Logic of Medicine*. Johns Hopkins University Press: Baltimore.

Offer, D. & Sabshin, M. (1966). *Normality: Theoretical and Clinical Concepts of Mental Health*. Basic Books: New York.

Reed, T. E. (1952). Red hair colour as a genetical character. *Annals of Eugenics* **17**, 115–139.

Reider, N. (1950). The concept of normality. *Psychoanalytical Quarterly* **19**, 43–51.

Sabshin, M. (1967). Psychiatric perspectives on normality. *Archives of General Psychiatry* **17**, 258–264.

Whitehead, A. N. (1925). *Science and the Modern World*. Macmillan: New York.

Psychological Medicine, 1972, **2**, 205–207

Psyche and history

Addressing the American Historical Association in 1958, William L. Langer emphasized that the psychological effects of the Black Death were a significant historical phenomenon and he proposed that the matter be studied by the methods of psychoanalysis. Since then the psychological aspects of historical events and personages have increasingly attracted attention, indeed to such an extent that this area of interest has received a specific designation, 'psychohistory'. As this interest has grown two problem areas have come under investigation.

One area encompasses the psychological impact of disease, particularly that produced by major or recurrent epidemics. This problem is important, not only in its own right, but also because it is a part of the larger problem of the affective history of societies and communities. Actually, the historical investigation of such problems is not completely new. One need only recall Hecker's (1832) study of the medieval dance frenzy, Crawfurd's study of 1914 on plague and pestilence in literature and art, and D'Irsay's examination in 1927 of defence reactions during the Black Death. Nonetheless, such studies were sporadic, so that a large and potentially important area of research still remains to be worked.

Useful approaches to this problem area have more recently come from several different directions. One has been the use of pictorial evidence to demonstrate a change in the psychological state of a social group over a period of time. Millard Meiss, in his study of painting in Florence and Siena after the Black Death, showed that changes in art which occurred after the epidemic were due to the establishment of a new state of mind among the people of these cities (Meiss, 1951). Employing a similar approach, but on a much larger scale, and utilizing a wide range of literary and visual sources, Alberto Tenenti (1957) explored psychological attitudes toward life and death in Italy and France during the Renaissance.

More provocative is the work of René Baehrel (1951), who pointed out that from a psychological viewpoint the period during which an epidemic prevails is a period of fear, of anxiety, and may be compared with and studied like periods of revolutionary terror. Indeed, Baehrel suggested that psychological attitudes developed in earlier epidemics and famine periods were latently available during the terror of the French Revolution. Moreover, he also argued that in such psychological climates social class antagonisms, religious animosities, and other hostile attitudes towards individuals and groups may be activated and realized in violent behaviour. This thesis had already been illustrated by Seraphine Guerchberg (1948) in her study of the controversy over the alleged plague sowers and the massacre of Jews on this ground at the time of the Black Death.

The broad framework within which studies, such as those of Baehrel and Tenenti, must be seen and from which they derive in part was set forth in 1941 by the French historian, Lucien Febvre. In this programmatic statement he urged historians to turn their attention to the emotional life of men in their social environment and to reconstruct it on the basis of its manifestations as indicated by available evidence. The evidence might be provided by a variety of sources, not only written records. For example, one might study how words were used at different periods, what words were available to what groups, and the like. A second source suggested by Febvre was iconography; a third was literature; and still another was provided by legal cases and documents. In short, any evidence that throws light on individual and collective psychology. In this sense Febvre envisaged a history of love, of pity, of cruelty, of death. How this programme was actually applied may be seen in his masterly work on the religion of Rabelais, where he showed on the basis of empirical evidence what sixteenth-century men could have experienced and considered thinkable in relation to the supernatural (Febvre, 1942). This is psychohistory on a conscious level, where the historian is aware that analysis of the manifest content of ideas and beliefs and of the modes of expression, the intensity of emotional relationships, and the selective valuation placed on different kinds of relationships reflects a certain psychological organization. Such aspects are indicative of the psychological make-up up and modes of behaviour of individuals and groups in relation to the larger structure of social and cultural life. Historical periods are characterized by different sensibilities—that is, modes of feeling shared in varying degree by those living at a particular time. An awareness that the personal and the public interpenetrate within the framework of society must underlie any endeavour to understand these psychological aspects. Individuals and groups cannot be divorced from the larger institutions within which they carry on their lives, since it is within this framework that their psychologies are formulated. The way in which an individual in a given historical period perceives his world, the feeling he has about it, depends on his interests, beliefs, and values, on the intricate connections between his inner life, his life-pattern, and the specific social and cultural conditions which he encounters in his environment. This characteristic mode of perceiving and feeling which we call sensibility is an expression of the way in which the personality integrates these diverse elements. Such relationships are as complex for groups as they are for individuals. In any given historical period, a society or a group within it may exhibit a characteristic pattern of emotional attitudes. A prevalent psychological orientation of this kind, which by analogy with Whitehead's idea of a climate of opinion can be called an emotional climate, develops out of social and cultural conditions specific to a society or group and is related to its historical development. Numerous individual sensibilities contribute to an emotional climate, and in turn the prevalence of such a complex of feelings tends to stimulate individuals and groups to perceive their socio-cultural environment, the various aspects of society, along certain lines and to act in characteristic ways.[1]

Against this background may be set the other current psychohistorical area of interest, the use of psychological models to understand historical individuals, particularly leaders of various types in terms of the interplay between public performance and private personality. This endeavour has also had earlier antecedents in the form of so-called pathographies—for example, Möbius's case history of Rousseau (Möbius, 1889), and Lange's of Hölderlin (Lange, 1909). Indeed, Jaspers tried to show how the neurotic drives of his subjects contributed to their creative accomplishments (Jaspers, 1922). These biographical studies were in essence case histories undertaken by psychiatrists or those with psychiatric orientations. Freud's discoveries and ideas were applied very early to biographical material, indeed by Freud himself as in *Eine Kindheitserinnerung des Leonardo da Vinci* and other contributions. Most of these early contributions were relatively crude and were frequently vitiated by the fallacy of unilateralism—that is, by an effort to establish a one to one relationship between traumatic early experiences and later behaviour, as for instance in the Bullitt-Freud analysis of Woodrow Wilson. Probably the most successful practitioner so far has been Erik Erikson with his studies of Luther and Gandhi (Erikson, 1958, 1969, respectively). But Erikson's work illustrates both some possibilities and limitations. Two points will clarify the limitations. Erikson begins his study of Luther with a story of the young monk having had a fit, a story for which there is no good evidence. Nevertheless, he used the story, justifying his practice on the ground that if it didn't happen, it as good as happened. But unfortunately Erikson gives no criteria indicating when and where he would admit rumour and legend as evidence, and when he would not. Another point is Erikson's emphasis on Luther's anality, apparently overlooking the fact that the whole tone of life and its expression in the sixteenth century was coarse. Cursing, belching, farting, gluttony, and rude behaviour were common at all levels of society, the highest as well as the lowest, certainly in Germany if one is to judge from the testimony of visitors such as Machiavelli in 1508.

There is no doubt that psychohistorical studies in the biographical area offer rich potentialities, and there are a few outstanding contributions, such as Starobinski's elegant and subtle analysis of the tensions in Rousseau's personality and their relation to his ideas and activities (Starobinski, 1958). However, if the potentialities of psychohistory are to be realized, certain points must be emphasized.

[1]For a development of these concepts and their application as analytic tools, see Rosen, G. (1967).

In modern history and biography, the study of process is pre-eminent. We want to see the character forming, its singularities taking shape in relation to the inner drives and compulsions. The task of the historian is to represent convincingly internal processes, pressures, and changes and thus to map out the elements that produced the phenomenon he confronts. To do this it is necessary first of all to be aware of the historical period. It is not enough to know about Luther; one must also know the sixteenth century and its varied aspects.

One must also beware of the reductionist fallacy—that is, not to reduce an individual to his psychic traumata and weaknesses. This is one of Erikson's considerable achievements, his portrayal of Luther's transformation of his weakness into spiritual power which enabled so many of his contemporaries to identify with him.

Historians have available to them a field of high interest in the investigation of collective and individual psychology in relation to historical developments. Huizinga showed some 40 years ago that the fifteenth century in Europe was a period of melancholy and morbid introspection, but he saw this as a phenomenon of cultural history. But we may also look at it as a problem of psychopathology in a period of cultural change, in which individuals and groups participated. These are some of the possibilities that exist for those who wish to study such problems (Rosen, 1968).

GEORGE ROSEN

REFERENCES

Baehrel, R. (1951). Épidémie et terreur: Histoire et sociologie, *Annales Historiques de la Révolution Française*, **23,** 113–146.

Crawfurd, R. H. P. (1914). *Plague and Pestilence in Literature and Art*. Clarendon Press: Oxford.

D'Irsay, S. (1927). Defence reactions during the Black Death, 1348–1349. *Annals of Medical History*, **9,** 169–179.

Erikson, E. H. (1958). *Young Man Luther. A Study in Psychoanalysis and History*. W. W. Norton: New York.

Erikson, E. H. (1969). *Gandhi's Truth: On the Origins of Militant Nonviolence*. W. W. Norton: New York.

Febvre, L. (1941). La sensibilité et l'histoire, *Annales d'Histoire Sociale*, **3,** 5–20.

Febvre, L. (1942). *Le Problème de l'Incroyance au XVIe Siècle, la Religion de Rabelais*. Édition revue. Michel: Paris, 1962 (originally published 1942).

Guerchberg, S. (1948). La controverse sur les prétendus semeurs de la "Peste Noire", d'après les traités de peste de l'époque. *Revue des Études Juives*, N.S., **8,** 3–40.

Hecker, J. F. K. (1832). *Die Tanzwuth, eine Volkskrankheit im Mittelalter*. T. C. F. Enslin: Berlin.

Jaspers, K. (1922). *Strindberg und Van Gogh. Versuch einer pathographischen Analyse unter vergleichender Heranziehung von Swedenborg und Hölderlin*. E. Bircher: Leipzig.

Lange, W. (1909). *Hölderlin, eine Pathographie mit zwölf Schriftproben und einer Stammtafel*. F. Enke: Stuttgart.

Langer, W. L. (1958). The next assignment. *American Historical Review*, **63,** 283–304.

Meiss, M. (1951). *Painting in Florence and Siena after the Black Death*. Princeton University Press: Princeton, N.J.

Möbius, P. J. (1889). *J. J. Rousseau's Krankheitsgeschichte*. F. C. W. Vogel: Leipzig.

Rosen, G. (1967). Emotion and sensibility in ages of anxiety; a comparative historical review. *American Journal of Psychiatry*, **124,** 771–784, 1967.

Rosen, G. (1968). *Madness in Society. Chapters in the Historical Sociology of Mental Illness*. Routledge: London.

Starobinski, J. (1958). *Jean-Jacques Rousseau, la Transparence et l'Obstacle*. Plon: Paris.

Tenenti, A. (1957). *Il Senso della Morte e l'Amore della Vita nel Rinascimento. Francia e Italia*. Einaudi: Torino.

Psychological Medicine, 1975, **5**, 113–124

Culture and schizophrenia[1]

The cross-cultural study of schizophrenia is not a new avenue of research. It was opened almost simultaneously with the early formulations of the concept of schizophrenia and developed in the spirit of a recognition of the relationship between psychopathological phenomena and the sociocultural context, exemplified by the classical studies of Durkheim. Some of the founders of modern European psychiatry visited what were then regarded as 'exotic' cultures and returned with observations which on the whole tended to strengthen their theoretical formulations which were based originally on patient populations in European institutions (for example, Kraepelin in Java, 1904; Bleuler in India, 1930). In spite of a great number of insightful and penetrating observations, the methodological aspects of the early research in schizophrenia in different cultures have been criticized for a number of reasons: observers' limited periods of contact with the foreign culture, frequent reliance on evidence that was no better than anecdotal, 'Eurocentric' assessment of the cultural background against which the features of the disorder were described, and lack of uniformity in the diagnostic criteria of schizophrenia.

The period between the two world wars was characterized by marked advances in cultural anthropology which resulted in attempts at theoretical formulations of the relationship between psychological adjustment and some essential elements of culture. However, there was only a limited degree of collaboration between this discipline and psychiatry, and conspicuously little was added to the knowledge on schizophrenia. At the same time, empirical studies of the ecology of mental disorder utilizing an epidemiological approach—for example, Faris and Dunham's (1939) study of mental illness in Chicago and Ödegaard's (1932) study of psychiatric morbidity among Norwegian immigrants in the USA—were marking milestones on a road which was to attract increasing attention in the decades after the second world war.

The influence of the environment on the disease process had long been recognized by clinical psychiatrists in the individual case, but the impact of these studies consisted in the convincing demonstration that ecological factors were consistently and significantly associated with certain disease characteristics in large populations of schizophrenic patients. The systematic inclusion of an ecological and cultural dimension in the study of schizophrenia in recent decades has been the result of a need that has been appreciated mostly by epidemiologically-oriented psychiatrists. It has led to a renewed interest in the closer collaboration between psychiatry and the social sciences. The leading part in this alliance is now sometimes played by the psychiatric epidemiologist and sometimes by the sociologist or cultural anthropologist: this explains the differences of emphasis in a number of studies and the broad spectrum of theoretical approaches, ranging from a recognition of schizophrenia as a biologically founded disease entity, a result of faulty interpersonal relationships (Bateson *et al.*, 1956), a product of social labelling (Scheff, 1966), or an artefact of society's repressive structure (Laing, 1967).

Most psychiatrists now accept the assumption that the study of the cultural aspects of schizophrenia can provide important clues to the nature of this disorder—that is, its aetiology, pathology, and response to treatment. Before attempting to examine how well this assumption is supported by the known facts, however, we must refer briefly to two difficulties inherent in this kind of inquiry.

In the first place, the scope and content of the concept of culture are difficult to define. Quoting

[1]This editorial is a shortened version of a contribution to a symposium on the biological and behavioural aspects of schizophrenia that was organized by the Interdisciplinary Society of Biological Psychiatry, and held in Amsterdam, 13 September 1974. A full account of the proceedings will be published by De Erven Bohn Publishers, Amsterdam. We are grateful to them and to the editor, Professor Herman M. van Praag, for permission to publish this paper.

Kroeber and Kluchhohn, Lewis (1965) noted that there existed 160 definitions of culture in English. Definitions like that provided by Walter (1952): 'culture is the learned ways of acting and thinking which provide for each individual ready-made and tested solutions for vital life problems . . .' offer little guidance to the variety of meanings, implicitly or explicitly invested in the term culture as used in empirical research. The boundaries between culture, social structure, and economic organization are difficult to demarcate, and in many instances such a demarcation may not be necessary. Moreover, while culture, subculture, social structure, and economic organization are undoubtedly forces influencing man's 'ways of acting and thinking', so also is the physical environment (external and internal) and, especially where the study of disease is concerned, its influence may be so closely interwoven as to render its exclusion from cross-cultural research undesirable. Therefore, at the present stage of our knowledge, it would be premature to pursue too rigorously the differences between cross- or transcultural, multi-ethnic, comparative and generally ecological approaches to mental illness.

Secondly, the differences in the definition and description of schizophrenia should be kept in mind in evaluating findings from cross-cultural research. Most psychiatrists today agree on the core definitions of the disorder given by Kraepelin and Bleuler but there still are significant disagreements on its boundaries, and this can lead to exaggerated differences in the frequency with which the diagnosis is made, as was clearly shown in the US/UK Diagnostic Study (Cooper *et al.*, 1972). In the absence of external criteria for verification, the diagnosis of schizophrenia depends almost entirely on clinical observation and examination which, in cross-cultural research, present serious additional difficulties. The WHO Programme A on standardization of psychiatric diagnosis, classification, and statistics, during which psychiatrists from many countries participated in diagnostic case exercises, outlined areas of agreement as well as of disagreement in making a diagnosis of schizophrenia and other disorders (Shepherd *et al.*, 1968). According to a number of studies (reviewed by Zubin, 1967) the reliability of the diagnosis of schizophrenia, even within one country, can vary significantly. A wider acceptance of the *International Classification of Diseases* and the accompanying *Glossary* of psychiatric disorders will hopefully increase international agreement on the diagnosis of schizophrenia but, at present, the results of studies of schizophrenia in different cultures should be approached with due caution, unless a clear operational definition of the disorder is given. A method of tackling this type of difficulty has been developed in the WHO *Report of the International Pilot Study of Schizophrenia* (IPSS) (1973).

The main findings of transcultural research in schizophrenia can be summarized in terms of (1) incidence and prevalence of the disorder; (2) symptomatology; and (3) course and outcome. Before reviewing these findings, however, we would mention the historical perspective applied to cultural research, and those observations which relate to cultural change.

SCHIZOPHRENIA IN HISTORICAL PERSPECTIVE

Although, according to Zubin (1968), a description of schizophrenia can be found in the ancient Indian text of *Caraka Samhita*, dated 3300 years ago, Jaspers (1963) noted that 'so far as we know schizophrenias were never of importance in the Middle Ages, while in the last few centuries it was precisely these that took striking effect . . .'. The scarcity and the questionable validity of early descriptions of schizophrenia have recently revived hypotheses of a viral origin of the disorder, relating the increased incidence of schizophrenia to the effects of the mass introduction of smallpox vaccination (Torrey and Peterson, 1973).

Retrospective historical studies of schizophrenia necessarily cover a limited time span and usually do not go back further than the 19th century. This limitation is imposed by the difficulty in identifying schizophrenia among the psychotic states that had been described before the diagnostic criteria were laid down for the several syndromes incorporated later into the disease entity of dementia praecox.

In their study of the admissions for psychoses in Massachusetts in 1840–44 and 1940, Goldhamer and Marshall (1953) concluded that the age-specific rates of hospital admissions for schizophrenia did not change significantly over a period of 100 years. By contrast, the prevalence ratio increased markedly, due to the ageing of the population and changing admission policies. In a similar study, carried out in Budapest and comparing the hospitalized psychoses in 1910 and 1960, Varga (1966) noted that both in 1910 and 1960 about one-quarter of the hospitalized patients suffered from schizophrenia but that the proportion of the paranoid forms was smaller in 1910. The schizophrenics at the beginning of the century were characterized by more florid symptomatology than in 1960, but the percentage of severely deteriorating cases in 1910 (16.7%) was not greater than in the 1960 sample. Varya failed to find evidence of an association between schizophrenia and 'social circumstances' in 1910 and concluded that there was 'more similarity than difference' between schizophrenic psychoses occurring in the two different historical periods.

The results of studies such as Goldhamer and Marshall's or Varga's should be approached with caution. The similarities found between rates for schizophrenia across two points in time may well be merely a reflection of the persisting attitude of the psychiatrists toward this disorder or of the stability of the admission policies with regard to schizophrenic patients. The importance of these factors in the evaluation of changes of the rates for psychosis over time has been demonstrated by Shepherd (1957).

SCHIZOPHRENIA AND CULTURAL CHANGE

The occurrence of psychoses among migrants has often been quoted as an example of the mental health hazards associated with change of the cultural environment. However, since Ödegaard's classical study which demonstrated an increased risk of schizophrenia among Norwegian immigrants to the US as compared with the corresponding rate in Norway (Ödegaard, 1932), few studies have produced clear evidence that migration *per se* is associated with a heightened expectancy of schizophrenia and other psychoses. This suggests that some kind of selection may have been responsible for Ödegaard's positive findings. Thus, in a study of all immigrants from Finland, West-, South-, and East-Europe, and a sample of Swedes who contacted the psychiatric services in a Swedish town during six months in 1971, the prevalence of schizophrenia among the migrants was, in fact, lower (4%) than among the sample of the natives (7%), although the former had a higher rate of psychoneurotic disorder (Haavio-Mannila, 1974).

A number of studies have demonstrated that schizophrenic patients tend to concentrate in urban areas (Bloom, 1968) and in city districts of specified socioeconomic characteristics (Faris and Dunham, 1939; Hare, 1956) but the evidence that the processes of urbanization and modernization have as their by-product a higher incidence of schizophrenia is not conclusive. Fifteen years after their initial survey, Lin *et al.* (1969) found a significant increase in the total prevalence of mental disorders in Taiwan (from 9.4 per 1,000 to 17.2 per 1,000). The rate for psychoses, however, showed no increase and there was even a decrease in the frequency of schizophrenia.

The significance of these negative findings is difficult to assess in the light of suggestions (for example, the Papua New Guinea study—Torrey *et al.*, 1974) that the risk for schizophrenia is increased for those rare populations where 'Westernization' interrupts a pre-existing relative cultural isolation.

SCHIZOPHRENIA IN DIFFERENT CULTURES

There are a great number of observations on the occurrence and symptomatology of schizophrenia in different cultures but relatively few studies qualify as truly comparative or cross-cultural.

PREVALENCE AND INCIDENCE

Some of the reported findings in epidemiological surveys of the prevalence of schizophrenia in different cultures are presented in summary form in the Table.

With few exceptions—for example, the very high rate found by Böök (1961) in a Northern Swedish community and the low rate reported by Eaton and Weil (1955) for the Hutterite sect—the data on

TABLE

EPIDEMIOLOGICAL SURVEY DATA ON PREVALENCE OF SCHIZOPHRENIA IN DIFFERENT CULTURES

Country	*Investigator*	*Year of survey*	*Population studied*	*Prevalence (per 1,000)*
S. Korea	Yoo	1956–60	11,974 (rural)	3.8
China	Lin	1946–48	19,931 (mixed)	2.1
Japan	Uchimura*	1940	8,330 (rural)	3.8
	Tsugawa*	1941	2,712 (urban)	2.2
	National Survey	1954	total (census)	2.3
India	Dube	1970	(mixed)	2.17
Iran	Bash and Bash-Liechti	1972	(rural)	2.0–2.1
USA	Lemkau*	1936	55,129 (urban)	2.9
	Roth*	1938	24,804 (rural)	1.7
	Eaton and Weil	1956	8,542 (rural)	1.1
Denmark	Strömgren*	1935	45,930 (rural)	3.3
	Juel-Nielsen and Strömgren	1962	total (census)	1.5
Norway	Bremer*	1944	1,325 (rural)	4.5
Sweden	Böök	1953–54	8,651 (rural)	10.8
	Sjögren	1944	8,736 (rural)	4.6
Germany	Brugger*	1929	37,561 (rural)	1.9
	Brugger*	1930–31	8,628 (rural)	2.5
England	L. Wing *et al.*	1966	175,304 (urban)	3.4
Scotland	Mayer-Gross	1948	56,231 (mixed)	4.2
USSR	Zharikov	1972	175,783 (urban)	5.1†
	Krasik	1965	(urban)	3.1
			(rural)	2.6
Bulgaria	Jablensky *et al.*	1972	140,758 (urban)	2.8

*Quoted from Lin (1960).
†Per 1,000 aged 16+.

the prevalence of schizophrenia appear to be very similar in different cultures.[2] However, the significance of this seeming similarity cannot be assessed without more knowledge concerning the methods, the diagnostic criteria, and the demographic characteristics of the populations on which the surveys were based. Thus, the proportion of patients diagnosed as schizophrenic out of the total reported prevalence of psychiatric disorders in several Asian countries varies between 19.5 and 63.8% (Wulff, 1967). Moreover, similar overall prevalence rates may mask important differences in the incidence, age, and sex distribution of the disorder.

In their survey of mental illness among Formosan aborigines as compared with the Chinese in Taiwan, Rin and Lin (1962) found that, although the life-time prevalence of all mental disorders (except epilepsy) among the aborigines was the same as among the Chinese, the rate for schizophrenia in the former was lower than in the Chinese. Murphy and Raman (1971), in a study of first admissions for schizophrenia in Mauritius, found that the age-specific incidence rates for the total population of the island were very close to those reported in England and Wales.[3] However, there were significant differences between the three major cultural groups on the island—that is, the Indian Moslems, the Hindu Indians, and the non-Indians—the Moslems having the lowest, and the non-Indians the highest incidence rates. A recent study in Papua New Guinea (Torrey *et al.*, 1974) reported a very low prevalence of schizophrenia among the native population, but of special interest were the significant differences in prevalence between geographical regions (.10 and .56 per 1,000) in which the population had had different amounts of contact with Western culture and civilization.

Striking inter-regional differences in the frequency of schizophrenia have also been reported in

[2] Few data are available on the prevalence of schizophrenia in Africa. Tooth (1950) found only 33 cases of schizophrenia in two provinces of the Gold Coast. According to Lambo (1960), out of 906 patients treated at Aro Hospital (Nigeria) in 1957–58, 48.4% were diagnosed as schizophrenic. Leighton *et al.* (1963) described a prevalence of schizophrenia of almost 10 per 1,000 in their study of psychiatric disorders among the Yoruba but their sample was very small (262 cases).

[3] The admission rate for schizophrenia in many communities equals, for practical purposes, population survey results (Ödegaard, 1952).

Europe (for example, in Croatia, Yugoslavia (Crocetti *et al.*, 1971)). Finally, there are several reports of surveys in developing countries which failed to identify schizophrenic patients among the populations studied. Thus, Giel and van Liujk (1969–70) interviewed a sample of 370 in a small Ethiopian village and found a 9.1% prevalence of psychiatric disorders. None of the 36 cases was diagnosed as schizophrenia, but this may have been a consequence of the small sample size or of other relevant factors. Such reports cannot be interpreted as lending support to the assumption that some populations may be free of schizophrenic disorders.

In summary, the existing data on the prevalence and incidence of schizophrenia in different cultures and different subcultures are not conclusive. Differences in the rates of occurrence of the disorder reported in populations of particular epidemiological interest (for example, ecological or genetic isolates, junctions between different cultural influences) have led to a revival of interest in the old question about 'diseases of civilization', to reservations regarding the belief 'that schizophrenia is a universal disorder that occurs with approximately the same prevalence in all societies known to man' and to suggestions that 'schizophrenia may be more common among societies that have had greater exposure to Western influences' (Torrey *et al.*, 1974).

SYMPTOMATOLOGY

Both similarities and differences are reported in the literature with regard to the clinical manifestations of schizophrenia, and it seems that selective emphasis on either could find factual support. According to Murphy and Raman (1971), the symptomatology of the patients in their Mauritius sample corresponded to what is regarded as schizophrenic symptomatology elsewhere. Describing psychoses among the Aivilik Eskimos, Carpenter (1953) wrote that the cases of schizophrenia he observed 'parallel standard Western forms of catatonic schizophrenia'. Pfeiffer (1967), drawing from his long-term observations in Indonesia, concluded that 'the disease pictures are essentially the same as in Central Europe' but nevertheless described in detail at least five characteristic differences: (1) the frequent occurrence of excited-confusional initial states; (2) an admixture of manic features; (3) the rare occurrence of typical catatonic states; (4) the low proportion of paranoid schizophrenic syndromes; and (5) the rarity of systematized delusions. Very similar findings were reported by Wulff (1967) in Vietnam. Lambo (1965) described in Nigeria a characteristic symptom-complex consisting of anxiety, depression, vague hypochondriacal symptoms, bizarre magico-mystical ideas, episodic twilight or confusional states, atypical depersonalization phenomena, emotional lability, and retrospective falsification of hallucinatory experiences. This symptom pattern was the most frequent presenting picture of schizophrenia among the non-literate rural Yoruba, while the literate and urban schizophrenic patients of the same ethnic stock tended to develop symptom patterns approximating to the types described in Europe. Differences in symptom patterns have also been described between Japanese and Caucasian patients (Katz and Sanborn, 1973) and between Japanese and Filipino patients (Enright and Jaeckle, 1963) in Hawaii. Differences of a similar extent have been reported to exist between schizophrenics of Irish and Italian origin in the USA (Opler and Singer, 1956).

Symptomatological differences are probably reflected in the frequency with which certain subtypes of schizophrenia are diagnosed in different cultures. Thus, in Pfeiffer's material, 60.3% of the cases were diagnosed as hebephrenic, 27.2% as catatonic, and only 11.9% as paranoid. Again, out of 74 schizophrenics on a census study in Papeete, Polynesia, 57 had an 'unspecified' form of the disorder, five were catatonic, four hebephrenic, and four paranoid (Bonnaud, 1970).

The question of the relative frequency in different cultures of certain symptoms regarded as characteristic of schizophrenia is of a particular interest. Both Pfeiffer (1967) and Wulff (1967) stress the relative rarity of Schneider's 'first-rank symptoms'[4] in South-East Asia. According to Wulff, the criteria for formal thought disorder are almost never applicable to Vietnamese patients because of cultural factors, or because of the different structure of the language. In Nigerian schizophrenics, the

[4]Auditory hallucinations in the third person discussing the patient; hearing one's own thoughts aloud; experiences of 'thought-broadcasting', 'thought-insertion' or 'thought-withdrawal'; delusions of control.

distinction between primary delusions and their secondary pathoplastic elaboration may be very difficult in practice (Lambo, 1965). Symptoms which in European studies have been described as characteristic of schizophrenia but rare in occurrence—for example, olfactory or haptic hallucinations—seem to be frequent and less 'pathognomonic' in patients from developing countries. By contrast, visual hallucinations, seldom regarded as characteristic of, or frequent in, schizophrenia, are more common among African schizophrenics. Social withdrawal and emotional flattening, both accepted as important symptomatic facets of schizophrenia in the European tradition, appear to be less frequent in some cultures—for example, among the Bahians in Brazil (Stainbrook, 1952), or quite frequent in others (India, Mauritius, Japan) but of less ominous prognostic significance. The frequent occurrence of confusion, visual hallucinations, emotional lability, and disturbances of motility in acute schizophrenic states in cultures as wide apart as Nigeria and Indonesia makes the differential diagnosis from organic disorders a particularly difficult task. It is interesting to note here Lambo's observations (1965) that demonstrable organic disease—for example, trypanosomiasis—in Africa is usually of a slow and insidious onset and in its early stages may mimic the Western stereotype of deteriorating schizophrenia.

The similarities and differences between schizophrenic symptomatology across cultures can be illustrated by two studies in which a more systematic cross-cultural approach was utilized. First, Lorr and Klett (1969) applied their factor-analytically derived typology of psychotic syndromes in a study of a total of 1,100 psychotic patients sampled from six countries (England, France, Germany, Italy, Japan, and Sweden) and came to the conclusion that, allowing for certain variations, the same original six psychotic types could be found among the patients in each country. Secondly, in a questionnaire survey, designed to tap psychiatrists' impressions of the clinical manifestations of schizophrenia in 27 countries, Murphy *et al.* (1963) found (1) that, despite some variation, there was a 'common, agreed method of viewing and reporting on schizophrenia' among psychiatrists from different cultural backgrounds, probably reflecting the common factors between the several psychiatric schools of thought in which the participants in the exercise had been trained, but (2) that 'doubt has been thrown on the picutre which Euro-American psychiatry has built up of the schizophrenic process'. This doubt was the result of the significant differences they observed in the frequency with which certain manifestations of schizophrenia were reported in the different cultures. Thus, visual and tactile hallucinations were most frequently reported in Africa and the Near East, social and emotional withdrawal in Japanese and Okinawan patients, catatonic negativism and stereotypy in East Indian and South American patients. Other differences—for example, the frequency of occurrence of paranoid delusions, delusions of grandeur, and depersonalization—appeared to be more related to differences between urban and rural environments rather than to gross cultural entities.

In summary, most studies indicate that the majority of clinical symptoms and signs commonly associated with schizophrenia can be found to occur in a great variety of cultures but the relative frequency and predominant content of some symptoms vary markedly from one culture to another.

COURSE AND OUTCOME

Several studies indicate that there may be significant differences in the course and outcome of schizophrenic disorders between different cultures and that these differences generally point to a distinction between patients identified in the developing and the developed countries.

The frequency of an acute onset of the psychosis has been noted, among others, by Lambo (1960, 1965) in Africa, Pfeiffer (1967) in Indonesia, and Wulff (1967) in Vietnam. In their study of mental illness among Formosan aborigines, Rin and Lin (1962) observed that 'the psychotic cases tend to follow a relatively favourable clinical course and prognosis, and the schizophrenic reaction was no exception in this regard. If left alone untreated in the aborigine communities, a large proportion of schizophrenic cases recovered within two years'. In the Mauritius study (Raman and Murphy, 1972) a 12 year follow-up of 215 first admissions for schizophrenia showed that 60% of the patients were functioning normally and had suffered no relapses since leaving hospital: the proportion of such cases in a five year follow-up in England and Wales was about 40% (Brown *et al.*, 1966).

It is important to note that prognostic indicators commonly held as predictors of good or poor outcome in schizophrenia—for example, mode of onset, presence of confusional and affective features, etc.—failed to discriminate between types of outcome in the Mauritius sample. On the other hand, the presence of physical illness—for example, malnutrition or anaemia, or psychosomatic symptoms in the initial stage of schizophrenia—appeared to be associated with a trend towards chronicity.

Pfeiffer's observation (1967) that in Indonesia 'chronic defect states . . . appear to be no less frequent than in Europe and essentially correspond to the usual forms' is in agreement with Raman and Murphy's finding that in Mauritius the proportion of deteriorating patients was approximately the same as in England and Wales. The results of these studies suggest that, although in all the cultures in which comparisons were made a roughly similar proportion of schizophrenic illnesses run a deteriorating, chronic course, there is a relative excess of patients in developing countries in whom the disorder has an extremely good prognosis, even if left untreated.

The results from the two year follow-up of the International Pilot Study of Schizophrenia (IPSS) are still being analysed but they seem to indicate that there are differences in the course and outcome of schizophrenic psychoses in the nine countries that were included—Colombia, Czechoslovakia, Denmark, India, Nigeria, Formosa, the Union of Soviet Socialist Republics, the United Kingdom, and the United States of America. The differences, although not all were significant, point to a trend toward a larger proportion of illnesses with a better outcome and milder course in the patients from developing countries as compared with those from developed nations. The significance of this finding and its relationship to other variables within each culture remain to be investigated; the results of the five year follow-up may throw additional light on this phenomenon.

PROSPECTS FOR RESEARCH

There is little doubt that nowadays the study of the cultural aspects of mental disorder should no longer be compared with a botanist's interest in exotic flowers. The expansion of international communication, including exchange of information on health and disease, stimulates eagerness in different societies to learn from each other and makes international comparisons increasingly feasible. In the field of psychiatry the dissatisfaction with the slow progress and the meagre yield of the search for causes of some major disorders, such as schizophrenia, exerts an additional pressure toward widening the scope and framework of research in the hope that important clues may be hidden somewhere beyond any single cultural horizon.

While this may be a legitimate expectation, its realization encounters a number of methodological obstacles which, unless overcome, lead to a state succinctly summarized by Pepper and Redlich (1961):

'Many cross-cultural studies tend to be hopeless conglomerations of disparate observations. Without more systematic and standardised methods of reporting results, it seems premature at this point to hope that factors of universal significance in the aetiology of mental disorders (non-"culture-bound") will be separated out by such studies'.

The observation and description of the minutiae of psychopathology in different cultures and subcultures can be carried on *ad infinitum* without contributing any substance to scientific knowledge in psychiatry, unless a general strategy is defined on the basis of a recognition of the relevance of cross-cultural research to the broad major issues in psychiatry. In this context, the main value of the cross-cultural approach is essentially comparative. It enables the investigator to study, in the setting of a 'natural experiment', the interplay of a wide array of factors—biological, physical, and behavioural—in the variations in the manifestations of mental illness which are due to environmental factors and which can provide valuable guidance to biologically-oriented research in psychiatry. At the same time, a better knowledge of the mechanism through which the environment operates, and of its effects on mental disorder, may eventually help identify those segments of the environment which are amenable to preventive or therapeutic modification.

There are at least three groups of methodological questions related to the cross-cultural approach to mental disorders and, more specifically, to the cross-cultural study of schizophrenia:

1. How should culture be defined and measured? Which classes of psychological phenomena, in health and disease, can be related to cultural differences and which cannot?
2. How should behaviour and its changes be measured reliably? How can schizophrenia be defined operationally and its manifestations be measured?
3. How can the paradigm of the controlled experiment or observation be applied in a transcultural context? How can the rate of occurrence and the manifestations of schizophrenia in different cultures be measured? Which factors should be kept under control?

Even though none of the above questions can be answered adequately at present, a critical examination of the state of the field may point to approaches for future research.

DEFINITION OF CULTURE

Culture is an ill-defined, molar concept, flexible enough to embrace anything from child-rearing practices and kinship systems to the preferred size of automobiles in a given part of the world. Without questioning the value of much cultural-anthropological research for an understanding of the influence of traditional social factors in shaping behaviour patterns in certain isolated and stagnant societies, one is left with the impression that the word 'culture' is overused, as a blanket term, to cover and often to obscure a number of economic, political, social, biological, and physical-environmental factors which can be associated with psychological disturbance. Culture is clearly a multivariate entity, and its study in relation to mental disorder requires both operational definitions of its components and measuring instruments to supersede the uncontrolled observations and anecdotal evidence that are often used by anthropologists.

Progress has been made in studying the relationships between the occurrence of psychosis and some variables belonging to culture. There is a good deal of highly sophisticated research on the associations between schizophrenic and social stratification (Hollingshead and Redlich, 1958; Goldberg and Morrison, 1963), urban ecology (Faris and Dunham, 1939; Hare, 1956; Bloom, 1968; Bagley *et al.*, 1973), and life events and stress (Birley and Brown, 1970). However, there is so far little to suggest a specific link between schizophrenia and such traditional foci of interest in cultural anthropology as the kinship system, child-rearing practices, and prescientific beliefs. The hypothesis of a regression in schizophrenia to archaic forms of thinking and communication which parallel 'normal' phenomena in a 'primitive' society has found little factual support. Attempts to explain the allegedly high frequency of schizophrenia in East Asia as a result of the 'Eastern way of life which is rigidly hierarchical and formal and which prizes and rewards introversion'; the frequency of catatonic states in India as due to the Indian's 'traditional tendency to reject society and the postures adopted by certain types of sanyasi or yogi'; or the 'barrenness of the clinical picture' in Africans by 'the paucity of their cultural and intellectual resources and their difficulties in dealing with abstractions' (Wittkower and Rin, 1965) can hardly be regarded as scientific and are reminiscent of value-judgments which should belong to the past.

Cultures may not be as different as is often assumed in cross-cultural research. Some anthropologists (Hallowell, 1965) believe that the weight of evidence points to a basic unity of man across cultures which is reflected in common personality types, common basic strategies for dealing with stress, and common basic forms of psychological disturbance. This is supported by empirical evidence from recent cross-cultural studies, such as Inkeles' study of the 'syndrome of modernity' in six different parts of the world (1973) and by a mass of psychiatric research which stresses the 'cultural invariance in primary symptomatology' (Zubin and Kietzman, 1966) or the 'worldwide similarity of relationships between psychopathological syndromes and social class' (Dohrenwend and Dohrenwend, 1967).

On the other hand, variations within a particular culture may be as large as the differences between cultures. This important aspect of the problem has received comparatively little attention in past research, much of which has been oriented primarily toward enunciating cross-cultural differences. If a multivariate approach to the study of culture and mental disorder is to be utilized, then a wide range of variables should be identified and defined, extending from social and economic factors or types of stress and stress-reducing devices characteristic of specified segments of the society, to infant mortality, gene pools, or degrees of exposure to noxious environmental agents. Appropriate measuring tools for these variables can be developed, at different levels of universality—'culture-bound', 'culture-fair', and 'culture-free' according to Zubin (1967). Approaches of this kind have been used in a number of studies (Venables and Wing, 1962; Rin *et al.*, 1966; Murphy, 1968), which have attempted to link epidemiological or clinical findings to specific measurable social and biological variables.

FORM, CONTENT, AND CAUSATION

The study of the variations in the occurrence and manifestations of schizophrenia, including variations in a cross-cultural context, depends to a significant degree on two kinds of important theoretical distinctions inherent in classical European psychiatry; between form and content of psychopathological phenomena (Jaspers, 1963) and between pathogenic and pathoplastic factors in causation (Birnbaum, 1974). These distinctions form a logical frame of reference that has been applied in many studies which have indicated a cross-cultural similarity in the basic forms of symptomatology of schizophrenia (possibly pointing to a common pathogeny) and a cultural variability in the content of symptoms, accountable for by the operation of cultural pathoplastic factors.

This standpoint has been criticized by those research workers who stand closer to the theory of cultural relativism and believe that each culture produces its own forms of disturbance. According to this view, similarities in the forms of symptomatology in schizophrenia are only superficial and disappear on closer scrutiny, since 'the usefulness of the Kraepelinian diagnostic system and its derivatives is limited by its culturally narrow origins' (Enright and Jaeckle, 1963). Such an argument can be answered in the words of a Nigerian faith-healer who, when asked by a well-known psychiatrist (Leighton, 1965) why he used the words 'delusions' and 'hallucinations' in describing one of his patients, replied:

> 'Well, when this man came here he was standing right where you see him now and he thought he was in Abeokuta . . . he thought I was his uncle and he thought God was speaking to him from the clouds. Now I don't know what you call that in the United States, but here we consider that these are hallucinations and delusions!'

The literature on the cross-cultural aspects of schizophrenia contains no evidence that in any culture does this disorder manifest forms of symptomatology which cannot be accounted for by the definition and classification of schizophrenia as laid down by Kraepelin and Bleuler. Moreover, regardless of differences in the 'baseline criteria of normality and abnormality' in different cultures (Katz and Sanborn, 1973), the evidence suggests that psychopathological behaviour is reliably recognized by the members of each culture (Kiev, 1972). This may not always apply to individual symptoms—for example, hearing 'voices' can be a 'normal' experience in certain subcultural groups—but even in such settings the total 'Gestalt' of psychopathological disturbance is recognized by the members of the group.

The results of recent studies—for example, the IPSS—suggest that it may be possible to develop a transculturally applicable definition of the syndrome of schizophrenia, compatible with the 'classical' concept of the disorder, and based on symptoms which are universally found and least dependent on the psychiatrists' own cultural and personal bias. The application of this definition would in no way diminish the importance of studying pathoplastic influences on the content or threshold of symptoms. If this definition could be supplemented further by cross-culturally applicable measures of primary versus secondary handicaps in schizophrenia (Wing and Brown, 1970), it would represent a major step forward in the methodology of epidemiologically-oriented cross-cultural research in schizophrenia.

METHODS

Even if a reliable operational definition of schizophrenia is available, and even if measurable variables are specified within a given cultural context, cross-cultural research may still yield uncertain results, unless the essential conditions of the controlled experiment or observation are met in the design of the study.

The present methodologies of cross-cultural research are far removed from the simplicity of design characteristic of the laboratory experiment, which may never be fully attainable in so highly complex a field. However, the consistent application of the epidemiological method in cross-cultural studies may be the best approximation to the paradigm of the controlled observation. The need for standardized and reliable assessment in psychiatric epidemiological research requires the development of a set of cross-culturally applicable methods, a set of cross-culturally applicable instruments, and the training of research workers capable of utilizing them in a comparable and reliable way (Sartorius, 1973).

For example, the method of case-finding, which is a recurrent methodological problem even in studies in the developed parts of the world, can present serious difficulties in many developing countries where population registers are incomplete or non-existent and where many psychotic patients never come to medical attention. The difficulty is well-illustrated by the phenomenon of the African 'vagrant psychotics' who eventually escape the net of epidemiological surveys, however thoroughly organized after the usual European or American model (Harding, 1973).

Another source of difficulties is associated with the techniques of observation and interviewing. Even allowing for linguistic problems, the interviewing technique itself should be carefully examined for its applicability in settings where, for example, the patient may expect to be told, rather than asked, by the medical man about his problems. It may be advantageous if the patient is approached by a research worker from his own culture, and the standardization of research instruments should go hand in hand with the training of psychiatrists from various cultures in the use of such instruments.

If the concept of culture embraces a great variety of factors then many different kinds of hypotheses can be evoked to explain and test further the significance of such findings as the reported differences in incidence and prevalence, symptomatology, course, and outcome of schizophrenia in various cultures. Thus, a difference in the incidence rate, if valid, could be due to demographic factors—for example, population in a high-risk age-group; genetic factors, environmental factors—for example, hypothesized viruses; or social factors which affect pathoplastically the rate of clinical manifestation of mild or latent forms of the disorder.

The number of possible explanations for differences in prevalence can be even greater. A variety of social factors have been shown in previous studies to affect the course of schizophrenic illnesses, and some cultures may be able to provide more readily appropriate social niches for persons suffering from the primary handicaps of schizophrenia, thus attenuating the severity of the resulting secondary handicaps. On the other hand, the greater proportion of schizophrenic disorders having a milder course and better prognosis in certain cultures may be associated with an increased infant mortality for carriers of the severe, and presumably genetically-founded, forms of the disease.

Hypotheses of this type are related to the notion of schizophrenia as a biologically rooted disease, but it should be equally possible to test, in a cross-cultural context, hypotheses of schizophrenia as a learned response to psychosocial stress. A methodology of cross-cultural research in schizophrenia, relying on an epidemiological approach and approximating as an equivalent to the famous Koch's postulates, would appear to be a promising strategy, open to extensions into the fields of both the social sciences and biological psychiatry.

Finally, improvements are needed in the way of reporting research findings. Few reports give adequate attention to the description of study design or population characteristics and methods, and results are not always presented in a form which would permit of reanalysis or replication. Secondary analysis or reanalysis of data in the light of new findings or new hypotheses can be an important research tool in the field of cross-cultural psychiatry where replication of studies is too costly or difficult to organize. A systematic re-evaluation of the field, or the 'study of studies', could constitute a significant aid to this objective.

A. JABLENSKY AND N. SARTORIUS

The paragraph on the International Pilot Study of Schizophrenia is based on the authors' participation in that study, a project sponsored by W.H.O., and funded by W.H.O., the National Institute of Mental Health (U.S.), and the participating field research centres. (For list of all investigators and staff see W.H.O. (1973)).

REFERENCES

Bagley, C., Jacobson, S., and Palmer, C. (1973). Social structure and the ecological distribution of mental illness, suicide, and delinquency. *Psychological Medicine*, **3**, 177–187.

Bash, K. W., and Bash-Liechti, J. (1972). Psychiatrische Epidemiologie in Iran. In *Perspektiven der heutigen Psychiatrie*. Ed.: H. E. Ehrhardt. Gerhards: Frankfurt.

Bateson, G., Jackson, D. D., Haley, J., and Weakland, J. (1956). Toward a theory of schizophrenia. *Behavioral Science*, **1**, 251–264.

Birley, J. L. T., and Brown, G. W. (1970). Crises and life changes preceding the onset of relapse of acute schizophrenia: clinical aspects. *British Journal of Psychiatry*, **116**, 327–333.

Birnbaum, K. (1974). The making of a psychosis. In *Themes and Variations in European Psychiatry*, pp. 197–238. Edited by S. R. Hirsch and M. Shepherd. Wright: Bristol.

Bleuler, E. (1930). Quoted from Wulff, E. (1967).

Bloom, B. L. (1968). An ecological analysis of psychiatric hospitalizations. *Multivariate Behavioral Research*, **3**, 423–463.

Böök, J. A. (1961). Genetical etiology in mental illness. In *Causes of Mental Disorders: A Review of Epidemiological Knowledge, 1959*, pp. 14–50. Proceedings of a round table, New York, 1959. Milbank Memorial Fund: New York.

Bonnaud, M. (1970). Enquête sur la santé mentale en Polynesie française. *Annales Médico-Psychologiques*, **128**, I, 375–421.

Brown, G. W., Bone, M., Dalison, B., and Wing, J. K. (1966). *Schizophrenia and Social Care*. Maudsley Monogr. 17. O.U.P.: London.

Carpenter, E. S. (1953). Witch-fear among the Aivilik Eskimos. *American Journal of Psychiatry*, **110**, 194–199.

Cooper, J. E., Kendell, R. E., Gurland, B. J., Sharpe, L., Copeland, J. R. M., and Simon, R. (1972). *Psychiatric Diagnosis in New York and London*. Maudsley Monographs No. 20. Oxford University Press: London.

Crocetti, G. M., Lemkau, P. V., Kulčar, Ž, and Kesić, B. (1971). Selected aspects of the epidemiology of psychoses in Croatia, Yugoslavia. 3. *American Journal of Epidemiology*, **94**, 126–134.

Dohrenwend, B. S., and Dohrenwend, B. P. (1967). Field studies of social factors in relation to three types of psychological disorder. *Journal of Abnormal Psychology*, **72**, 369–378.

Dube, K. C. (1970). A study of prevalence and biosocial variables in mental illness in a rural and an urban community in Uttar Pradesh—India. *Acta Psychiatrica Scandinavica*, **46**, 327–359.

Eaton, J. W., and Weil, R. J. (1955). *Culture and Mental Disorders*. Free Press: Glencoe, Ill.

Enright, J. B., and Jaeckle, W. R. (1963). Psychiatric symptoms and diagnosis in two subcultures. *International Journal of Social Psychiatry*, **9**, 12–17.

Faris, R. E. L., and Dunham, H. W. (1939). *Mental Disorders in Urban Areas*. University of Chicago Press: Chicago.

Giel, R., and Liujk, J. N., van (1969/70). Psychiatric morbidity in a rural village in South-Western Ethiopia. *International Journal of Social Psychiatry*, **16**, 63–71.

Goldberg, E. M., and Morrison, S. L. (1963). Schizophrenia and social class. *British Journal of Psychiatry*, **109**, 785.

Goldhamer, H., and Marshall, A. W. (1953). *Psychosis and Civilization*. Free Press: Glencoe, Ill.

Haavio-Mannila, E., and Stenius, K. (1974). *Mental Health Problems and New Ethnic Minorities in Sweden*. Research Report No. 202. Institute of Sociology, University of Helsinki: Helsinki.

Hallowell, A. I. (1965). Hominid evolution, cultural adaptation and mental dysfunctioning. In *Transcultural Psychiatry*, pp. 26–61. Edited by A. V. S. de Reuck and R. Potter. CIBA Foundation Symposium. Churchill: London.

Harding, T. (1973). Psychosis in a rural West African community. *Social Psychiatry*, **8**, 198–203.

Hare, E. H. (1956). Mental illness and social conditions in Bristol. *Journal of Mental Science*, **102**, 349–357.

Hollingshead, A. B., and Redlich, F. C. (1958). *Social Class and Mental Illness*. Wiley: New York.

Inkeles, A. (1973). Six-country study on the effects of modernization. In *International Collaboration in Mental Health*. Edited by B. S. Brown and E. F. Torrey. U.S. Department of Health, Education, and Welfare. Publications No. 73-9120. Government Printing Office: Washington.

Jablensky, A., Temkov, I., and Boyadjieva, M. (1974). *Prevalence of Mental Disorders and Patterns of Psychiatric Care in an Urban Area*. (To be published.)

Jaspers, K. (1963). *General Psychopathology*, 7th edn. Manchester University Press: Manchester.

Juel-Nielsen, N., and Strömgren, E. (1963). Five years later. A comparison between census studies of patients in psychiatric institutions in Denmark in 1957 and 1972. *Acta Jutlandica*, **35**.

Katz, M. M., and Sanborn, K. O. (1973). Multiethnic studies of psychopathology and normality in Hawaii. In *International Collaboration in Mental Health*. Edited by B. S. Brown and E. F. Torrey. U.S. Department of Health, Education, and Welfare. Publications No. 73-9120. Government Printing Office: Washington.

Kiev, A. (1972). *Transcultural Psychiatry*. Penguin: London.

Kraepelin, E. (1904). Comparative psychiatry. In Hirsch, S. R., and Shepherd, M. (eds.) (1974). *Themes and Variations in European psychiatry*. Wright: Bristol.

Krasik, E. D. (1965). The comparative epidemiology of schizophrenia in towns and in rural areas. *Zhurnal Nevropatologii i psikhiatrii*, **65**, 608–616.

Laing, R. D. (1967). *The Politics of Experience*. Penguin: Harmondsworth.

Lambo, T. A. (1960). Further neuropsychiatric observations in Nigeria. *British Medical Journal*, **2**, 1696–1704.

Lambo, T. A. (1965). Schizophrenic and borderline states. In *Transcultural Psychiatry*, pp. 62–83. Edited by A. V. S. de Reuck, and R. Porter. CIBA Foundation Symposium. Churchill: London.

Leighton, A. H. (1965). Cultural change and psychiatric disorder. In *Transcultural Psychiatry*, pp. 216–235. Edited by A. V. S. de Reuck and R. Porter. CIBA Foundation Symposium. Churchill: London.

Leighton, A. H., Lambo, T. A., Hughes, C. C., Leighton, D. C., Murphy, J. M., and Macklin, D. B. (1963). *Psychiatric Disorder Among the Yoruba.* Cornell University Press: Ithaca, New York.

Lewis, Sir A. (1965). Chairman's opening remarks. In *Transcultural Psychiatry*, pp. 1–3. Edited by A. V. S. de Reuck and R. Porter. CIBA Foundation Symposium, Churchill: London.

Lin, T. (1959). Effects of urbanization on mental health. *International Social Science Journal*, **11**, 24–33.

Lin, T. (1960). *Reality and Vision: A Report of the First Asian Seminar on Mental Health and Family Life.* Bureau of Printing: Manila.

Lin, T., Rin, H., Yeh, E., Hsu, C., and Chu, H. (1969). Mental disorders in Taiwan, fifteen years later; a preliminary report. In *Mental Health Research in Asia and the Pacific*, pp. 66–91. Edited by W. Caudill and T. Lin. East-West Center Press: Honolulu.

Lorr, M., and Klett, C. J. (1969). Psychotic behavioral types. A cross-cultural comparison. *Archives of General Psychiatry*, **20**, 592–597.

Mayer-Gross, W. (1948). Mental health survey in a rural area. A preliminary report. *Eugenics Review*, **40**, 140–148.

Murphy, H. B. M. (1968). Cultural factors in the genesis of schizophrenia. In *Transmission of Schizophrenia*, pp. 137–153. Edited by D. Rosenthal and S. S. Kety. Pergamon Press: Oxford.

Murphy, H. B. M., and Raman, A. C. (1971). The chronicity of schizophrenia in indigenous tropical peoples. Results of a twelve-year follow-up survey in Mauritius. *British Journal of Psychiatry*, **118**, 489–497.

Murphy, H. B. M., Wittkower, E. D., Fried, J., and Ellenberger, H. (1963). A cross-cultural survey of schizophrenic symptomatology. *International Journal of Social Psychiatry*, **9**, 237–249.

Nationwide Prevalence Survey of Mental Disorders in Japan (1954). Japan. Ministry of Health and Welfare: Tokyo.

Ödegaard, Ö. (1932). Emigration and insanity: a study of mental disease among Norwegian-born population in Minnesota. *Acta Psychiatrica et Neurologica Scandinavica*, Suppl. 4.

Ödegaard, Ö. (1952). The incidence of mental diseases as measured by census investigations versus admission statistics. *Psychiatric Quarterly*, **26**, 212–218.

Opler, M. K., and Singer, J. L. (1956). Ethnic differences in behavior and psychopathology: Italian and Irish. *International Journal of Social Psychiatry*, **2**, 11–23.

Pepper, M. P., and Redlich, F. C. (1961). Social psychiatry. *American Journal of Psychiatry*, **117**, 610–615.

Pfeiffer, W. M. (1967). Psychiatrische Besonderheiten in Indonesien. In *Beiträge zur vergleichenden Psychiatrie*, pp. 102–142. Edited by N. Petrilowitsch. *Aktuelle Fragen des Psychiatrie und Neurologie*, Vol. 5, Bibliotheca Psychiatrica et Neurologica, No. 132. Karger: Basel, New York.

Raman, A. C., and Murphy, H. B. M. (1972). Failure of traditional prognostic indicators in Afro-Asian psychotics: results of a long-term follow-up survey. *Journal of Nervous and Mental Disease*, **154**, 238–247.

Rin, H., Chu, H.-M., and Lin, T. (1966). Psychophysiological reactions of a rural and suburban population in Taiwan. *Acta Psychiatrica Scandinavica*, **42**, 410–473.

Rin, H., and Lin, T.-Y. (1962). Mental illness among Formosan aborigines as compared with the Chinese in Taiwan. *Journal of Mental Science*, **108**, 134–146.

Sartorius, N. (1973). Culture and the epidemiology of depression. *Psychiatria, Neurologia et Neurochirurgia*, **76**, 479–487.

Scheff, T. J. (1966). *Being Mentally Ill.* Aldine: Chicago.

Shepherd, M. (1957). *A Study of the Major Psychoses in an English County.* Maudsley Monographs No. 3. Chapman and Hall: London.

Shepherd, M., Brooke, E. M., Cooper, S. E., and Lin, T. (1968). An experimental approach to psychiatric diagnosis. An international study. *Acta Psychiatrica Scandinavica*, **441**, Suppl. 201.

Stainbrook, E. (1952). Some characteristics of the psychopathology of schizophrenic behavior in Bahian society. *American Journal of Psychiatry*, **109**, 330–335.

Tooth, G. (1950). *Studies in Mental Illness in the Gold Coast.* Colonial Research Publications No. 6. HMSO: London.

Torrey, E. F. (1973). Is schizophrenia universal? An open question. *Schizophrenia Bulletin*, No. 7, 53–59.

Torrey, E. F., and Peterson, M. R. (1973). Slow and latent viruses in schizophrenia. *Lancet*, **2**, 22–24.

Torrey, R. F., Torrey, B. B., and Burton-Bradley, B. G. (1974). The epidemiology of schizophrenia in Papua New Guinea. *American Journal of Psychiatry*, **131**, 567–573.

Varga, E. (1966). *Changes in the Symptomatology of Psychotic Patterns.* Akadémiai Kiadó: Budapest.

Venables, P. H., and Wing, J. K. (1962). Level of arousal and the subclassification of schizophrenia. *Archives of General Psychiatry*, **7**, 114–119.

Walter, P. A. F. (1952). *Race and Culture Relations.* McGraw-Hill: New York.

Wing, J. K., and Brown, G. W. (1970). *Institutionalism and Schizophrenia.* Cambridge University Press: London.

Wing, J. K., Cooper, J. E., and Sartorius, N. (1974). *Measurement and Classification of Psychiatric Symptoms.* Cambridge University Press: London.

Wing, L., Wing, J. K., Hailey, A., Bahn, A. K., Smith, H. E., and Baldwin, J. A. (1967). The use of psychiatric services in three urban areas: an international case register study. *Social Psychiatry*, **2**, 158–167.

Wittkower, E. D. (1969). Perspectives of transcultural psychiatry. *International Journal of Psychiatry*, **8**, 811–824.

Wittkower, E. D., and Rin, H. (1965). Transcultural psychiatry. *Archives of General Psychiatry*, **13**, 397–394.

World Health Organization (1973). *Report of the International Pilot Study of Schizophrenia*, vol. 1. WHO: Geneva.

Wulff, E. (1967). Psychiatrischer Bericht aus Vietnam. In *Beiträge sur vergleichenden Psychiatrie*, pp. 1–84. Edited by N. Petrilowitsch. *Aktuelle Fragen des Psychiatrie und Neurologie*, vol. 5. Bibliothea Psychiatrica et Neurologica, No. 132. Karger: Basel/New York, 1–84.

Yoo, P. S. (1962). Mental disorders in Korean rural communities. In *Proceedings, Third World Congress of Psychiatry*, Montreal, 1961. Vol. 2, pp. 1305–1309. McGill University Press: Montreal.

Zharikov, N. M. (1972). Epidemiology of schizophrenia. In *Schizofreniya. Mul' ti distsiplinarnoe Issledovanie*, pp. 186–224. Edited by A. V. Snezhnevskii. Meditsina: Moscow.

Zubin, J. (1967). Classification of the behavior disorders. *Annual Review of Psychology*, **18**, 373–406.

Zubin, J. (1968). *Classification of Human Behavior.* Paper read before the Canadian Psychological Association Symposium on Measurement, Classification and Prediction of Human Behaviour (mimeograph), Calgary, Alberta, 1968.

Zubin, J., and Kietzman, M. L. (1966). A cross-cultural approach to classification in schizophrenia and other mental disorders. In *Psychopathology of Schizophrenia*, pp. 482–514. Edited by P. H. Hoch and J. Zubin. Grune and Stratton: New York.

Psychological Medicine, 1976, 6, 7–13

Hallucinations

Hallucinatory phenomena were recognized as long ago as the 4th century by Macarus and, until fairly recent times, were generally credited with occult significance which gave rise to a belief in the magical powers of the percipient. Such experiences have had a considerable effect on the lives of the hallucinators – the hysterical crisis of Paul (who saw Jesus in a vision) was instrumental in his acceptance of the new faith; Socrates had his 'daemon' which warned and guided him from within; while Joan of Arc's visions and voices played a memorable role in altering the course of history. But it was the decline of the demoniacal model during the 18th and 19th centuries and its replacement by the medical model in the realm of insanity which led to a more objective evaluation of hallucinatory significance and an increasing concern with phenomenology and definition.

The definition of a true hallucination has posed problems, both of inclusion and exclusion. On the one hand, observers have been keen to reach agreement on a set of positive defining criteria, while on the other to distinguish true hallucinations from similar kinds of non-veridical perceptual experience. The latter concern has given rise to the differentiation of true hallucinations from illusion (Esquirol, 1838), from pseudohallucinations (Kandinsky, 1885), from hypnagogic images (Maury, 1848) and from a large variety of other types of mental imagery. Horowitz (1970) has proposed that various kinds of hallucinatory and imagery experiences can be distinguished and classified on four dimensions: in terms of their vividness, the context in which they occur, their content, and the degree of interaction with veridical perception.

From the viewpoint of positive defining criteria of a true hallucination, three such criteria would probably be considered essential by modern observers: namely (1) percept-like experience in the absence of an external stimulus, (2) percept-like experience which has the full force and impact of a real perception, and (3) percept-like experience which is unwilled, occurs spontaneously and cannot be readily controlled by the percipient. Each of these three criteria also serves to differentiate a true hallucination from other types of similar experience. The criterion of 'absence of an external basis' is an obvious one and has been included in nearly every definition of the phenomenon since Esquirol. It serves to separate the different experiences of hallucination and illusion. The second criterion concerning the realistic nature of the experience has gained prominence in recent times. Jaspers (1911, 1963) distinguished true hallucinations from imagery and pseudo-hallucinations on the grounds that the latter occur in 'inner subjective space' while the former have an objective reality of their own. Sedman (1966) used similar criteria in distinguishing 'inner voices' which are a form of pseudo-hallucination from those that can be considered true hallucinations. In a series of recent phenomenological studies, Aggernaes (1972*a*, *b*; Aggernaes & Myeborg, 1972) has shown that hallucinatory experiences can be reliably classified on seven specific and relatively subtle dimensions of reality characteristics, including that of involuntarity. Moreover, he has demonstrated that the true hallucinations of chronic schizophrenic patients are akin to actual perceptions in having positive reality characteristics and in being clearly discriminable from imagined objects and people. The third criterion of 'lack of control' on the part of the percipient is important for differentiating hallucinatory experiences from examples of memory and imagination imagery. The latter have been discussed at length by Richardson (1969).

HALLUCINATIONS IN NORMAL INDIVIDUALS

It has long been recognized that hallucination-like experiences can occur in normal healthy individuals under certain conditions. Sir Francis Galton (1883), who collected a series of such examples from his colleagues and relatives, noted that fasting, lack of sleep and solitary musing were often 'conducive to visions'. The relationship of such experiences to severe food and water deprivation has become a matter of common, universally accepted folklore: the severely dehydrated refugee crawling across the desert under a blazing hot sun is expected to hallucinate an oasis. Some less extreme examples of such a relationship have been described and discussed by Forrer (1960), who concluded: 'The circumstance of hunger and thirst which accompanied each benign hallucination suggests an ultimate physiological origin for the phenomenon itself.' There are two particular circumstances, thought to be conducive to the production of hallucinations in normal individuals, which have received particular attention in recent times: namely sensory deprivation and hallucinogenic drugs.

Sensory deprivation procedures involve an attempt to minimize as far as possible all external sensory stimulation or to reduce the patterning of such stimulation without abolishing it completely (the latter procedure being generally referred to as perceptual deprivation). The first report of such a procedure, which emanated from McGill University (Bexton *et al.*, 1954), indicated that hallucinations were experienced by nearly all individuals subjected to it. However, it has become clear that the definition of a hallucination employed in this and most of the other early studies was fairly loose and included many kinds of perceptual and imagery experiences. Zuckerman & Cohen (1964) carried out a systematic survey of approximately 40 sensory deprivation studies in which adequate and clear information had been provided concerning the nature of hallucinatory-like reports. They opted to use the more neutral terminology of Murphy *et al.* (1962), who refer to such visual experiences as 'reported visual sensations' (RVS) and such auditory experiences as 'reported auditory sensations' (RAS). Furthermore, since both kinds of experience can run the whole gamut from meaningless sensations such as flashes of light, spots, simple geometric patterns, etc., to meaningful integrated scenes, they subdivided both report categories into type A (meaningless sensations) and type B (meaningful, integrated sensations). The general impression they give is that the type B reports come far closer to true hallucinatory experiences than those of type A, although the criterion of a complete reality experience may still be lacking in many of them. The median percentage incidence of the two kinds of type B reports was: RVS, 19%; RAS, 15%. However, the actual incidence of true hallucinations as opposed to illusions, imagery and pseudo-hallucinations may be even lower, as is suggested by the study of Leff (1968). One of the interesting features observed in many of the sensory deprivation studies is that of a clear progression over time from type A to type B reports although the total number of reports does not necessarily increase with the length of the isolation period.

The hallucinogenic effects of drugs such as psilocybin, mescalin and LSD-25 have aroused considerable interest among investigators in the hope that they would provide an ideal model for studying the functional psychoses. Most of the work in this area has therefore involved phenomenological comparison between the drug-induced and the spontaneously occurring psychotic state. Such comparisons have tended to highlight their differences rather than their similarities. Most observers agree that the perceptual disturbances induced by ingestion of mescaline and LSD-25 are predominantly visual in nature, reports of auditory experiences being particularly rare (Bliss & Clark, 1962; Feinberg, 1962; Malitz *et al.*, 1962); the reverse is generally held to be true for schizophrenia.

The visual perceptual disturbances reported after administration of these drugs show a similar variation to those encountered with sensory deprivation. They appear to range along a continuum from simple, meaningless and unstructured sensations (e.g. distortions of the colour, shape and size of objects), through more structured simple sensations which Klüver (1942) described as being invariably present and referred to as 'form-constants' (e.g. various geometric shapes, lattice-work, cobwebs, etc.), to the experience of meaningful and integrated objects and scenes. As with sensory deprivation, many investigators have observed a progression in the complexity of visual disturbances over time and in relation to dosage level. However, it is the former two kinds of experience which predominate in the drug-induced state, the experience of meaningful and integrated perceptions having a relatively low incidence. As with sensory deprivation, the experience of true hallucination under mescalin and LSD-5 intoxication is probably fairly infrequent.

Another point of difference between drug-induced and schizophrenic hallucinations has been uncovered by Aggernaes (1972*b*). He has demonstrated that, whereas the hallucinations of chronic schizophrenic patients have relatively clear-cut, stable and positive reality characteristics akin to those of actual perceptions, the reality characteristics of LSD hallucinations are more ephemeral and unstable. There is, however, some evidence of overlap between the two kinds of experience. Langs & Barr (1968) found that, while the experiential reports and behaviour of normal subjects receiving LSD in no way resembled those of an undifferentiated schizophrenic group, approximately 25% of the LSD subjects exhibited similar experiences to a paranoid schizophrenic subgroup. This LSD subgroup was characterized on personality tests and questionnaires as having 'paranoid tendencies'. Langs & Barr summarized this important finding in the following terms: 'The drug response appears, then, to be an extension of pre-existing tendencies, expressed openly in the altered state.'

HALLUCINATIONS IN ORGANIC DISORDERS

Hallucinations occur in a wide range of physical and organic diseases, occasionally on their own but more commonly as part of a generalized psychotic state. Although no single, therapeutically created lesion, reported by the neurosurgical community, has been found to be invariably and exclusively associated with the production of hallucinatory activity, various sources of evidence suggest that the temporal cortex and related structures may play a more important role than others.

One piece of evidence comes from the clinical examination of patients with focal epileptic lesions. Hallucinations are frequently present in temporal lobe epilepsy, during either the aura or the attack itself, while being relatively uncommon in epileptic states of other origin. As with the hallucinatory experiences which can be induced in normal individuals, those of temporal lobe epilepsy vary in structure and complexity from simple, elementary sensations and patterns to those of more meaningful and integrated percepts. In general it appears that the more posterior the lesion in the temporal cortex, the more complex and structured the hallucinatory experience. (Mayer-Gross *et al.*, 1969).

A second source of evidence comes from the study of drug/lesion interactions. Baldwin *et al.* (1959) administered LSD-25 to a group of chimpanzees, with the consequent production of bizarre, psychotic-like episodes in the animals. These episodes were not affected by lobectomies, either unilateral or bilateral, of the frontal, parietal or occipital lobes, nor by unilateral temporal lobectomies. But they did not occur after bilateral temporal lobectomies. The existence of an intact temporal cortex (although not necessarily a healthy one) appeared to be required for the production of psychotic-like behaviour, presumably including some hallucinatory activity.

The third source of evidence, and the one which has inspired the greatest amount of interest, comes from studies involving direct electrical stimulation of the human brain under local anaesthesia. Penfield and his associates (Penfield & Rasmussen, 1950; Penfield & Jasper, 1954; Penfield & Perot, 1963) have observed that meaningful visual and auditory hallucinations occurred only with electrical stimulation in or near the temporal lobe. Similar results have been obtained by other workers (Mahl *et al.*, 1964; Horowitz & Adams, 1970). Furthermore, a similar response has been observed in one ethically questionable study (Ishibashi *et al.*, 1964) in anatomically healthy brains as opposed to those of patients undergoing surgery for intractable temporal lobe epilepsy.

One important feature of these direct electrical stimulation studies is that hallucinatory experiences cannot be induced in all patients. In fact only 40 out of a total of 520 of Penfield's epileptic patients (i.e. 7·7%) reported such experiences. Nor can hallucinations be reliably produced by repeated stimulation of identical structures in the same patients (e.g. Horowitz & Adams, 1970). This kind of observation is seemingly incompatible with Penfield's thesis that the mechanism is a normal one involving the direct activation of stored records. The alternative explanation offered by other workers (e.g. Mahl), namely that of an indirect effect mediated by an altered state of consciousness, would seem at present to be more likely.

HALLUCINATIONS IN FUNCTIONAL PSYCHOTIC DISORDERS

While hallucinations are known to occur in all the major functional psychotic states, it is generally believed that the phenomenological characteristics of such hallucinations vary according to the diagnostic category of the patient and that, as a result, the nature of the hallucinatory experience has a particular diagnostic significance. A number of statements are often made to this effect. First, that auditory hallucinations are common in schizophrenia while visual hallucinations are rare. The evidence from systematic investigations is overwhelming in favour of this proposition. Secondly, that the opposite pattern is true for patients suffering from affective disorders and organic brain syndromes: and, thirdly, that auditory hallucinations generally, and certain types in particular, are characteristic of schizophrenia to the point of being pathognomic. The evidence relating to these latter two contentions is conflicting.

A number of American studies have produced evidence which is contrary to both the modality-specific and form specific notions of hallucinations in schizophrenia and the affective disorders (Goodwin *et al.*, 1971). On the other hand, the ongoing World Health Organization study of schizophrenia (WHO, 1973) has shown that there is a high incidence of auditory hallucinations among a core or central group of schizophrenic patients (74%) in general, and that two of Schneider's first rank types in particular (i.e. third-person voices and running commentaries) are highly discriminatory for a diagnosis of schizophrenia. This conflict between findings may be a function of two factors. First, it may stem from the broader conception of schizophrenia and the narrower conception of affective disorder employed in the United States compared with Europe (see Cooper *et al.*, 1969). Alternatively, it may depend on whether the conception of schizophrenia employed in diagnosis is fundamentally that of Schneider (1959) or that of Bleuler (1911). If the Schneiderian conception is adopted, in which certain forms of auditory hallucinations are considered first-rank symptoms, then a high correlation between these and a diagnosis of schizophrenia is to be expected. If, on the other hand, Bleuler's conception involving auditory hallucinations as accessory symptoms is used, then the correlation between the type of hallucination and the diagnosis of schizophrenia is likely to be somewhat diluted.

THEORIES OF THE HALLUCINATORY MECHANISM

Many theories have been proposed to account for the appearance in consciousness of hallucinatory-like phenomena, including dreams. These range from purely psychoanalytic conceptions such as 'regression', on the one hand, to fairly specific neurophysiological conceptions on the other. A few of the more general, explicitly stated models will now be considered.

One such model is the 'neurophysiological dissociation' theory of Marrazzi. Using electrodes to measure evoked cortical potentials in the exposed cortex of the cat, Marrazzi (1962) found that LSD-25 produced inhibition of the association areas without affecting the primary visual cortex. On this basis he proposed that hallucinogenic drugs have their effect by producing a functional dissociation between the primary receiving cortex and the association areas, this loss of control of the latter over the former being responsible for the hallucinatory experience. In more recent studies, Marrazzi and his coworkers have been able to quantify the behavioural effects of this functional dissociation in both the visual system (Marrazzi, 1970) and the auditory system (Marrazzi *et al.*, 1972) in man, and to show that the effect can be nullified by the prior administration of chlorpromazine.

A somewhat similar theory to that of Marrazzi is the 'perceptual release' theory. This was first postulated by Hughlings Jackson, who considered all hallucinatory phenomena as stemming from the loss of control of one area of the brain (an inhibitory mechanism) over the rest. Jackson's theory has been updated and further developed by West (1962) into a general theory to account for a whole range of non-veridical percept-like experiences, including dreams, hypnagogic and hypnopompic imagery, hallucinations and delirium. The essential assumptions of West's theory are first, that percept-like experiences are based on neural traces, templates or engrams which are the permanent record of past experience in the brain (Penfield & Perot, 1963); secondly, following the Gestalt notion of a continual and dynamic organization of memory traces, that these templates or engrams are woven into the basic material of fantasies, dreams and hallucinations; and thirdly, that the end-product of this reorganized experience is normally prevented from emerging into consciousness by the presence of effective, external sensory input, but that release into consciousness can occur under certain specific conditions. These conditions involve the existence of a level of arousal sufficient to permit awareness, combined with impairment of effective sensory input.

While West's theory is a purely psychological one, it differs from that of Marrazzi in at least two other important respects. First, in making arousal level a central concept, West is presumably according an important role to subcortical structures, especially those of the reticular system. In contrast, Marrazzi's theory limits the area of dysfunction to structures within the cortex itself. Secondly, unlike Marrazzi, West accords a central role in his theory to the disequilibrium between external sensory input and internal input from within.

In Fischer's 'sensory/motor ratio' theory this concept of a disequilibrium between internal and external sensory input has been made both the necessary and sufficient condition for the occurrence of hallucinations. Fischer (1969) defined hallucinations as 'intensively active sensations with blocked peripheral, voluntary motor-manifestations'. This proposal was based on the observation that in the hallucinogenic-drug-induced state and during REM sleep, cortical activity and awareness are increased while voluntary motor activity is greatly diminished or inhibited completely. This led to the theory that the hallucinated state is characterized by increased sensory awareness combined with decreased motor responsiveness: a high sensory/motor ratio. Fischer and his colleagues (Fischer *et al.* 1970) went on to develop an operational definition of this sensory/motor ratio in terms of handwriting area (the sensory component) and handwriting pressure (the motor component). In a series of studies involving the administration of psilocybin to college students, these workers found that the sensory/motor ratio is generally increased at drug peak and then decreases again as the drug effect diminishes; that the effect increases with dosage level; and that the effect is greater in subjects who are categorized as 'perceivers' than in those categorized as 'judgers'. Fischer suggests that the important inhibitory effect of voluntary motor activity resides in its function of providing a reality check on the experiences of the individual. Moreover, he suggests that some individuals are able to counteract the hallucinogenic drug effect by increasing their voluntary motor activity, while others are not. Fischer's theory therefore differs from West's mainly in terms of this conception of the inhibitory process: while it must be an active process for Fischer, for West a purely passive receipt of external sensory input is sufficient to prevent the emergence of hallucinatory experience in consciousness.

FURTHER RESEARCH DIRECTIONS

There are three particular areas within the realm of hallucinatory processes and experience which are badly in need of further elaboration and exploration. First, there is a dearth of information concerning the precise mechanisms (biochemical, physiological and psychological) underlying the spontaneously occuring hallucinations of functional psychotic and organic patients. There is some suggestion that physiological arousal may be an important factor in this respect. For example, Alpert *et al.* (1970) demonstrated that hallucinatory experiences could be induced in alcoholic patients with a prior history of such experiences, by means of ditran administration: and, more importantly, that the occurrence of hallucinations coincided in time with a state of increased physiological arousal induced by the drug. In a similar vein, Allen & Agus (1968) reported that they could reliably induce hallucinations in two schizophrenic patients with a hallucinatory history by getting them to hyperventilate, i.e. by artificially manipulating their respiration rate. The author of this editorial (Slade, 1972, 1973) has observed in two schizophrenic patients that the occurrence of their auditory hallucinations was temporally related to increases in self-rated emotional arousal (i.e. tension, anxiety, etc.).

A second area of importance, much neglected both experimentally and theoretically, is that concerning the nature of hallucinatory predisposing factors. One of the most outstanding features of the literature on hallucinations, including those experimentally induced in normals as well as those spontaneously occurring in pathological states, is the fact of individual differences. Some people experience hallucinations under specifiable conditions, while others do not. This provides a clear and strong indication that there must be constitutional factors which predispose some individuals to such experiences. The appropriate research paradigm for investigating such factors would seem to involve the comparison of a group of patients having a history of hallucinations with another group without such a history but matched in terms of all other relevant symptoms. Although this paradigm is an obvious one, very few studies of this type have been carried out. A notable exception is the recent study of Mintz & Alpert (1972). They found that their group of auditory hallucinators differed from non-hallucinating patients and normal controls on two measures: one involving vividness of auditory imagery, the other involving poor reality-testing in the auditory modality. They therefore concluded that a combination of vivid imagery allied with defective reality-testing may provide the predispositional basis for hallucinatory experiences.

A final important area for further research is that concerning the precise factors which determine the modality, form and content of a hallucinatory experience. While phenomenological studies have a significant role to play here, experimental investigations of hypothesized factors are also likely to be crucial.

PETER SLADE

REFERENCES

Aggernaes, A. (1972*a*). The experienced reality of hallucinations and other psychological phenomena. *Acta Psychiatrica Scandinavica* **48**, 220–238.

Aggernaes, A. (1972*b*). The difference between the experienced reality of hallucinations in young drug abusers and schizophrenic patients. *Acta Psychiatrica Scandinavica* **48**, 287–299.

Aggernaes, A. & Nyeborg, O. (1972). The reliability of different aspects of the experienced reality of hallucinations in clear states of consciousness. *Acta Psychiatrica Scandinavica* **48**, 239–252.

Allen, T. E. & Agus, B. (1968). Hyperventilation leading to hallucinations. *American Journal of Psychiatry* **125**, 632–637.

Alpert, M., Angrist, B., Diamond, F. & Gershon, S. (1970). Comparsion of ditran intoxication and acute alcohol psychoses. In W. Keup (ed.), *Origin and Mechanisms of Hallucinations*. Plenum Press: New York.

Baldwin, M., Lewis, S. A. & Bach, S. A. (1959). The effects of lysergic acid after cerebral ablation. *Neurology* **9**, 469–474.

Bexton, W. H., Heron, W. & Scott, T. H. (1954). Effects of decreased variation in the sensory environment. *Canadian Journal of Psychology* **8**, 70–76.

Bleuler, E. (1911). *Dementia Praecox or the Group of Schizophrenias*. International Universities Press: New York, 1950.

Bliss, E. L. & Clark, K. D. (1962). Visual hallucinations. In L. J. West (ed.), *Hallucinations*. Grune & Stratton: New York.

Cooper, J. E., Kendell, R. E., Gurland, B. J., Sartorius, N. & Farkas, T. (1969). Cross-national study of diagnosis of mental disorders: some results from the first comparative investigation. *American Journal of Psychiatry* **125**, suppl., 21–29.

Esquirol, J. E. D. (1838). *Les Maladies mentales*. Baillière: Paris.

Feinberg, I. (1962). A comparison of the visual hallucinations in schizophrenia with those induced by mescaline and LSD-25. In L. J. West (ed.), *Hallucinations*. Grune & Stratton: New York.

Fischer, R. (1969). The perception–hallucination continuum. *Diseases of the Nervous System* **30**, 161–171.

Fischer, R., Kappeler, T., Wisecup, P. & Thatcher, K. (1970). Personality trait dependent performance under psilocybin. *Diseases of the Nervous System* **31**, 91–101.

Forrer, G. R. (1960). Benign auditory and visual hallucinations. *Archives of General Psychiatry* **3**, 95–98.

Galton, F. (1883). *Inquiries into the Human Faculty and Its Development*. Macmillan: London.

Goodwin, D. W., Alderson, P. & Rosenthal, R. (1971). Clinical significance of hallucinations in psychiatric disorders: a study of 116 hallucinatory patients. *Archives of General Psychiatry* **24**, 76–80.

Horowitz, M. J. (1970). *Image Formation and Cognition*. Appleton-Century-Crofts: New York.

Horowitz, M. J. & Adams, J. E. (1970). Hallucinations on brain stimulation: evidence for revision of the Penfield hypothesis. In W. Keup (ed.), *Origin and Mechanisms of Hallucinations*. Plenum Press: New York.

Ishibashi, T., Hori, H., Endo, K. & Sato, T. (1964). Hallucinations produced by electrical stimulation of the temporal lobes in schizophrenic patients. *Tohuku Journal of Experimental Medicine* **82**, 124–139.

Jaspers, K. (1911). Die Trugwahrnehmungen. *Zeitschrift für die gesamte Neurologie und Psychiatrie* **4**, 289–354.

Jaspers, K. (1963). *General Psychopathology*. Manchester University Press: Manchester.

Kandinsky, V. (1885). *Kritische und klinische Betrachtungen im Gebiete der Sinnestäuschungen*. Friedländer: Berlin.

Klüver, H. (1942). Mechanisms of hallucinations. In Q. McNemar & M. A. Merrill (eds.), *Studies in Personality*. McGraw-Hill: New York.

Langs, R. J. & Barr, H. L. (1968). Lysergic acid diethylamide (LSD-25) and schizophrenic reactions: a comparative study. *Journal of Nervous and Mental Disease* **147**, 163–172.

Leff, J. P. (1968). Perceptual phenomena and personality in sensory deprivation. *British Journal of Psychiatry* **114**, 1499–1508.

Mahl, G. F., Rothenberg, A., Delgado, J. M. R. & Hamlin, H. (1964). Psychological responses in the human to intracerebral electrical stimulation. *Psychosomatic Medicine* **26**, 337–368.

Malitz, S., Wilkens, B. & Esecover, H. (1962). A comparison of drug-induced hallucinations with those seen in spontaneously occurring psychoses. In L. J. West (ed.), *Hallucinations*. Grune & Stratton: New York.

Marrazzi, A. S. (1962). Pharmacodynamics of hallucination. In L. J. West (ed.), *Hallucinations*. Grune & Stratton: New York.

Marrazzi, A. S. (1970). A neuropharmacologically based concept of hallucination and its clinical application. In W. Keup (ed.), *Origin and Mechanisms of Hallucinations*. Plenum Press: New York.

Marrazzi, A. S., Woodruff, S. & Kennedy, D. (1972). Perceptual challenge to measure illness and therapy. *American Journal of Psychiatry* **128**, 886–890.

Maury, A. (1848). Des hallucinations hypnagogiques de système nerveux. *Annales Médico-Psychologiques* **11**, 26–40.

Mayer-Gross, W., Slater, E. & Roth, M. (1969). *Clinical Psychiatry*, 3rd ed. Baillière, Tindall & Cassell: London.

Mintz, S. & Alpert, W. (1972). Imagery vividness, reality-testing and schizophrenic hallucinations. *Journal of Abnormal Psychology* **79**, 310–316.

Murphy, D. B., Myers, T. I. & Smith, S. (1962). Reported visual sensation as a function of sustained sensory deprivation and social isolation. *U.S.A. Leadership HRU Draft Research Report*. Presidio of Monterey (Pioneer VI).

Penfield, W. & Jasper, H. (1954). *Epilepsy and the Functional Anatomy of the Human Brain*. Little, Brown: Boston.

Penfield, W. & Perot, P. (1963). The brain's record of auditory and visual experience: a final summary and discussion. *Brain* **86**, 595–696.

Penfield, W. & Rasmussen, T. (1950). *The Cerebral Cortex of Man*. Macmillan: New York.

Richardson, A. (1969). *Mental Imagery*. Routledge & Kegan Paul: London.

Schneider, K. (1959). *Clinical Psychopathology*. Grune & Stratton: New York.

Sedman, G. (1966). 'Inner voices': phenomenological and clinical aspects. *British Journal of Psychiatry* **112**, 485–490.

Slade, P. D. (1972). The effects of systematic desensitization on auditory hallucinations. *Behaviour Research and Therapy* **10**, 85–91.

Slade, P. D. (1973). The psychological investigation and treatment of auditory hallucinations: a second case report. *British Journal of Medical Psychology* **46**, 293–296.

West, L. J. (1962). A general theory of hallucinations and dreams. In L. J. West (ed.), *Hallucinations*. Grune & Stratton: New York.

World Health Organization (1973). *International Pilot Study of Schizophrenia*, vol. 1. WHO: Geneva.

Zuckerman, M. & Cohen, N. (1964). Sources of reports of visual and auditory sensations in perceptual-isolation experiments. *Psychological Bulletin* **62**, 1–20.

Psychological Medicine, 1977, **7**, 363–367

The present status of anorexia nervosa[1]

During the past decade there has been a spate of research articles on anorexia nervosa. One reason for this is probably that the illness has been recognized much more frequently in recent years (Theander, 1970) or perhaps that it has actually increased in its incidence (Kendell *et al.* 1973). There is also the advantage that anorexia nervosa is one of the few psychiatric disorders that lends itself readily to being accorded clear-cut diagnostic criteria. These have been expressed in terms of necessary criteria where all the stipulated requirements must be satisfied (Russell, 1970), or in terms of quantitative criteria where a given proportion of possible abnormalities or a certain degree of disturbance, such as the amount of weight loss, should be present (Feighner *et al.* 1972). The former approach would appear to be preferable, but the latter can at least serve the purpose of providing operational definitions of value in clinical research. Finally, anorexia nervosa allows the researcher to study simultaneously disturbances of mental and bodily function, so enabling him to observe their complex interaction. It is appropriate, therefore, to refer in turn to studies that have concentrated on the psychological aspects of the illness and on its physical aspects. An attempt will also be made to synthesize the findings of these studies – by no means an easy task.

Evidence for anorexia nervosa having a psychological origin is not hard to come by. The patients tell us that they do not eat normally because they are fearful of becoming fat or of losing control over eating, or that they experience unpleasant feelings of guilt after having eaten. In 1962 Hilde Bruch suggested that these patients show a disturbance of their body image marked by indifference to their emaciation which they defend as normal and right. She has pointed out that the denial of their thinness is pathognomonic of anorexia nervosa (Bruch, 1974). Recently, experimental evidence has supported the presence of a perceptual disorder. Wasted patients, when asked to estimate their body size, tend to indicate that they see themselves as wider than they actually are, and wider indeed than the configuration of a normally proportioned woman. Different methods of measurement have been used: a size-estimation bar carrying lights whose separation was taken as the estimate of body width (Slade & Russell, 1973) or the presentation to the patients of photographs of themselves enlarged or diminished by means of a special lens (Meyer & Tuchelt-Gallwitz, 1968; Garner *et al.* 1977). In general, there has been agreement that patients with anorexia nervosa see themselves as abnormally wide and fat (Crisp & Kalucy, 1974; Goldberg *et al.* 1977). Some investigators have found that the perceptual disturbance is sensitive to the patient's eating pattern and becomes worse after a meal (Crisp & Kalucy, 1974). Others report that the disturbance becomes diminished if the patient gains weight as a result of treatment (Slade & Russell, 1973): herein lies the paradox that gaining weight has the effect of reducing the patient's view of herself as a fat person. In another experimental study, patients with anorexia nervosa were found, in contrast with normal subjects, to vary their food intake according to their own awareness of body size: when they were deceived into believing that they had gained weight, they ate less, and *vice versa* (Russell *et al.* 1975). It was concluded that in these patients body weight is not regulated readily by normal physiological mechanisms but is more at the mercy of external cues of body size. The findings of these studies may be combined. Food intake in anorexia nervosa is unduly dependent on the patient's awareness of her body size; as this awareness is a distorted one in the direction of seeing herself as unduly large, it follows that the patient will starve herself in an attempt to return to what she considers to be more normal proportions. Yet the starvation and weight loss may worsen the distorted awareness of herself. Here, therefore, is a basis for the self-perpetuation of anorexia nervosa. Thus, clinical observations supplemented by experimental studies confirm – if any confirmation was needed – that abnormal attitudes to eating and body size are responsible for the illness or at least for its perpetuation. Such a view has been prevalent since the first descriptions of anorexia nervosa which was attributed by Gull in 1874 to a morbid state of mind.

[1] Address for correspondence: Professor G. F. M. Russell, Royal Free Hospital, Pond St., London NW3 2QG.

As regards the physical aspects of anorexia nervosa the hypothesis has been put forward that the illness is in part due to a disorder of hypothalamic function (Russell, 1965, 1972*a*). Support for this hypothesis has come from a number of studies which have been concerned with the control of water balance, thermo-regulation, and especially the endocrine status of patients with anorexia nervosa (Warren & Vande Wiele, 1973; Mecklenburg *et al.* 1974; Boyar *et al.* 1974; Garfinkel *et al.* 1977). The question is a complicated one. It is probably fair to consider several of the bodily disturbances found in malnourished patients with anorexia nervosa as depending for their pathogenesis on a disorder of hypothalamic function. But most of these disturbances are a direct consequence of the patient's malnutrition, and clear up rapidly if she can be persuaded to return to a healthy weight or if she recovers spontaneously. For example, elevated blood levels of growth hormone, originally observed by Landon *et al.* (1966), have been shown by Brown *et al.* (1977) to return rapidly to normal in patients whose caloric intake has improved. On the other hand, defects of thermo-regulation persist longer and require that the patient's weight returns fully to normal, but in this example also it is probable that the defects of temperature control are directly caused by malnutrition, including the loss of protective subcutaneous fat (Wakeling & Russell, 1970). Much more interesting are the observations that correction of the patient's weight loss fails, in the short term at least, to reverse the intricate hormonal disturbances affecting the hypothalamic–pituitary–gonadal axis. In normal subjects there is a complex circular interaction between the hypothalamus, the anterior pituitary and the gonads. Gonadotrophin-releasing hormones originate from the hypothalamus and discharge the gonadotrophins (luteinizing hormone (LH) and follicle-stimulating hormone (FSH)) from the anterior pituitary gland. The gonadotrophins cause oestrogens and progesterone to be secreted by the ovaries. Oestrogens and progesterone in turn exert negative and positive feedback effects on the hypothalamus and the anterior pituitary. In severe anorexia nervosa, urinary and blood levels of gonadotrophins (FSH and LH) and oestrogens are always low or undetectable (Russell *et al.* 1965; Bell *et al.* 1966; Crisp *et al.* 1973). Moreover, there is evidence of a diminished release of LH following the administration of one of the following substances: synthetic gonadotrophin-releasing hormone, clomiphene (a synthetic drug used in the treatment of anovular infertility), or ethinyl oestradiol. Under appropriate circumstances these substances are likely to cause elevation of blood LH levels in normal menstruating women. Synthetic gonadotrophin-releasing hormone discharges FSH and LH if these are present in the anterior pituitary stores. Clomiphene is thought to act by blocking the negative feedback effects of oestrogens on the hypothalamus. Ethinyl oestradiol owes its effect to a positive feedback action that is only evident after a short (3-day) course of the drug, a negative feedback effect predominating during the actual period of its administration. In the undernourished patient all these responses are absent or much diminished. If, however, the patient can be persuaded to eat so that her weight returns to normal, many of these hormonal disturbances are gradually reversed. For example, urinary and blood levels of gonadotrophins (LH and FSH) and oestrogens gradually rise (Russell & Beardwood, 1968; Crisp *et al.* 1973). On the other hand, these levels do not readily fluctuate in a cyclical fashion such as would herald a resumption of regular menstruation. Among the tests of responsiveness of LH to different substances, the action of gonadotrophin-releasing hormone is most readily restored to normal, establishing that there is a rapid return of the functional capacity of the anterior pituitary (Sherman *et al.* 1975; Brown *et al.* 1977). The response to clomiphene may also return (Marshall & Russell Fraser, 1971; Beumont *et al.* 1973; Wakeling *et al.* 1976; Brown *et al.* 1977), but some patients show only an incomplete response even though their weight has been restored to normal (Wakeling *et al.* 1976). The most significant findings are the negative and positive feedback effects of administered oestrogen on LH-release in patients whose weight has become normal. Although the negative feedback effects are soon restored, the positive feedback release of LH following a 3-day course of ethinyl oestradiol returns in only a small proportion of the patients (Wakeling *et al.* 1977*a*, 1977*b*). This finding indicates a more persistent abnormality in the hypothalamic regulation of gonadotrophin release, and confirms an earlier view that the specific endocrine disturbance in anorexia nervosa is dependent only in part on the patient's loss of weight and malnutrition (Russell & Beardwood, 1968).

The research findings on disturbances of the hypothalamic–pituitary–gonadal axis assume a

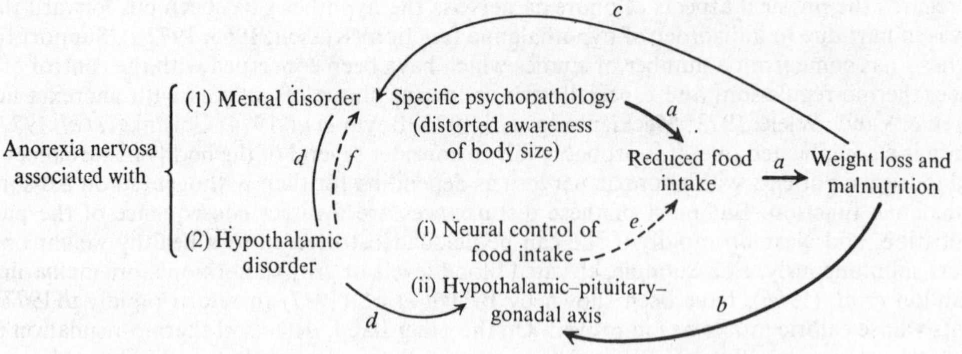

FIG. 1.

considerable significance, for they cannot simply be interpreted as a consequence of the malnutrition of anorexia nervosa. They must indicate a more fundamental disorder of hypothalamic function. Moreover, they are directly relevant to a salient clinical phenomenon, namely the cessation of spontaneous menstruation, which is one of the necessary diagnostic features of anorexia nervosa. Finally, these findings are in keeping with early clinical observations that amenorrhoea may be an early event in the course of the illness preceding any loss of weight (Kay & Leigh, 1954), and persisting in a minority of patients in spite of maintaining a normal weight over a period of several months or even years. A cautionary note must be sounded. An individual patient's responsiveness of LH to clomiphene or ethinyl oestradiol has been of little value in predicting the outcome of her illness. It may have served to predict the imminence of a return of menstruation, but no more than this. Neither does it seem to be correlated with the patient's psychological recovery, a full LH response to administered oestrogen being compatible with persistence of the mental disturbances characteristic of anorexia nervosa.

How do recent researches help us to decide whether a disorder of hypothalamic function is relevant to the genesis of anorexia nervosa? What follows is necessarily a simplistic discussion of a most baffling problem. Endocrinologists, who have the merit of seeing the issues in black-and-white terms, have put forward 3 possibilities (Mecklenberg *et al.* 1974):

(1) weight loss 'damages' the hypothalamus;

(2) the mental disturbance, or those events that are considered of psychogenic importance ('psychic stress'), interfere with hypothalamic function;

(3) the endocrine manifestations and the psychopathological features are relatively independent expressions of a primary hypothalamic defect of unknown aetiology.

At the risk of appearing even more naïve, but in an attempt to clarify the issues and to sum up the evidence so far, a flow diagram (Fig. 1) is presented which emphasizes the circular interactions between the psychological disorder, the endocrine disturbances and the malnutrition. The thickness of the lines reflects the weight of evidence supporting each interaction. Firmly established is the pathway that attributes to the mental disorder the reduced food intake and loss of weight (*a*), which in turn cause the endocrine disturbance and amenorrhoea (*b*). It is also probable that the weight loss and malnutrition aggravate the mental disorder in the manner discussed earlier (*c*). The literature on the effects of emotional upheavals and mental illness in causing amenorrhoea also supports a direct pathway between mental and hypothalamic disorders in anorexia nervosa (*d*) (Drew, 1961; Russell, 1972*b*). Next, there is a possible link between a disorder in the hypothalamic control of food intake and the food refusal characteristic of anorexia nervosa (*e*). It was this possibility which gave rise to the original hypothesis of anorexia nervosa being caused by a disorder of hypothalamic function. A final postulated link (*f*) is that representing the neural effects of a hypothalamic disorder in moulding the patient's mental functions so as to give rise to her abnormal attitudes to eating, body size and sexuality. These last two links (*e* and *f*) are the weakest ones in the chain, for there is as yet no direct evidence in support of them. What is clear, however, is that self-perpetuating disturbances play an important part in anorexia nervosa.

In the absence of established causes and specific treatments, our therapeutic endeavours must depend on the interruption of these vicious circles. Short-term successes are most readily achieved by restoring body weight to normal and thus correcting malnutrition and its consequences (Russell, 1977). Even so, a substantial proportion of patients relapse, so that the regime of refeeding must be repeated on one or more occasions (Morgan & Russell, 1975). It may be possible to reduce the number of relapses and shorten the overall course of the illness by means of skilled psychotherapy aimed at the psychopathology that is characteristic of anorexia nervosa (Thomä, 1967; Bruch, 1974), but it would be gratifying if a well-designed study established the efficacy of this treatment.

GERALD RUSSELL

REFERENCES

Bell, E. T., Harkness, R. A., Loraine, J. A. & Russell, G. F. M. (1966). Hormone assay studies in patients with anorexia nervosa. *Acta Endocrinologica* **51**, 140–148.

Beumont, P. J. V., Carr, P. J. & Gelder, M. G. (1973). Plasma levels of luteinizing hormone and of immunoreactive oestrogens (oestradiol) in anorexia nervosa: response to clomiphene citrate. *Psychological Medicine* **3**, 495–501.

Boyar, R. M., Katz, J., Finkelstein, J. W., Kapen, S., Weiner, H., Weitzman, E. D. & Hellman, L. (1974). Anorexia nervosa: immaturity of the 24-hour luteinizing hormone secretory pattern. *New England Journal of Medicine* **291**, 861–865.

Brown, G. M., Garfinkel, P. E., Jeuniewic, N., Moldofsky, H. & Stancer, H. C. (1977). Endocrine profiles in anorexia nervosa. In *Anorexia Nervosa* (ed. R. A. Vigersky), pp. 123–135. Raven Press: New York (in the press).

Bruch, H. (1962). Perceptual and conceptual disturbances of anorexia nervosa. *Psychosomatic Medicine* **24**, 187–194.

Bruch, H. (1974). *Eating Disorders: Obesity, Anorexia Nervosa and the Person Within*. Routledge and Kegan Paul: London.

Crisp, A. H. & Kalucy, R. S. (1974). Aspects of the perceptual disorder in anorexia nervosa. *British Journal of Medical Psychology* **47**, 349–361.

Crisp, A. H., Mackinnon, P. C. B., Chen, C. & Corker, C. S. (1973). Observations of gonadotrophic and ovarian hormone activity during recovery from anorexia nervosa. *Postgraduate Medical Journal* **49**, 584–590.

Drew, F. L. (1961). The epidemiology of secondary amenorrhoea. *Journal of Chronic Diseases* **14**, 396–407.

Feighner, J. P., Robins, E., Guze, S. B., Woodruff, R. A., Winokur, G. & Munoz, R. (1972). Diagnostic criteria for use in psychiatric research. *Archives of General Psychiatry* **26**, 57–63.

Garfinkel, P. E., Moldofsky, H. & Garner, D. M. (1977). The outcome of anorexia nervosa: significance of clinical features, body image and behaviour modification. In *Anorexia Nervosa* (ed. R. A. Vigersky), pp. 315–329. Raven Press: New York (in the press).

Garner, D. M., Garfinkel, P. E., Stancer, H. C. & Moldofsky, H. (1977). Body image disturbances in anorexia nervosa and obesity. In *Anorexia Nervosa* (ed. R. A. Vigersky), pp. 27–30. Raven Press: New York (in the press).

Goldberg, S. C., Halmi, K. A., Casper, R., Eckert, E. & Davis, J. M. (1977). Pretreatment predictors of weight gain in anorexia nervosa. In *Anorexia Nervosa* (ed. R. A. Vigersky), pp. 31–41. Raven Press: New York (in the press).

Gull, W. (1874). Anorexia nervosa (apepsia hysterica, anorexia hysterica). *Transactions of the Clinical Society of London* **7**, 22–28.

Kay, D. W. K. & Leigh, D. (1954). The natural history, treatment and prognosis of anorexia nervosa, based on a study of 38 patients. *Journal of Mental Science* **100**, 411–431.

Kendell, R. E., Hall, D. J., Hailey, A. & Babigian, H. M. (1973). The epidemiology of anorexia nervosa. *Psychological Medicine* **3**, 200–203.

Landon, J., Greenwood, F. C., Stamp, T. C. B. & Wynn, V. (1966). The plasma sugar, free fatty acid, cortisol and growth hormone response to insulin, and the comparison of this procedure with other tests of pituitary and adrenal function. II. In patients with hypothalamic or pituitary dysfunction or anorexia nervosa. *Journal of Clinical Investigation* **45**, 437–449.

Marshall, J. C. & Russell Fraser, T. (1971). Amenorrhoea in anorexia nervosa: assessment and treatment with clomiphene citrate. *British Medical Journal* iv, 590–592.

Mecklenburg, R. S., Loriaux, D. L., Thompson, R. H., Andersen, A. E. & Lipsett, M. B. (1974). Hypothalamic dysfunction in patients with anorexia nervosa. *Medicine* **53**, 147–159.

Meyer, J. E. & Tuchelt-Gallwitz, A. (1968). A study on social image, body image and the problem of psychogenetic factors in obesity. *Comprehensive Psychiatry* **9**, 148–154.

Morgan, H. G. & Russell, G. F. M. (1975). Value of family background and clinical features as predictors of long-term outcome in anorexia nervosa: four-year follow-up study of 41 patients. *Psychological Medicine* **5**, 355–371.

Russell, G. F. M. (1965). Metabolic aspects of anorexia nervosa. *Proceedings of the Royal Society of Medicine* **58**, 811–814.

Russell, G. F. M. (1970). Anorexia nervosa: its identity as an illness and its treatment. In *Modern Trends in Psychological Medicine*, vol. 2 (ed. J. Harding Price), pp. 131–164. Butterworths: London.

Russell, G. F. M. (1972*a*). Premenstrual tension and 'psychogenic' amenorrhoea: psycho-physical interactions. *Journal of Psychosomatic Research* **16**, 279–287.

Russell, G. F. M. (1972*b*). Psychological and nutritional factors in disturbances of menstrual function and ovulation. *Postgraduate Medical Journal* **48**, 10–13.

Russell, G. F. M. (1977). General management of anorexia nervosa and difficulties in assessing the efficacy of treatment. In *Anorexia Nervosa* (ed. R. A. Vigersky), pp. 277–289. Raven Press: New York (in the press).

Russell, G. F. M. & Beardwood, C. J. (1968). The feeding disorders, with particular reference to anorexia nervosa and its associated gonadotrophin changes. In *Endocrinology and Human Behaviour* (ed. R. P. Michael), pp. 310–329. Oxford University Press: London.

Russell, G. F. M., Loraine, J. A., Bell, E. T. & Harkness, R. A. (1965). Gonadotrophin and oestrogen excretion in patients with anorexia nervosa. *Journal of Psychosomatic Research* **9**, 79–85.

Russell, G. F. M., Campbell, P. G. & Slade, P. D. (1975). Experimental studies on the nature of the psychological disorder in anorexia nervosa. *Psychoneuroendocrinology* **1**, 45–56.

Sherman, B. M., Halmi, K. A. & Zamudio, R. (1975). LH and FSH response to gonadotrophin-releasing hormone in anorexia nervosa: effect of nutritional rehabilitation. *Journal of Clinical Endocrinology and Metabolism* **41**, 135–142.

Slade, P. D. & Russell, G. F. M. (1973). Awareness of body dimensions in anorexia nervosa: cross-sectional and longitudinal studies. *Psychological Medicine* 3, 188–199.

Theander, S. (1970). Anorexia nervosa: a psychiatric investigation of 94 female cases. *Acta Psychiatrica Scandinavica*, Supplement 214.

Thomä, H. (1967). *Anorexia Nervosa* (trans. G. Brydone). International University Press: New York.

Wakeling, A. & Russell, G. F. M. (1970). Disturbances in the regulation of body temperature in anorexia nervosa. *Psychological Medicine* **1**, 30–39.

Wakeling, A., Marshall, J. C., Beardwood, C. J., De Souza, V. F. A. & Russell, G. F. M. (1976). The effects of clomiphene citrate on the hypothalamic–pituitary–gonadal axis in anorexia nervosa. *Psychological Medicine* **6**, 371–380.

Wakeling, A., De Souza, V. F. A. & Beardwood, C. J. (1977*a*). Assessment of the negative and positive feedback effects of administered oestrogen on gonadotrophin release in patients with anorexia nervosa. *Psychological Medicine* **7**, 397–405.

Wakeling, A., De Souza, V. F. A. & Beardwood, C. J. (1977*b*). The effects of administered oestrogen on luteinizing hormone release in subjects with anorexia nervosa in acute and recovery stages. In *Anorexia Nervosa* (ed. R. A. Vigersky), pp. 199–209. Raven Press: New York (in the press).

Warren, M. P. & Vande Wiele, R. L. (1973). Clinical and metabolic features of anorexia nervosa. *American Journal of Obstetrics and Gynaecology* **117**, 435–449.

Psychological Medicine, 1978, **8**, 353–356

Research into the dementias[1]

Attempting to establish priorities in medical research is usually a thankless exercise. Research prospers through personal commitment rather than collectively perceived need, and individual inspiration when available stands to achieve immensely more than carefully conceived scientific policies. There is a place, nonetheless, for drawing attention to neglected areas, stressing problems of outstanding need, and highlighting organizational blocks and barriers which may be impeding the natural development of a subject. Such issues are particularly germane when several disciplines have a central part to play in achieving progress and must work in close liaison with one another.

These may be considered among the main reasons for focusing attention on biomedical research in the dementias as the Medical Research Council has done in a recent report (Medical Research Council, 1977). The pamphlet aims to chart problem areas and avenues for useful research into this distressing class of illnesses, and to consider strategies for facilitating enquiries by clinicians and laboratory workers.

The need for such work is abundantly obvious. The presenile dementias are major tragedies; and the senile dementias so ubiquitous that they threaten constantly to overwhelm the treatment and caring services. Yet these mysterious conditions have traditionally been by-passed by medical research in favour of topics more immediately attractive. Despite the lure of a visible pathology, the fundamentals of causation have only sporadically been explored, and the rich clinical material everywhere available has usually been seriously neglected. Much of the blame doubtless lies in the parallels that have been drawn between the common forms of dementia in the elderly and the processes of 'natural senescence' – sterile conceptions of 'abiotrophy' or 'premature ageing' have served to deflect endeavour, and only recently have more hopeful and testable hypotheses begun to be explored. Patterns of patient care have further conspired to impede progress. Responsibility is shared among several clinical disciplines. Patients tend to be cared for in units remote from teaching hospitals and academic centres so that opportunities for intensive study become immensely hard to achieve. Demarcation disputes, and the business of trying to cope, are more liable to surround the aged dement than processes of scientific enquiry.

Need and neglect alone, however, cannot promise a useful yield. Before accepting the dementias as suitable targets for intensive research we will need more encouragement to proceed. Thus, we may note that strong reasons can be marshalled against the simple ageing hypothesis. Epidemiological evidence shows that, even in extreme old age, the majority of persons retain their intellectual competence. It now seems likely that parenchymatous senile dementia is analogous in virtually all respects to Alzheimer's disease occurring at a very much younger age. A pathologically accelerated ageing process may indeed be involved, but the pathogenic factor could be toxic, biochemical or quite other in nature.

Moreover, we have witnessed examples of what may come to light when other 'degenerative' conditions are studied by modern techniques of biological enquiry. Parkinson's disease now has not only a respectable biochemical basis but a reasonably effective replacement therapy. Creutzfeldt–Jakob disease, itself traditionally included among the presenile dementias, has firmly joined the ranks of transmissible, and presumably agent-mediated, disorders. Attention therefore naturally turns towards attempts at unravelling the basis of the Alzheimer type of dementia, by far the commonest of the primary dementing illnesses. A cursory survey shows no dearth of avenues for study.

[1] Address for correspondence: Dr W. A. Lishman, Institute of Psychiatry, De Crespigny Park, Denmark Hill, London SE5 8AF.

Quantitative histology, biochemistry and experimental pathology have obvious parts to play; histochemistry, immunology and cytology are also implicated.

The traditionally static techniques of neuropathology are being supplemented by more dynamic conceptions and a more discriminating approach to the meaning of long-hallowed changes. A main task is to determine what are the significant tissue elements involved in the disease and how far these diverge from age-dependent changes. The degree of development of senile plaques, for example, has proved to correlate closely with the severity of the dementing process (Blessed *et al.* 1968; Tomlinson *et al.* 1970). But it is far from clear whether neuronal loss itself is so related, or indeed whether it is significantly more advanced in dementia than in age-matched controls. Careful cell (and synapse) counting by automated techniques can hope to clarify this issue and help decide whether or not we are dealing with a primarily neuronal disease. The phenomena represented by the neurofibrillary tangles in cell bodies and the senile plaques are also intriguing. Do the tangles embarrass cell function and axoplasmic transport? What is the origin of the plaques? Senile plaques consist of damaged neuritic terminals along with the formation of amyloid. Their frequent proximity to blood vessels and their amyloid content could betray a metabolic or immunological origin, with degeneration starting at the periphery of the neurone and spreading back to involve the cell bodies later. The demonstration that plaques can be induced in animals by infecting mice with the scrapie agent (Wisniewski *et al.* 1975) sharpens the need to gain further clarity on such issues.

Biochemical analysis of brain tissue provides a complementary approach. The discovery that a wide range of reliable neurochemical results can be obtained on autopsy material has led to the urgent need for establishing 'brain banks' which could greatly facilitate enquiries. Findings to date include loss of a specific brain protein (neuronin S-6) in the cortex (Bowen *et al.* 1973), and evidence that tangle-bearing neurones contain a new protein of abnormal type (Iqbal *et al.* 1974). A report of increased aluminium content in the brain in Alzheimer's disease is particularly intriguing (Crapper *et al.* 1973), since aluminium is known experimentally to be capable of inducing a form of neurofibrillary change in animals.

By far the most promising biochemical approach, however, is the study of enzymes involved in synaptic transmission. This reflects the functional competence of the elements which remain, and allows a search for selective loss in functional subsystems. Following the leads obtained in Huntington's chorea, of reduced GABA and glutamic acid decarboxylase in the basal ganglia (Perry *et al.* 1973; Bird & Iversen, 1974), equivalent studies are now the focus of interest in presenile and senile dementia of the Alzheimer type. Investigations from several centres are combining to suggest a widespread deficiency in the cholinergic system, affecting many parts of the cortex and the hippocampus severely (Davies, 1977; Perry *et al.* 1977; Spillane *et al.* 1977; White *et al.* 1977). The enzymes responsible for the synthesis of acetylcholine (choline acetyl transferase) and for its degradation (acetylcholinesterase) have been found to be remarkably deficient, while the density of receptor binding sites appears to remain relatively normal, implying that replacement therapy may conceivably be effective. Such findings will, of course, require substantiation. Opportunities for artefacts are numerous – the agonal state of the patient, the procedures used prior to collection of samples, even the time of day of death are variables to be monitored closely. The cholinergic deficiencies may be only one of many interacting biochemical abnormalities. Nevertheless, trials of choline or its analogues, or other means of potentiating cholinergic mechanisms, would seem well justified and are already under way.

The established transmissibility of Creutzfeldt–Jakob disease, and growing awareness of 'slow viruses' in relation to other neurological diseases, naturally raises the possibility that these too may be implicated in Alzheimer's/senile dementia. The evidence so far is, however, slender. Traub *et al.* (1977) review the experience to date from Gajdusek's laboratory. Out of 35 cases of Alzheimer's disease, 3 have transmitted to experimental animals. All, however, have produced on transmission the picture of spongiform encephalopathy which is one of the main characteristics of Creutzfeldt–Jakob disease; they do not produce the histological picture of Alzheimer's disease. Two were examples of the rare familial variant of Alzheimer's dementia and all were atypical in one way or another. There is also the possibility that the Creutzfeldt–Jakob agent may sometimes have occurred as a secondary pathogen in a brain already damaged by Alzheimer's disease. Again the area is one for continuing vigilance. Quite apart from any potential treatment outcome, it will be important to learn whether risk attaches to cortical biopsies in the general run of demented patients. A considerable scare has already been raised by evidence of surgical transmission of the Creutzfeldt–Jakob agent – first by corneal transplant in one case (Duffy *et al.* 1974), and more recently by the insertion of possibly infected silver electrodes into the brains of 2 young epileptic patients (Bernoulli *et al.* 1977).

The above are but examples of several lines of approach to the fundamentals of causation. It would be tempting to pin one's hopes on a few such areas alone and endow them with special priority for the investment of resources. Such a course of action might conceivably pay off if the gods were willing. But the field is so much on the threshold of discoveries and so replete with uncertainties that it would seem wise to keep several options open. Thus, the MRC report has recognized the need for encouraging a broad range of research enterprises, at least until such time as developments tip the scales in one direction or another.

Meanwhile clinicians, including clinical psychologists, have much to do. Diagnostic practices require continuing attention, nosology badly needs refinement, and treatment approaches could even now be extended. Surveys have shown the considerable yield of treatable pathologies when various populations of patients with the syndrome of dementia are comprehensively screened. Marsden & Harrison (1972) found that 15% of 106 patients admitted to hospital with presumptive diagnoses of presenile or senile dementia had conditions amenable to treatment. Smith *et al.* (1976) estimated the figure at 20%. Psychiatric conditions, especially depressive illness and severe neurotic disorders, can constitute a substantial source of error, as witnessed by follow-up studies of patients diagnosed as suffering from presenile dementia in psychiatric units (Nott & Fleminger, 1975; Ron *et al.* 1978). The significance and the measurement of cerebral atrophy, in different age groups and in a variety of settings, needs thorough reappraisal, and computerized axial tomography is now at hand to allow this to be done.

Nosological confusions are rife and present major barriers to other areas of research. The distinctions during life between arteriopathic and parenchymatous forms of dementia are still far from certain, likewise distinctions between several subvarieties of the latter. The status of 'simple' presenile dementia has not been resolved; and parenchymatous senile dementia may yet prove to consist of more than one pathological entity. The requirements here are clear-cut – follow-up of adequate numbers of patients, studied intensively during life, then with full neuropathological and neurochemical examination after death. The further key question of the precise extent of the distinctions between dementia and 'normal' senescence will almost certainly require longitudinal community surveys of the elderly, so that early patterns of cognitive failure can be charted and followed with time. These latter enterprises would have an additional value in allowing comprehensive assessment of antecedents, precipitants, and the role of somatic pathologies in relation to dementia. Nosological groundwork of this nature may seem relatively unexciting, but we shall ignore such basic matters at great cost. A firm nosology would bring multiple lasting benefits – in allowing the discernment of clinical associations of the various disorders, clarifying the picture of genetics, speeding the pay-off from laboratory work, and streamlining trials of treatment.

Treatment is unfortunately the poor relation in most discussions of the primary dementias. Of the numerous substances claimed to improve cognitive functioning, whether by improved blood flow or enhanced cell metabolism, none appear to be truly useful. Trials may show slight measurable gains, chiefly in social functioning, but this can often be obtained by the sensitive use of standard psychotropic medication. It may be expected, however, that offshoots of the biochemical developments mentioned above will burgeon, and the pharmaceutical industry is no doubt watching such matters closely. It would seem a sound investment now to devote considerable energy into improving means of monitoring the progress of patients with dementia. We need clearer delineation of core areas of disability, and careful selection of the parameters and methods most suited for measuring change. Conventional psychometric tests are clearly unsatisfactory for the purpose. Measures of information processing or simple tests of mental speed and flexibility could perhaps prove far superior.

There is abundant room too for working towards more skilful use of existing methods of management. Demented patients survive for many years, both in the community and in institutions; we must aim to promote the optimum quality of life that is possible for them, and to ease the burden on relatives, attendants and resources. The determinants of key symptoms such as restlessness, for example, could repay detailed study, likewise psychosocial means for delaying the downward curve to total dependence. There are encouraging indications that lee-way exists at many stages of the disorder for promoting the optimum use of residual functions, avoiding confrontations with failure, and helping the patient to cope with his own diminishing resources. Systematic research is needed to show what types of disability respond best and to what particular forms of psychological and social intervention. Miller (1977) has drawn together the scattered evidence on such matters, and on the value that could accrue from devising supportive 'prosthetic' environments. Health services research is also extensively implicated. Evaluation of patterns and models of care, and acceptance that several such models are needed, will be an essential prelude to more rational and satisfactory services.

Research into the dementias is clearly a multi-faceted enterprise. Both fundamental and applied components require to be carefully nurtured, and the former perhaps need very specially to be safeguarded. It is sobering to think how difficult it would have been, a decade or two ago, to write in much detail about such matters. It will be interesting, a decade from now, to see whether present aspirations have proved illusory, or whether substantial advances will, in fact, have been achieved.

W. A. LISHMAN

REFERENCES

Bernoulli, C., Siegfried, J., Baumgartner, G., Regli, F., Rabinowicz, T., Gajdusek, D. C. & Gibbs, C. J. (1977). Danger of accidental person-to-person transmission of Creutzfeldt–Jakob disease by surgery. *Lancet* i, 478–479.

Bird, E. D. & Iversen, L. L. (1974). Huntington's chorea – post-mortem measurement of glutamic acid decarboxylase, choline acetyltransferase and dopamine in basal ganglia. *Brain* **97**, 457–472.

Blessed, G., Tomlinson, B. E. & Roth, M. (1968). The association between quantitative measures of dementia and of senile change in the cerebral grey matter of elderly subjects. *British Journal of Psychiatry* **114**, 797–811.

Bowen, D. M., Smith, C. B. & Davison, A. N. (1973). Molecular changes in senile dementia. *Brain* **96**, 849–856.

Crapper, D. R., Krishnan, S. S. & Dalton, A. J. (1973). Brain aluminium distribution in Alzheimer's disease and experimental neurofibrillary degeneration. *Science* **180**, 511–513.

Davies, P. (1977). Cholinergic mechanisms in Alzheimer's disease. *British Journal of Psychiatry* **131**, 318–319.

Duffy, P., Wolf, J., Collins, G., De Voe, A. G., Streeten, B. & Cowen, D. (1974). Possible person-to-person transmission of Creutzfeldt–Jakob disease. *New England Journal of Medicine* **290**, 692–693.

Iqbal, K., Wisniewski, H. M., Shelanski, M. L., Brostoff, S., Liwnicz, B. H. & Terry, R. D. (1974). Protein changes in senile dementia. *Brain Research* **77**, 337–343.

Marsden, C. D. & Harrison, M. J. G. (1972). Outcome of investigation of patients with presenile dementia. *British Medical Journal* ii, 249–252.

Medical Research Council (1977). *Senile and Presenile Dementias.* A Report of the MRC Subcommittee, compiled by W. A. Lishman. Medical Research Council: London.

Miller, E. (1977). *Abnormal Ageing: The Psychology of Senile and Presenile Dementia.* Wiley: London.

Nott, P. N. & Fleminger, J. J. (1975). Presenile dementia: the difficulties of early diagnosis. *Acta Psychiatrica Scandinavica* **51**, 210–217.

Perry, E. K., Gibson, P. H., Blessed, G., Perry, R. H. & Tomlinson, B. E. (1977). Neurotransmitter enzyme abnormalities in senile dementia. *Journal of the Neurological Sciences* **34**, 247–265.

Perry, T. L., Hansen, S. & Kloster, M. (1973). Huntington's chorea: deficiency of γ-aminobutyric acid in brain. *New England Journal of Medicine* **288**, 337–342.

Ron, M. A., Toone, B. K., Garralda, E. & Lishman, W. A. (1978). Diagnostic accuracy in presenile dementia (Submitted for publication.)

Smith, J. S., Kiloh, L. G., Ratnavale, G. S. & Grant, D. A. (1976). The investigation of dementia: the results in 100 consecutive admissions. *Medical Journal of Australia* **2**, 403–405.

Spillane, J. A., White, P., Goodhardt, M. J., Flack, R. H. A., Bowen, D. M. & Davison, A. N. (1977). Selective vulnerability of neurones in organic dementia. *Nature* **266**, 558–559.

Tomlinson, B. E., Blessed, G. & Roth, M. (1970). Observations on the brains of demented old people. *Journal of the Neurological Sciences* **11**, 205–242.

Traub, R., Gajdusek, D. C. & Gibbs, C. J. (1977). Transmissible virus dementia: the relation of transmissible spongiform encephalopathy to Creutzfeldt–Jakob disease. In *Aging and Dementia* (ed. W. Lynn Smith and M. Kinsbourne), ch. 5. SP Books Division of Spectrum Publications Inc: New York.

White, P., Hiley, C. R., Goodhardt, M. J., Carrasco, L. H., Keet, J. P., Williams, I. E. I. & Bowen, D. M. (1977). Neocortical cholinergic neurones in elderly people. *Lancet* i, 668–669.

Wisniewski, H. M., Bruce, M. E. & Fraser, H. (1975). Infectious aetiology of neuritic (senile) plaques in mice. *Science* **190**, 1108–1110.

Psychological Medicine 1979, **9**, 401–408

The scientific status of electro-convulsive therapy[1]

Electro-convulsive therapy (ECT) has been available for just over 40 years, whereas neuroleptic drugs have recently celebrated their 25th anniversary. Yet much more is known of the magnitude and scope of effectiveness, the mechanism of action, and even the adverse effects, of neuroleptic drugs in the treatment of schizophrenia than of electro-convulsive therapy in depression. Research on drug therapy of schizophrenia has advanced rapidly in the past 15 years while clinical research on ECT has progressed little. Until recently, basic research on possible mechanisms of action was also very limited.

It seems unlikely that this state of affairs presages the demise of convulsant therapy as a major treatment modality. Despite criticisms from a number of sources, most psychiatrists remain convinced that ECT has a unique place in the treatment of depression. Yet it is an entirely empirical treatment. In this respect it is far from unique in medicine; but it must be unusual for a treatment to remain widely used and so little understood for so long a period.

Advances in understanding mechanisms of action are desirable but many purely clinical questions remain unanswered. The Department of Health and Social Security and the Royal College of Psychiatrists are ascertaining the extent to which ECT is now used in British hospitals. It seems possible that a number of smaller projects, if properly designed, could provide answers to some outstanding questions concerning the scope and indications for this treatment. Such answers might substantially influence current practice, based as it is on information from trials carried out when antidepressant medications were relatively new, and to a large extent upon the individual clinician's intuition.

EFFECTIVENESS IN DEPRESSION

In an attempt to obtain an overall view of the effectiveness of ECT in comparison with other therapies, Wechsler *et al.* (1965) summarized 153 studies published between 1958 and 1963 in American, British and Canadian journals, involving a total of 5864 patients. They present the figures shown in Table 1.

Since many studies were uncontrolled, and these studies showed higher rates of improvement than those with a control group, these figures almost certainly exaggerate the effectiveness of antidepressant treatments, including ECT. More cogent perhaps is the contrast which these authors were able to demonstrate in the findings of studies dealing with depressions of recent onset and those which included mainly chronic depressions (but also some schizophrenic patients) (see Table 2). The superiority of both drugs and ECT over placebo is much less in the latter group.

No firm conclusions can be drawn from a literature survey. Patient selection is uncontrolled and many studies in which ECT was compared directly with other treatments included small numbers of patients. The soundest basis for an assessment of the efficacy of ECT are 2 major controlled trials completed in the early 1960s. The first (Greenblatt *et al.* 1962, 1964), in the United States, included 281 patients, and the second (Medical Research Council, 1965), in the United Kingdom, included 259 patients. Both were multicentre studies and included groups treated with placebo, imipramine and a monoamine oxidase inhibitor, as well as ECT. The age range of the American study (16–70 years) was wider than of the MRC trial (40–69 years), and it seems likely that the range of clinical features qualifying for admission (including groups labelled psychoneurotic depressive reaction, and

[1] Address for correspondence: Dr T. J. Crow, Division of Psychiatry, Clinical Research Centre, Northwick Park Hospital, Watford Road, Harrow, Middlesex HA1 3UJ.

Table 1.

	No. studies	Mean % improvement
MAOIs	76	50·4
Tricyclics	55	64·8
Placebo	25	23·2
ECT	9	72·0

Table 2.

	Mean % improvement	
	Depressions of recent onset	Chronic depressions
All drugs	61·7	31·9
Placebo	23·7	20·7
ECT	86·1	36·7

Table 3.

	Greenblatt *et al.* (1964) moderate to marked improvement (%)		MRC (1965) no or only slight symptoms (%)
ECT	92	ECT	71
Imipramine 200–250 mg daily	74	Imipramine 200 mg daily	52
Placebo	69	Placebo	39
MAOI:		MAOI:	
Phenelzine 15–60 mg daily	79	Phenelzine 60 mg daily	30
Isocarboxazid 40–50 mg daily	56	—	—

schizophrenic reaction depressed as well as manic depressive, depressed and involutional psychotic reaction) was also somewhat broader in the American trial. The treatment period was longer in the American trial (8 weeks including at least 9 ECT in the ECT group) than in the MRC trial (3½ weeks, including 4–8 treatments). These differences must be borne in mind, but a comparison of the main findings at the end of the treatment period is instructive (Table 3).

In the American trial ECT was superior to each of the other treatments and placebo at the 1 % level of significance or beyond, and in the UK study ECT was superior to imipramine (on the above assessments) at the 5 % level and to other treatments at a higher level of significance.

The findings of these 2 studies are similar and establish ECT as a highly effective treatment of depressive illness that appears to be acting more rapidly than what most clinicians would regard as adequate doses of imipramine. Although there are trials (e.g. Fahy *et al.* 1963; Mcdonald *et al.* 1966) in which ECT has been compared with a tricyclic antidepressant and has not been found significantly better (although both treatments were superior to placebo), the numbers of patients were substantially smaller than in the 2 major trials and the differences were in favour of ECT. In a non-randomized comparison of ECT, imipramine and placebo, Wittenborn *et al.* (1962) concluded that imipramine might influence more aspects of behaviour than ECT, but such an advantage has not been documented in more strictly controlled comparisons. Of some interest are the results of a study reported by Wilson *et al.* (1963) and analysed in 2 parts: in the first phase ECT was found to be superior to imipramine 150–200 mg daily; in the second phase, when the dose of imipramine was increased to 250 mg daily, the response to these 2 treatments was similar. The numbers of patients were insufficient to draw firm conclusions, but the findings do raise the possibility that there are regimes of tricyclic medication which can produce results similar to those achieved with ECT.

In general, the findings of other studies do not challenge the conclusions of the major studies that ECT has therapeutic effects in depression which are at least as good as those produced by other treatment methods and that the onset of the effect of ECT is more rapid. At the same time it should be emphasized that all those trials of ECT which have included such a group have shown substantial remission rates on placebo alone. For example, in the MRC (1965) trial the differences between ECT and other treatments diminished with length of follow-up, although the interpretation of these differences was complicated by the addition of other treatments after completion of the initial trial period.

MECHANISM OF THE ANTIDEPRESSANT EFFECT

It is widely assumed that it is the induction of convulsion which is responsible for the therapeutic effect. This question is of academic interest and also of practical importance since it seems highly likely that many of the adverse effects stem from the passage of current and the induction of fit. Therefore, if the treatment is to continue to be widely used on an empirical basis, it seems important to establish beyond all reasonable doubt what are and are not the essential ingredients. Clinicians need only remind themselves of the case of insulin coma therapy to realize that empirical treatments can be widely adopted, and accepted as self-evidently beneficial, before the real long-term benefits and hazards have been established in careful controlled studies. Although the major studies reviewed above demonstrate the effectiveness of the ECT procedure in depressive illness beyond reasonable doubt, it has to be considered that the therapeutic effect, or some part of the effect, is unrelated to the passage of current and the induction of fit.

Earlier attempts to establish this point by comparing ECT with 'pseudo-ECT' (i.e. anaesthesia without the shock, or with the shock modified in some way to avoid a fit) have yielded equivocal findings:

(*a*) Miller *et al.* (1953) compared ECT with anaesthesia alone, and with anaesthesia followed by sub-convulsive shock, in 40 patients with chronic schizophrenia, and observed no differences in response to the 3 treatments.

(*b*) Ulett *et al.* (1956) compared ECT with photoconvulsive and subconvulsive photic stimulation, and a control group, in 84 patients with a variety of depressive and schizophrenic symptoms. All patients were apparently sedated but not anaesthetized, and patients given photic stimulation were also given intravenous injections of the convulsant hexazol. There were rather large differences between groups in pre-treatment ratings, but improvement scores were greater in the photoconvulsive and ECT groups than in the other 2 groups. However, a χ^2 comparison of the ECT and placebo groups failed to reveal significant differences either at completion of the treatment or at follow-up (Costello, 1976).

(*c*) Brill *et al.* (1959) compared ECT administered in 3 different ways (without anaesthesia, with succinylcholine, and with thiopentone) with anaesthesia induced either by thiopentone or nitrous oxide (i.e. with anoxia), in 97 patients with schizophrenic and depressive reactions. Many patients were judged to be improved after each of these treatments but there were no significant differences between treatments. This remained true when the 30 patients with depression were separated from those 67 with schizophrenic illnesses.

(*d*) Cronholm & Ottosson (1960) compared 3 types of convulsive therapy in 65 patients with episodes of endogenous depression: (i) convulsions provoked by supraliminal stimulation, (ii) convulsions provoked by stimulation just above the convulsive threshold, and (iii) convulsions elicited by electrical stimulation but modified by intravenous lidocaine which reduces the duration and spread of seizure activity. It was argued that if therapeutic activity were dependent upon the convulsion it would be less in group (iii) than in the other 2 groups, whereas if it were dependent upon electrical stimulation *per se* the effect would be greater in group (i) than in groups (ii) and (iii).

In general, groups (i) and (ii) showed significantly greater improvements than group (iii). The results were therefore interpreted as consistent with the hypothesis that the convulsion is the essential element. The Cronholm & Ottosson result has often been regarded as the most convincing evidence for this viewpoint. However, there are aspects in the design of this study which make the conclusions less certain than would otherwise be the case. Although in the summary of their paper the patients are described as being allocated at random to the 3 treatments, the description of the procedure reveals that this was not so. Initially, patients were allocated alternately (i.e. not according to a random procedure) to groups (ii) and (iii). After 2 years it was decided to add group (i) (with supraliminal stimulation) and this group was then filled until it had reached the size of groups (ii) and (iii). Subsequently, patients were again allocated in sequence (i.e. not according to a random procedure) to the 3 groups. Although the authors present evidence that the 3 groups were comparable in initial severity, the design does allow for the entry of a systematic bias and cannot be regarded as blind. Moreover, 4 patients who relapsed after having been studied on one occasion were taken back into the trial.

(*e*) Robin & Harris (1962) reported that a group of 15 patients treated with ECT (bi-weekly, number not stated) and placebo tablets improved to a significantly greater extent, as assessed on a number of the components of the Hamilton rating scales and a global outcome assessment, than 16 patients treated with 'pseudo-ECT' and imipramine (dose not stated). However, few details of the conduct and analysis of this trial are presented and behaviour rating scales apparently did not distinguish between the groups.

Thus, while the findings of the studies of Cronholm & Ottosson (1960) and Robin & Harris (1962) are consistent with the view that the electrically induced convulsion is an important element in the therapeutic process, neither study is decisive and the negative findings of Brill *et al.* (1959), who did find a therapeutic effect in their rather heterogeneous group of patients but found it unrelated to the convulsion, remain to be explained.

Two recent studies have attempted to resolve this issue:

(*a*) Freeman *et al.* (1978) randomly allocated 40 patients judged to be suitable for ECT to either 2 real ECTs or 2 'pseudo-ECTs'. Subsequently, all patients received real ECT. The dependent variables were ratings after the first 2 treatments and at weekly intervals thereafter, and the number of ECTs judged necessary by the independent clinician. The findings were that the group treated with real ECT showed significantly more improvement on some, but not all, rating scales after 2 treatments, and were judged by the clinician to require fewer subsequent treatments to achieve a satisfactory response. Thus, the results were interpreted by the authors as demonstrating the superiority of the procedure including the convulsion.

However, interpretation of this study is complicated by the fact that treatment was discontinued for reasons other than a satisfactory response in 6 of the 20 cases treated initially with real ECT and only 2 of 20 of those treated with 'pseudo-ECT'. Since in the former group in 2 cases treatment was discontinued by the clinician's decision that the response to ECT was unsatisfactory (a possibility apparently not allowed for in the design), and 2 further cases refused further treatment because they felt it was not helping them, it appears that the assessment of the trial based on number of subsequent real ECTs required cannot be taken as decisive. The difference in ratings observed after 2 treatments are interesting, but it is surprising that significant differences between the groups were not observed at subsequent assessments. Clinical lore, and some trials in which serial assessments have been made (e.g. Cronholm & Ottosson, 1960; Herrington *et al.* 1974), suggest that the beneficial effects of ECT are rather slow to emerge.

(*b*) Lambourn & Gill (1978) randomly allocated 32 patients with depressive psychosis to unilateral pulse ECT (inducing a bilateral convulsion) and to a simulated procedure including anaesthesia but omitting the electrical stimulus. Outcome was assessed after 6 treatments (administered thrice weekly) and again 1 month later by the Hamilton (1960) rating scale, and was also assessed globally by the referring clinician, and in terms of subsequent treatments (ECT or antidepressants) required. The Hamilton overall ratings revealed no significant differences either after 6 treatments or 1 month later. One individual item (hypochondriasis) showed a significant change in favour of the ECT group and one (middle insomnia) a change in favour of the simulated ECT group. Neither the referring doctors' global assessment nor additional treatment distinguished the 2 groups.

Comparison of these 2 trials allows few firm conclusions to be drawn. While the study of Freeman *et al.* (1978) was interpreted as showing that even 2 real ECTs have a significantly better effect than 2 simulated ECTs, the Lambourn & Gill study with an apparently stronger design (6 real against 6 simulated ECTs) and follow-up at 1 month gives no support at all to this view. It might be argued that the use of unilateral rather than bilateral stimulation is a critical factor. However, bilateral convulsions were observed in their real ECT series by Lambourn & Gill, and such an interpretation would challenge the view of Cronholm & Ottosson that the convulsion is an important element in the therapeutic effect. It has been suggested (Freeman, 1978) that the patients in the Lambourn & Gill study were less depressed than those in the study of Freeman *et al.* (1978). However, pre-treatment Hamilton ratings in the 2 studies do not support this view. Thus, the findings of the Lambourn & Gill study do raise serious questions not only about the mechanism of action of ECT but also its efficacy in the form in which it is commonly administered. Not the least interesting of the findings is the magnitude of the overall improvement (a reduction in Hamilton score to 58 % after 6 simulated ECTs and to 19 % of pre-treatment values 1 month after the end of the trial) in patients receiving no electrical shock.

It is sometimes argued (e.g. Kendell, 1978) that the fact that other methods of inducing a convulsion, e.g. by flurothyl (Laurell, 1970) or by photo-convulsant methods (Ulett *et al.* 1956), are also effective in the treatment of depression suggests that the convulsive activity, rather than any other component of the procedure, is the therapeutic element. However, what has been demonstrated is that these other therapies in certain circumstances are not significantly less effective than ECT, and this is not necessarily the same thing as to demonstrate that by themselves they have antidepressant activity. This is certainly a possibility, but it is in any case not difficult to suggest elements other than the convulsion which these procedures have in common with ECT which may be relevant to the therapeutic effect. For example, Lowinger & Dobie (1969) have described how, at least in an out-patient setting, response to placebo appears to be influenced by expectations of staff concerning the effects of treatment. When staff believe that high dose treatment is being given, patients on placebo tablets appear to do better. Expectations presumably determine the subsequent intensity of staff involvement in assessment and therapy.

ANIMAL EXPERIMENTS

At the same time that there has been a quickening of interest in the mechanism of action in depression there has been increasing interest in the effects of repeated convulsions in animal experiments. While such experiments may not directly illuminate the antidepressant effect, they do make it plausible that treatments which parallel the clinical mode of administration have specific behavioural and neurochemical effects. For example, Modigh (1975) observed that, after a course of 7 daily electro-convulsive shocks, but not after a single shock, mice show increased locomotor activity when this was assessed 3 and 6 days after the last shock. Groups of mice showed enhanced locomotor responses to the drugs apomorphine and clonidine, agonists of the post-synaptic dopamine and noradrenaline receptors respectively, after reserpine pre-treatment. These results are interpreted as suggesting that electroconvulsive shock enhances the sensitivity of catecholamine receptors or of some structure associated with these receptors. Similar findings were reported by Evans *et al.* (1976) with respect to the stimulating effects of a combination of tranylcypromine and L-dopa, which might be expected to activate catecholaminergic mechanisms, and also with a combination of L-tryptophan and tranyl-cypromine, which probably acts mainly upon serotonergic processes. In this case also a post-synaptic site of action was suggested by the finding that enhanced responsiveness following electroshock was elicited by 5-methoxy-*N*-*N*-dimethyltryptamine, an agent which may be a serotonin receptor agonist.

These experimentally induced changes resemble the therapeutic effect in that they occur only following a succession of spaced shocks, and also in that they do not occur with peripheral electrical stimulation or with a series of shocks at hourly intervals (Costain *et al.* 1978). Similar changes are seen following convulsions induced by flurothyl (Green, 1978).

It has become possible to examine whether these changes occur at the level of the receptor with the development of ligand-binding assays. Cross *et al.* (1979) found that neither dopamine nor serotonin receptors showed significant changes in number following repeated spaced electroshock treatment in rats. Dopamine and serotonin turnover are probably unchanged (Modigh, 1976; Evans *et al.* 1976), but there may be a sustained increase in noradrenaline turnover (Modigh, 1976). The mechanism of this effect and its relationship to the behavioural changes observed in animal experiments remains to be determined.

LONG-TERM EFFECTS

Few controlled studies have examined the long-term effects, whether beneficial or adverse, of electroconvulsive therapy. The possible long-term benefits of ECT are emphasized by an analysis of follow-up studies of depression (Avery & Winokur, 1976) in which series of patients treated with convulsive therapy are compared with groups treated with antidepressant drugs and with neither ECT nor antidepressant medication. Avery & Winokur combine an analysis of the literature with the results of their own retrospective study to support the argument that the increased mortality of depressed patients can be reduced by convulsive or adequate antidepressant treatment. In these authors' own study the mortality of the group treated with ECT was significantly lower in a 3-year follow-up than that of groups who received inadequate antidepressant therapy or no antidepressants and no ECT. Non-suicidal deaths and particularly myocardial infarctions were significantly more frequent in the inadequately treated group, and the differences were greater among men and in the older age groups. Avery & Winokur (1978) also found that suicidal attempts were less frequently seen in patients treated with ECT than in those treated with antidepressants, and this was true in patients both with and without a history of suicidal attempts.

Concern about the possible adverse effects of ECT has focused on whether a component of the well-known impairment of memory persists in the long term. Assessment of this possibility is complicated by the observation (Sternberg & Jarvik, 1976) that memory functions are impaired by depression itself and improve with improvements in mental state. Some memory deficits which follow ECT may be attributable to inadequate response rather than to the effects of treatment itself. Thus, Cronholm & Ottosson (1963) found that patients who showed the most improvement following ECT experienced least subjective memory impairment.

Memory impairment is probably related to the number of shocks given. Squire & Miller (1974) found that the ability to retain new material for 24 hours was more impaired after the fourth than after the first shock treatment. After a number of shock treatments there is an impairment of ability to recall events from the remote past (Squire, 1975) and this impairment does not change in the 24 hours following the last treatment.

The question of the precise duration of objective memory loss following ECT, and the possibility that there may be relatively long-term or even permanent losses, has been too little investigated. Some of the difficulties mentioned above of separating deficits attributable to depression from those due to ECT, the difficulty of assessing premorbid performance, and the problem of obtaining appropriate control groups, may account for discrepancies in the literature. Thus, Bidder *et al.* (1970) estimated that performance had returned to pre-ECT levels within 30 days, but Halliday *et al* (1968) presented evidence for a deficit on some non-verbal learning tasks at 3 months. In an attempt to answer this question, Squire & Chace (1975) applied a battery of tests of delayed and remote memory to groups of patients who had received bilateral and unilateral ECT or other treatments for depression 6–9 months previously. They obtained no evidence for specific learning deficits attributable to ECT, although persons who had received bilateral ECT rated their memory as impaired significantly more often than did those in other follow-up groups. The authors suggest that this may indicate either that the subjects were aware of a deficit below the level of sensitivity of the tests, or that the experience of bilateral ECT had made the subjects more alert to subsequent memory failures, and thus led them to underestimate their memory abilities. The objective tests were selected for their range and sensitivity in testing memory functions and the results are, in general, reassuring. However, some disquieting findings remain. Thus, Cronin *et al.* (1970) found that unilateral non-dominant ECT produced less impairment than either bilateral or unilateral dominant ECT on the modified word learning test and the Wechsler memory scales; these differences were as marked 4–6 weeks after a course of 8 ECTs as after the eighth treatment. In a study of the cognitive status of patients who had been subjected to cingulotomy, Teuber *et al.* (1976) found that the subjects who had previously received more than 50 ECTs were more impaired than those who had received either no ECT or who had received less than 50 previous ECTs on tests of verbal and non-verbal fluency, delayed alternation, tactual maze learning, and some other recall and recognition tests. It is possible that those who had received more ECT were suffering from more severe illnesses, but these data draw attention to the importance of further investigations of the effects of repeated courses of ECT.

OUTSTANDING ISSUES

The largest and most carefully conducted studies have demonstrated ECT to be a most effective and rapid treatment of depressive illness. However, examination of the literature reveals that the widely held view that the convulsion is a necessary component of the therapeutic effect has never been unequivocally established. The importance of this issue is re-emphasized by the apparently contradictory findings of 2 recent studies, and is highlighted by recent advances in neurochemistry which have made possible detailed investigations of the effects of repeated electroshock on neurotransmitter function. A comparison of the clinical and chemical effects of therapeutically active drugs and ECT could substantially elucidate the mechanisms of affective change.

The major outstanding issues for research on ECT are:

(i) The question of whether the fit is indeed the critical component of the therapeutic effect as suggested by Cronholm & Ottosson, or whether, as suggested by the work of Brill *et al.* (1959) and Lambourn & Gill (1978), other components of the procedure make a substantial contribution.

(ii) The possible long-term psychological effects of ECT.

(iii) The question of whether the effects of ECT are qualitatively different from those of available antidepressant medications. Further studies should include comparison of the treatments both with respect to the rapidity of the short-term response and, in view of the data recently presented by Avery & Winokur (1976, 1978), with respect to the long-term mortality from suicide and other causes.

(iv) The long-standing, but unanswered, issue of whether there are certain types of depression which respond only to ECT.

T. J. CROW

REFERENCES

Avery, D. & Winokur, G. (1976). Mortality in depressed patients treated with electroconvulsive therapy and antidepressants. *Archives of General Psychiatry* **33**, 1029–1037.

Avery, D. & Winokur, G. (1978). Suicide, attempted suicide, and relapse rates in depression: occurrence after ECT and antidepressant therapy. *Archives of General Psychiatry* **35**, 749–753.

Bidder, T. G., Strain, L. J. & Brunschwig, L. (1970). Bilateral and unilateral ECT. Follow-up study and critique. *American Journal of Psychiatry* **127**, 737–745.

Brill, N. Q., Crumpton, E., Eiduson, S., Grayson, H. M., Hellman, L. I. & Richards, P. A. (1959). Relative effectiveness of various components of electroconvulsive therapy. *Archives of Neurology and Psychiatry* **81**, 627–635.

Costain, D. W., Grahame-Smith, D. G. & Green, A. R. (1978). Relevance of the enhanced 5-hydroxytryptamine behavioural responses in rats to electroconvulsive therapy. *British Journal of Pharmacology* **62**, 394P.

Costello, C. G. (1976). Electroconvulsive therapy: is further

investigation necessary? *Canadian Psychiatric Association Journal* **21**, 61–67.
Cronholm, B. & Ottosson, J. -O. (1960). Experimental studies of the therapeutic action of electroconvulsive therapy in endogenous depression. *Acta Psychiatrica Scandinavica* Suppl. 145, **35**, 69–101.
Cronholm, B. & Ottosson, J. -O. (1963). The experience of memory function after electroconvulsive therapy. *British Journal of Psychiatry* **109**, 251–258.
Cronin, D., Bodley, P., Potts, L., Mather, M. D., Gardner, R. K. & Tobin, J. C. (1970). Unilateral and bilateral ECT: a study of memory disturbance and relief from depression. *Journal of Neurology, Neurosurgery and Psychiatry* **33**, 705–713.
Cross, A. J., Deakin, J. F. W., Lofthouse, R., Longden, A., Owen, F. & Poulter, M. (1979). On the mechanism of action of electro-convulsive therapy: some behavioural and biochemical consequences of repeated electrically induced seizures in rats. *British Journal of Pharmacology* (in the press).
Evans, J., Grahame-Smith, D. G., Green, A. R. & Tordoff, A. F. C. (1976). Electroconvulsive shock increases the behavioural responses of rats to brain 5-hydroxytryptamine accumulation and central nervous system stimulant drugs. *British Journal of Pharmacology* **56**, 193–199.
Fahy, P., Imlah, N. & Harrington, J. (1963). A controlled comparison of electroconvulsive therapy, imipramine and thiopentone sleep in depression. *Journal of Neuropsychiatry* **4**, 310–314.
Freeman, C. P. (1978). How does ECT work? *Lancet* ii, 893–894.
Freeman, C. P., Basson, J. V. & Crighton, A. (1978). Double-blind controlled trial of electro-convulsive therapy (ECT) and simulated ECT in depressive illness. *Lancet* i, 738–740.
Green, A. R. (1978). Repeated exposure of rats to the convulsant agent flurothyl enhances 5-hydroxytryptamine and dopamine mediated behavioural responses. *British Journal of Pharmacology* **62**, 325–331.
Greenblatt, M., Grosser, G. H. & Wechsler, H. (1962). A comparative study of selected antidepressant medications and ECT. *American Journal of Psychiatry* **119**, 144–153.
Greenblatt, M., Grosser, G. H. & Wechsler, H. (1964). Differential response of hospitalized depressed patients to somatic therapy. *American Journal of Psychiatry* **120**, 935–943.
Halliday, A. M., Davison, K., Brown, M. W. & Kreeger, L. C. (1968). A comparison of the effects on depression and memory of bilateral ECT and unilateral ECT to the dominant and non-dominant hemispheres. *British Journal of Psychiatry* **114**, 997–1012.
Hamilton, M. (1960). A rating scale for depression. *Journal of Neurology, Neurosurgery and Psychiatry* **23**, 56–62.
Herrington, R. N., Bruce, A., Johnstone, E. C. & Lader, M. H. (1974). Comparative trial of L-tryptophan and ECT in severe depressive illness. *Lancet* ii, 731–734.
Kendell, R. E. (1978). Electroconvulsive therapy. *Journal of the Royal Society of Medicine* **71**, 319–321.
Lambourn, J. & Gill, D. (1978). A controlled comparison of simulated and real ECT. *British Journal of Psychiatry* **133**, 514–519.
Laurell, B. (1970). Comparison of electric and flurothyl convulsive therapy. II. Antidepressive effect. *Acta Psychiatrica Scandinavica* Suppl. 145, 22–35.
Lowinger, P. & Dobie, S. (1969). What makes the placebo work? A study of placebo response rates. *Archives of General Psychiatry* **20**, 84–88.
McDonald, I. M., Perkins, M., Marjerrison, G. & Podilsky, M. (1966). A controlled comparison of amitriptyline and electroconvulsive therapy in the treatment of depression. *American Journal of Psychiatry* **112**, 1427–1431.
Medical Research Council (1965). Report by Clinical Psychiatry Committee. Clinical trial of the treatment of depressive illness. *British Medical Journal* i, 881–886.
Miller, D. H., Clancy, J. & Cumming, E. (1953). A comparison between unidirectional current nonconvulsive electrical stimulation given with Reiter's machine, standard alternating current electroshock (Cerletti method), and pentothal in chronic schizophrenia. *American Journal of Psychiatry* **109**, 617–621.
Modigh, K. (1975). Electroconvulsive shock and postsynaptic catecholamine effects: increased psychomotor stimulant action of apomorphine and clonidine in reserpine pretreated mice by repeated ECT. *Journal of Neural Transactions* **36**, 19–32.
Modigh, K. (1976). Long-term effects of electroconvulsive shock therapy on synthesis, turnover and uptake of brain monoamines. *Psychopharmacology* **49**, 179–185.
Robin, A. A. & Harris, J. A. (1962). A controlled comparison of imipramine and electroplexy. *Journal of Mental Science* **106**, 217–219.
Squire, L. R. (1975). A stable impairment in remote memory following electroconvulsive therapy. *Neuropsychologia* **13**, 51–58.
Squire, L. R. & Chace, P. M. (1975). Memory functions six to nine months after electroconvulsive therapy. *Archives of General Psychiatry* **32**, 1557–1564.
Squire, L. R. & Miller, P. L. (1974). Diminution of anterograde amnesia following electroconvulsive therapy. *British Journal of Psychiatry* **125**, 490–495.
Sternberg, D. E. & Jarvik, M. E. (1976). Memory functions in depression. *Archives of General Psychiatry* **33**, 219–224.
Teuber, H. L., Corkin, S. & Twitchwell, T. E. (1976). A study of cingulotomy in man. A report to the National Commission for the Protection of Human Subjects of Biomedical and Behavioural Research.
Ulett, G. A., Smith, K. & Gleser, G. C. (1956). Evaluation of convulsive and subconvulsive shock therapies utilizing a control group. *American Journal of Psychiatry* **112**, 795–802.
Wechsler, H., Grosser, G. H. & Greenblatt, M. (1965). Research evaluating antidepressant medications on hospitalized mental patients: a survey of published reports during a five-year period. *Journal of Nervous and Mental Disease* **141**, 231–239.
Wilson, I. C., Vernon, J. T., Guin, T. & Sandifer, M. G. (1963). A controlled study of treatments of depression. *Journal of Neuropsychiatry* **4**, 331–337.
Wittenborn, J. R., Plante, M., Burgess, F. & Maurer, H. (1962). A comparison of imipramine, electroconvulsive therapy and placebo in the treatment of depressions. *Journal of Nervous and Mental Disease* **135**, 131–137.

Psychological Medicine, 1980, **10**, 603–606

Type A behaviour and ischaemic heart disease[1]

It is a common medical belief that psychosocial factors, in some form or another, contribute to the risk of developing ischaemic heart disease (IHD). Anecdotal evidence comes from many of the great figures of medical history. William Harvey described a coronary patient whose illness was the result of 'anger and indignation which he yet communicated to no one' (Leibowitz, 1970). John Hunter's angina was brought on by 'agitation of the mind' and he was reported to have died from an attack provoked by a particularly irritating hospital board meeting in 1793 (Home, 1794). In 1910, Osler described the typical coronary patient as 'the keen and ambitious man, the indicator of whose engine is always at full speed ahead' – a description very like that which has latterly been termed Type A behaviour.

Since Osler, there have accumulated many clinical and epidemiological reports relating psychosocial factors to ischaemic heart disease (e.g. see the reviews by Jenkins, 1971, 1976). These data are of varying quality and do not provide consistent evidence of a role in aetiology. Perhaps the strongest evidence for a causal link between psychosocial factors and ischaemic heart disease comes from the studies of Type A behaviour (Dembroski, 1977). We would do well, therefore, to examine critically the evidence on Type A behaviour with a number of questions in mind. Has a causal link been established? What is the magnitude of the association? To what extent do variations in the frequency of Type A behaviour account for variations in the occurrence of IHD?

First, what is Type A behaviour? One might have hoped for a definition – which we do not have. It is described as an 'action–emotion' complex (Rosenman, 1977) that is characterized by impatience, a sense of time-urgency, competitiveness, striving for achievement, aggressiveness, hyper-alertness, restlessness, explosive speech and abruptness of gesture. The techniques used for measurement do not clarify the issue very much. In their initial cross-sectional studies, Friedman and Rosenman used clinical judgements to classify people and demonstrated an association between Type A behaviour and ischaemic heart disease in both men and women (Friedman & Rosenman, 1959; Rosenman *et al.* 1961).

Subsequently, in a longitudinal study in California, they used a more formal version of clinical judgement. Type A behaviour was assessed by a structured interview. In classifying people, importance was placed not only on the content of the answers to the questions but on the individual's mannerisms and behaviour during the interview. This technique had the curious property that exactly 50% of the population at entry into their longitudinal study were classified as Type A, there being no reason *a priori* why this should be so. It is not clear which characteristics of Type A individuals should be considered as representing the crucial part of the behaviour pattern and which are merely associated characteristics. Nevertheless, this global classification into Type A or Type B was remarkably revealing. Over an $8\frac{1}{2}$ year follow-up period in the California study, Type A men had twice the incidence of ischaemic heart disease as Type B men (Rosenman *et al.* 1975).

For these studies to be replicated, reproducible measures of Type A behaviour had to be developed. Jenkins developed an elaborate questionnaire designed for self-administration – the Jenkins Activity Survey (JAS) – which was correlated with the structured interview (73% agreement) (Jenkins *et al.* 1967). Although the JAS assessment of Type A behaviour has been shown to be associated with IHD in cross-sectional studies (Jenkins, 1976), in Rosenman & Friedman's longitudinal study the JAS was less strongly associated with IHD incidence than was the structured interview (Jenkins *et al.* 1974). It seems that the JAS is missing some crucial component of the Type A behaviour pattern – either because of the way the questions were asked, or the way the questionnaire was scored, or possibly

[1] Address for correspondence: Dr Michael Marmot, Department of Medical Statistics and Epidemiology, London School of Hygiene and Tropical Medicine, Keppel Street, London WC1E 7HT.

because the subjects' mannerisms and style displayed in the structured interview are not well correlated with the answers to the questionnaire, but are correlated with the risk of disease.

Other approaches to measuring Type A behaviour have been made. In the Framingham Massachusetts Heart Study, a Type A scale was constructed from 10 questions that asked about presumed Type A characteristics. Men and women classified as Type A on this questionnaire have an increased prevalence and incidence of ischaemic heart disease (Haynes *et al.* 1978, 1980). In the UK, yet a fourth measure of Type A behaviour, the Bortner scale, has been shown in a case–control study to be associated with IHD (Heller, 1979). Other studies, while not specifically measuring Type A behaviour, have produced data consistent with the above (Jenkins, 1976).

The consistency of these results, while not clarifying our understanding of Type A behaviour, do increase the likelihood that it reflects characteristics that are causally related to ischaemic heart disease. There is some evidence both from an autopsy study (Friedman *et al.* 1968) and from studies of patients undergoing coronary angiography (Zyzanski *et al.* 1976; Blumenthal *et al.* 1978) that Type A behaviour may be related to the underlying process of atherosclerosis, i.e. to the chronic disease process.

There are plausible biological reasons why Type A behaviour might precipitate an acute myocardial infarction or sudden death. Type A subjects have been reported to have a faster clotting time than Type B (Friedman & Rosenman, 1959), increased platelet aggregation (Jenkins *et al.* 1975) and a higher urinary output of catecholamines during working hours (Friedman, 1977*a*) – although this latter finding has not been confirmed (DeBacker *et al.* 1979). Whether the association between IHD death and Type A behaviour (Friedman 1977*b*) is related to these mechanisms is not clear.

In the California study, Type A behaviour was related to new cases of myocardial infarction, to angina pectoris and to recurrent ischaemic heart disease. It does appear that the differences in risk of clinical IHD between Type As and Type Bs cannot be explained by differences in serum cholesterol, or blood pressure or in cigarette smoking (Rosenman *et al.* 1975). In other words, the epidemiological and clinical/laboratory evidence suggests that Type As may possibly be at higher risk because of a direct effect on the neuroendocrine system.

These studies have all been directed at discriminating one individual's disease risk from another's. A different kind of question is the extent to which variations in the frequency of Type A behaviour may explain group or population differences in the rate of occurrence of IHD.

It would indeed be an intriguing notion if, as has been suggested (Rosenman, 1977), the twentieth-century coronary epidemic is the result of an environment that has increased the prevalence of Type A behaviour; or if males have more IHD than females because of their greater tendency to be Type A; or if Italians, French and Japanese have low IHD rates because of their relative infrequency of Type A behaviour; or if clerical officers in the British civil service have a higher risk of IHD than their administrative superiors (Marmot *et al.* 1978) because the administrators are less likely to be Type A.

These are not easy questions to assess, first because only the most enthusiastic supporter of the Type A concept would suggest that all hitherto unexplained variations in the occurrence of IHD may be explained by variations in one single behaviour pattern. To put it in perspective, the risk of developing IHD in Type A individuals was marginally less than twice the risk in Type Bs after adjustment for other risk factors. Secondly, the testing of these assertions presupposes the existence of a measure of Type A behaviour that is not culturally, socially or sexually biased. The structured interview was developed for use in a study of employees of several corporations in California and, as Jenkins (1976) points out, initially most studies using the JAS did not include persons with low education, rural occupations, or aged over 65. Only one or two studies have included women. To show that men tend more often to be Type A than women (Waldron *et al.* 1977) or that Americans tend more to be Type A than Belgians (Kittel *et al.* 1978) is suggestive, but one would like to have confidence that the measure reflects the same thing in both sexes or cultures. For example, the JAS was used in a study of Japanese-Americans (Cohen, 1974). Their low Type A scores were consistent with their low rates of IHD compared with white Americans, but a factor analysis of the answers to the JAS questionnaire revealed that the questions clustered together in a different manner from that observed in the study of predominantly middle-class white Californians. There was the clear implication that the questionnaire responses did not mean the same thing in these two different cultures.

One approach to the cross-cultural validation of a Type A measure is to test predictive validity. If a measure of Type A behaviour is shown to be associated with IHD in different cultures, it increases one's confidence in the measure, although it does not necessarily imply that one may then use this measure to compare the frequency of Type A behaviour. A high/low dichotomy may successfully discriminate IHD cases from non-cases in different cultures, without the absolute levels of the scores having the same meaning. Nevertheless, there is evidence that Type A behaviour is associated with IHD in populations outside North America (Heller, 1979; Zyzanski, 1977).

We are thus at an interesting stage in the research on Type A behaviour. The balance of evidence points to a causal association with ischaemic heart disease, but the origin and nature of Type A behaviour have been described in only the vaguest terms. Attempts to demonstrate a dose–response relationship or to show that components of the Type A behaviour pattern are related to ischaemic heart disease have proved largely unsuccessful (Jenkins *et al.* 1967). More intensive research is now under way, aimed at better description of Type A behaviour.

It seems likely that further advances in our knowledge will come from studies now in progress that are attempting to relate Type A behaviour to risk of IHD and to other psychosocial factors in subjects other than middle-class white American men. It has been suggested that Type A behaviour is neither a personality pattern nor a reflection of a stressful environment, but a combination of the two. It may be that Type A behaviour is a middle-class American way of reacting. Reactions to a stressful environment in women, in working-class Englishmen, in Belgians or Swedes may take a form other than that typical of Type A behaviour, but the underlying notion still may be correct; i.e. that a failure to cope in an appropriate manner with a stressful environment predisposes to ischaemic heart disease. We need answers to the questions of what constitutes a 'stressful environment' or an appropriate manner of coping. The results of the research on Type A behaviour and ischaemic heart disease make it clear that it is worth seeking answers to these questions.

MICHAEL MARMOT

REFERENCES

Blumenthal, J. A., Williams, R. & Kong, Y. (1978). Type A behaviour and angiographically documented coronary disease. *Circulation* **58**, 634–639.

Cohen, J. B. (1974). Sociocultural change and behaviour patterns in disease etiology: an epidemiologic study of coronary disease among Japanese Americans. Unpublished doctoral dissertation: University of California, Berkeley.

DeBacker, G., Kornitzer, M. & Kittel, F. (1979). Relation between coronary-prone behaviour pattern, excretion of urinary catecholamines, heart rate, and heart rhythm. *Preventive Medicine* **8**, 14–22.

Dembroski, T. M. (ed.) (1977). *Proceedings of the Forum on Coronary-Prone Behaviour*. DHEW Publication no. (NIH) 78-1451. Washington, D.C.

Friedman, M. (1977*a*). Type A behaviour pattern: some of its pathophysiological components. *Bulletin of the New York Academy of Medicine* **53**, 593–604.

Friedman, M. (1977*b*). Type A behaviour: its possible relationship to pathogenetic processes responsible for coronary heart disease (a preliminary inquiry). In *Proceedings of the Forum on Coronary-Prone Behaviour* (ed. T. M. Dembroski), pp. 179–184. DHEW Publication no. (NIH) 78–1451. Washington, D. C.

Friedman, M. & Rosenman, R. H. (1959). Association of specific overt behaviour pattern with blood and cardiovascular findings. *Journal of the American Medical Association* **169**, 1286–1296.

Friedman, M., Rosenman, R. H. & Straus, R. (1968). The relationship of behaviour pattern A to the state of the coronary vasculature: a study of fifty-one autopsy subjects. *American Journal of Medicine* **44**, 525–537.

Haynes, S. G., Feinleib, M. & Levine, S. (1978). The relationship of psychosocial factors to coronary heart disease in the Framingham study. II. Prevalence of coronary heart disease. *American Journal of Epidemiology* **107**, 384–402.

Haynes, S. G., Feinleib, M. & Kannel, W. B. (1980). The relationship of psychosocial factors to coronary heart disease in the Framingham study. III. Eight-year incidence of coronary heart disease. *American Journal of Epidemiology* **111**, 37–58.

Heller, R. F. (1979). Type A behaviour and coronary heart disease. *British Medical Journal* ii, 368.

Home, E. (1794). A short account of the author's life by his brother-in-law, Everard Home. In *Cardiac Classics* (ed. F. A. Willius and T. E. Keys), pp. 269–275. C. V. Mosby: St Louis (1941).

Jenkins, C. D. (1971). Psychologic and social precursors of coronary disease. *New England Journal of Medicine* **284**, 244–255, 307–317.

Jenkins, C. D. (1976). Recent evidence supporting psychologic and social risk factors for coronary disease. *New England Journal of Medicine* **294**, 987–994, 1033–1038.

Jenkins, C. D., Rosenman, R. H. & Friedman, M. (1967). Development of an objective psychological test for the determination of the coronary-prone behaviour pattern in employed men. *Journal of Chronic Diseases* **20**, 371–379.

Jenkins, C. D., Rosenman, R. H. & Zyzanski, S. J. (1974). Prediction of clinical coronary heart disease by a test for the coronary-prone behavior pattern. *New England Journal of Medicine* **290**, 1271–1275.

Jenkins, C. D., Thomas, G. & Olewine, D. (1975). Blood platelet aggregation and personality traits. *Journal of Human Stress* **1**, 34–46.

Kittel, F., Kornitzer, M., Zyzanski, S. J., Jenkins, C. D., Rustin, R. M. & Degre, C. (1978). Two methods of assessing the Type A coronary-prone behaviour pattern in Belgium. *Journal of Chronic Diseases* **31**, 147–155.

Leibowitz, J. O. (1970). *The History of Coronary Heart Disease*. University of California Press: Berkeley.

Marmot, M. G., Rose, G., Shipley, M. & Hamilton, P. J. S. (1978). Employment grade and coronary heart disease in British civil servants. *Journal of Epidemiology and Community Health* **32**, 244–249.

Osler, W. (1910). The Lumleian Lectures on angina pectoris. *Lancet* i, 697–702, 839–844.

Rosenman, R. H. (1977). History and definition of the Type A coronary-prone behaviour pattern. In *Proceedings of the Forum on Coronary-Prone Behaviour* (ed. T. M. Dembroski), pp. 13–17. DHEW Publication no. (NIH) 78–1451. Washington, D.C.

Rosenman, R. H. & Friedman, M. (1961). Association of specific behaviour pattern in women with blood and cardiovascular findings. *Journal of the American Medical Association* **24**, 1173–1184.

Rosenman, R. H., Brand, R. J., Jenkins, C. D., Friedman, M., Straus, R. & Wurm, M. (1975). Coronary heart disease in the Western Collaborative Group Study. Final follow-up experience of 8½ years. *Journal of the American Medical Association* **233**, 872–877.

Waldron, I., Zyzanski, S. J., Shekelle, R. B., Jenkins, C. D. & Tannenbaum, S. (1977). The coronary-prone behaviour pattern in employed men and women. *Journal of Human Stress* **3**, 2–18.

Zyzanski, S. J. (1977). Associations of the coronary-prone pattern. In *Proceedings of the Forum on Coronary-Prone Behaviour* (ed. T. M. Dembroski), pp. 46–66. DHEW Publication no. (NIH) 78–1451. Washington, D.C.

Zyzanski, S. J., Jenkins, C. D. & Ryan, T. J. (1976). Psychological correlates of coronary angiographic findings. *Archives of Internal Medicine* **136**, 1234–1237.